Julian Kassen, M.D.
RUTGERS MEDICAL SCHOOL
INSTITUTE OF MENTAL HEALTH SCIENCES
UNIVERSITY HEIGHTS
PISCATAWAY, NJ 08554

The Child in His Family

THE IMPACT OF DISEASE AND DEATH

VOLUME 2

*YEARBOOK OF THE INTERNATIONAL ASSOCIATION
FOR CHILD PSYCHIATRY AND ALLIED PROFESSIONS*

EDITOR-IN-CHIEF—E. JAMES ANTHONY, M.D. (U.S.A.)

CO-EDITOR—CYRILLE KOUPERNIK, M.D. (FRANCE)

Volume 1   **The Child in His Family**

E. James Anthony and Cyrille Koupernik, Editors

Volume 2   **The Child in His Family:
The Impact of Disease and Death**

E. James Anthony and Cyrille Koupernik, Editors

The Child in His Family

THE IMPACT OF DISEASE AND DEATH

VOLUME 2

Edited by

E. JAMES ANTHONY, M.D.
St. Louis, Missouri, U.S.A.

and

CYRILLE KOUPERNIK, M.D.
Paris, France

A WILEY-INTERSCIENCE PUBLICATION

JOHN WILEY & SONS, New York • London • Sydney • Toronto

Library of Congress Cataloging in Publication Data:

Main entry under title:

The Child in his family.

(International yearbook for child psychiatry and allied disciplines, v. 2)
"Volume 2."
1. Sick children—Psychology. 2. Children and death. 3. Parent and child. I. Anthony, Elwyn James, ed. II. Koupernik, Cyrille, 1917–   ed.
III. Series.

RJ47.C43   155.9'37   72–11702
ISBN 0–471–03226–3

Printed in the United States of America

10 9 8 7 6 5 4 3 2

To Children in Their Families Everywhere and

more especially to *SASHA, STEPHANIE, SONIA, BRUNO, DANIEL, GEOFFREY, RACHEL, AND CHRISTOPHER*

Contributors

Kenneth S. Adam (M.D.), Assistant Director, Student Mental Health Service, McGill University, Montreal, Canada

Jean-Marc Alby (M.D.), Medecin-Assistant des Hopitaux de Paris, Service du Prof. Rene Wolfromm, Hopital Rotschild, Paris, France

Nicole Alby (Licenciee de Philosophie), Attachee de Psychologie, Service du Prof. Jean Bernard, Hopital Saint Louis, Paris, France

Dov R. Aleksandrowicz (M.D.), Staff Psychiatrist, The Menninger Foundation, Topeka, Kansas, U.S.A.

T. Asuni (M.A., M.D., D.PM.), Consultant Psychiatrist and Medical Superintendent, Neuro-Psychiatric Hospital, Aro, Abeokuta, Nigeria

Charles M. Binger (M.D.), Assistant Clinical Professor of Psychiatry, University of California, S. F. Clinical Coordinator of the Children's Service of the Langley Porter Neuropsychiatric Institute in San Francisco, Langley Porter Neuropsychiatric Institute, San Francisco, California, U.S.A.

John Bowlby (M.D., F.R.C. Psychiatrists), Consultant Psychiatrist, Tavistock Clinic, Tavistock Centre, London, England

Renato Castro de la Mata (M.D.), Chief Section of Social Psychiatry, Program of Community Medicine, Universidad, Peruana Cayetano, Heredia, Lima, Peru

Henri Collomb (M.D.), Professeur de Psychiatrie, Universite de Dakar, Dakar, Senegal, West Africa

Leon Cytryn (M.D.), Research Associate, Children's Hospital of the D.C., Associate Professor of Pediatric Psychiatry, The George Washington University School of Medicine, Washington, D.C., U.S.A.

Luis Estrada De Los Rios (Ph.D.), Chief, Service of Psychology, Hospital Del Empleado, Lima, Peru

Daniel Feinberg (M.D.), Clinical Instructor in Child Psychiatry, Albert Einstein College of Medicine, Bronx, New York; Supervising Psychiatrist, Center for Preventive Psychiatry, White Plains, New York, U.S.A.

Erna Furman (B.A. Hon.) (London), Assistant Clin. Professor in Child Therapy, Child Therapist, Cleveland Center for Research in Child Development and Dept. of Psychiatry, Case Western Reserve Medical School, Cleveland, Ohio, U.S.A.

Robert A. Furman (M.D.), Director, Cleveland Center for Research in Child Development, Cleveland, Ohio, U.S.A.

Edward H. Futterman (M.D.), Associate Professor of Psychiatry, The Abraham Lincoln School of Medicine, University of Illinois College of Medicine, Chicago, Illinois, U.S.A.

Michael Gourevitch (Docteur en Medecine), Medecin des Hopitaux Psychiatriques, Hopital Psychiatrique de Villejuif, Villejuif (Val-de-Marne) France

Geoffrey E. Gorer (M.D.), Haywards Heath, Sussex, England

Howard Hansen (M.D.), Associate Professor of Pediatrics and Psychiatry, University of Southern California School of Medicine, Los Angeles, California, U.S.A.

Patricia Hassakis (M.D.), Pediatrics, U.C.L.A. Department of Pediatrics, Los Angeles, California, U.S.A.

Dr. L. A. Hersov (M.D., M.R.C.P., F.R.C.Psych., D.P.M.), Consultant Physician, The Bethlem Royal Hospital and the Maudsley Hospital, London, England

Irwin Hoffman (A.B.), Instructor in Psychology, Department of Psychiatry, Abraham Lincoln School of Medicine, Chicago, Illinois, U.S.A.

Eliezer Ilan (M.A.), Director of Child Guidance Clinic, Senior Teacher, Ministry of Health, The Hebrew University, Jerusalem, Israel

Reimer Jensen (Cand. Psych.), Associate Professor, The Royal Danish School of Educational Studies, Copenhagen 2400 NV, Denmark

Judith S. Kestenberg (M.D.), Clinical Associate Professor, Dept. of Psychiatry, College of Medicine, Downstate Medical Center, Brooklyn, New York, U.S.A.

R. S. Khare (Ph.D.), Professor of Anthropology, University of Virginia, Charlottesville, Virginia, U.S.A.

Hilel Klein (M.D.), Medical Director, Eitanim Psychiatric Government Hospital, Jerusalem, Israel

Cyrille Koupernik (M.D.), Formerly Assistant des Hopitaux de Paris, Ittleson Visiting Lecturer; Psychiatrist, the American Hospital of Paris, 63, Bd. Victor-Hugo 92 Neuilly, Paris (80), France

Moses Laufer (M.Sc., Ph.D.), Director, Centre for the Study of Adolescence/ Brent Consultation Centre, London. Part-Time Staff, Hampstead Child-Therapy Clinic, London, England

Stanley J. Leiken (M.D.), Assistant Clinical Professor, Division of Child Psychiatry, Dept. of Child Psychiatry, U.C.L.A. Neuropsychiatric Institute, Los Angeles, California, U.S.A.

Serge Lebovici (M.D.), Director, Centre Alfred Binet, Paris 13, France

Reginald S. Lourie (M.D.), Professor of Child Health and Development and Psychiatry, George Washington University of Medicine, Washington, D.C., U.S.A.

Lee B. Macht (M.D.), Assistant Professor of Psychiatry, Harvard Medical School, Boston, Massachusetts, U.S.A.

John E. Mack (M.D.), Associate Professor of Psychiatry, Harvard Medical School, Boston, Massachusetts, U.S.A.

Alegria Majluf (M.S.), Advisor, Nursery School of Education Board, Ministry of Education, Lima, Peru

Peter Van P. Moore (M.D.), Research Associate, Children's Hospital of the D.C., Clinical Instructor of Psychiatry, The Georgetown University Medical School, Washington, D.C., U.S.A.

Joseph M. Natterson (M.D.), Associate Clinical Professor, Department of Psychiatry, USC School of Medicine, Los Angeles, California, U.S.A.

Phyllis Palgi (M.A.) (Soc.Sc.), Doctorant, Chief Anthropologist, Mental Health Division, Government of Israel, Lecturer, Department of Behavioral Sciences, Tel-Aviv University Medical School, Tel-Aviv, Israel

Norman D. Paul (M.D.), Family Psychiatrist, Harvard Medical School, Assistant Clinical Professor of Psychiatry, Cambridge, Mass., U.S.A.

Anna Potamianou (Ph.D.), In private practice; formerly the scientific Director of the Center for Mental Health and Research (1957–1968), Athens, Greece

J. Pouillon, Charge de conferences, Ecole pratique des hautes etudes (VIe section), Laboratoire D'Anthropologie Sociale, College de France, Paris, France

Ginette Raimbault (M.D.), Maltre de Recherche de l'Institut National de Sante et de Recherche Medicales (I.N.S.E.R.M.), Unite de Recherches Metaboliques (Prof. P. Royer, Hopital des Enfants, 149, rue de Sevres, 75 Paris (150 arr.), Paris 75, France

Nina Rausch de Traubenberg (Ph.D.), Maltre Assistant, Clinical Psychologist, Child Psychiatric Clinic-Hopital La Salpetriere, Paris, Universite Rene Descartes, Institut de Psychologie, 28 rue Serpente-Paris VI, Clinique de Psychiatrie Infantile, La Salpetriere, Paris XIII, Paris 75, Seine, France

Adolfo E. Rizzo (M.D.), Instructor in Clinical Child Psychiatry, Washington University Division of Child Psychiatry, St. Louis, Missouri, U.S.A.

Mary E. Robinson (Ph.D.), Research Associate, Children's Hospital of the D.C., Assistant Clinical Professor of Pediatrics (Child Development), The George Washington University School of Medicine, Washington, D.C., U.S.A.

Donald J. Scherl (M.D.), Assistant Professor of Psychiatry, Harvard Medical
    School, Boston, Massachusetts, U.S.A.

John E. Schowalter (M.D.), Director of Training and Associate Professor of
    Pediatrics & Psychiatry, Yale University Child Study Center, New
    Haven, Connecticut, U.S.A.

John J. Sigal (Ph.D.), Research Director, Institute of Community and
    Family Psychiatry, Jewish General Hospital, Montreal, Quebec,
    Canada

Maria A. Silva De Castro (M.D.), Assistant Professor, Universidad Peruana
    Cayetano Heredia, Lima, Peru

Albert J. Solnit (M.D.), Director, Child Study Center, Sterling Professor of
    Pediatrics and Psychiatry, Yale University, New Haven, Connecticut,
    U.S.A.

Joel Vernick (M.S.W.), Clinical Social Worker, National Institute of Child
    Health and Human Development, Bethesda, Maryland, U.S.A.

Miriam Williams (M.D., L.R.C.P. & S.E.), Psychoanalyst—Adult and
    Child, Los Angeles Psychoanalytic Institute (British Psa. Assoc.), Santa
    Monica, California, U.S.A.

Marilyn Winograd (M.A.), Director, Early Childhood Development Center,
    Evanston, Illinois, U.S.A.

W. H. G. Wolters (Drs.), Head Psycho-Social Department, Wilhelmina
    Children's Hospital, University of Utrecht, Utrecht, The Netherlands

Foreword

It is only a few years since Geoffrey Gorer, one of the contributors to this volume, remarked how in our generation death had replaced sex as the topic most heavily steeped in taboo. Now that taboo is lifting. The volume before us shows that a host of clinicians not only recognize the central role that death may play in the problems of our field but are already embarking on systematic studies to explore them.

The taboo on considering death, and especially the deaths of parents or children, is no accident. All partings are painful. What makes death so especially painful is that, whereas other partings may be reversed, the parting of death can never be; at least not on this earth. That is what creates difficulties for our patients. And that, too, is what creates difficulties for ourselves.

Once we are brave enough to study the ways in which ordinary people respond to a bereavement, we realize how ignorant we have hitherto been and how necessary it is to correct the norms and values of our western culture.

There is now abundant evidence to show that, at all ages short of old age, a bereaved person finds it almost impossible to believe that the loss has really occurred and is really permanent. As a result a great deal of time and thought is given to considering how the loss occurred, who may be to blame, and even how it can be reversed. Much behavior that, during a period of grief, is otherwise inexplicable can be understood as reflecting a search for the lost person. Much anger can be seen as directed against those who insist that the loss is permanent and who therefore will not encourage or participate in the search. During childhood these ideas and feelings are frequently conscious though perhaps not divulged to others. During adult life they may also be conscious, though in our culture they are often disguised. Some of the evidence on which these generalizations are based is presented in a paper on "Separation and Loss Within the Family" published in the first volume of the Yearbook. For example, on interviewing a group of 22 London widows at the end of their first year of bereavement, my colleague Colin Parkes found that over half of them still found it hard to accept the fact that their husbands were dead. Most of them still spent much time thinking about the past and still sometimes had a sense of their husband's nearby presence. The same is true of children after they have lost a parent, now well documented by Martha Wolfenstein.

In other cultures, the fact that widows and children have such thoughts and feelings is not only well recognized but culturally accepted. In Japan, for example, a widow is expected to create a small shrine in her living room at which her husband's spirit is deemed to reside and where she can consult him: "The lost object is not lost. The mourner can cling to the deceased, who has become an ancestor to be worshiped and fed, and with whom the mourner can share experiences and discuss eventful happenings."* This custom, our colleagues there believe, aids a widow come to terms with her loss.

It is of the utmost importance for Western culture that we should recognize that those thoughts and feelings are both general and typical, for it is only when we do so that we are in a position to help bereaved people recover from the blow. A new perspective calls, moreover, for a changed vocabulary. For example, the word "denial" is ill-chosen for talking about a bereaved person's hopes that all may not be lost. Denial is an egocentric word. It claims that the speaker is the arbiter of what is real and that anyone who disagrees with him is wrong. A better word is "disbelief." The more we respect how a person is feeling and thinking and are able to see things from his point of view the better able are we to help him.

Common experience suggests that it is only when a bereaved person— adult or child—can share his feelings with others that he can, in due course, get over the loss. Here again our cultural values can be a handicap. For so many of a bereaved person's feelings are apt to be regarded as unworthy and unmanly. They commonly comprise yearning for the impossible, intemperate anger, impotent weeping, and horror at the prospect of loneliness. All too often in western countries to express such feelings is to court criticism and contempt. It is therefore no wonder that so often they go unexpressed, and may later become unconscious.

Once the hopes and expectations that a bereaved person has of recovering the person lost become unconscious, they are very apt to become displaced or redirected towards others. A child is seen as the impersonation of a dead spouse and so is clung to; or a baby is held to be the reincarnation of a child who died, and so is expected to fulfill the dead child's destiny. Many of the papers in this volume discuss the clinical problems that stem from

*J. Yamamoto et al., Mourning in Japan, *Amer. Journal of Psychiatry.* Vol. 125 (1969), 1660–1665.

these inevitable but misdirected hopes of recovering someone loved who has gone.

This raises yet a further point—the need for clinicians to recognize that to make an affectional bond with another person, to be grieved and angry when it is broken, and to disbelieve that a loss can be permanent, is neither more nor less than an expression of our common humanity. To be attached to another human being is in no sense a sign of weakness, an attribute of infancy or childhood that an adult should be ashamed of, but an integral part of being a healthy man or woman. Because in misfortune it is healthy and natural to seek the presence and aid of another trusted person, the term "attachment" is far preferable to the traditional "dependency." For dependency is drenched in adverse value judgment; whereas we are all proud to be described as "attached," everyone feels humiliated to be called "dependent." In the same way to describe the weeping of grownups as a regression is not only probably mistaken on scientific grounds but reflects an attitude more likely to hinder a patient's recovery than to help him.

Failure in our culture to recognize attachment for what it is gives rise to many troubles. For example, a main reason why some people find expressing grief extremely difficult seems to be that the family in which they were brought up, and with which they may still mix, is one in which the attachment behavior of a child is regarded unsympathetically, and as something to be grown out of as quickly as possible. In such families, to cry or otherwise to protest at separation is apt to be dubbed babyish, and anger or jealousy as reprehensible. In such families, moreover, the more a child demands to be with his mother or his father the more he is told that such demands are silly and unjustified; the more he cries or throws a tantrum the more he is told he is babyish and "spoiled." As a result of being subjected to such pressures, moreover, he is likely to come to accept those standards for himself, to internalize them. As a result, to cry, to make demands and to feel angry because they are not met, will be judged by him as unjustified, babyish, and bad. And, so, when he suffers serious loss, instead of expressing the feelings that every bereaved person is filled with, he is inclined to stifle them. Furthermore, because his relatives, products of the same family culture, are likely to share the same critical outlook toward emotion and its expression, the very person who most needs understanding and encouragement is the one least likely to receive it.

These are large issues and also controversial ones. Many years will elapse before they are clarified and solutions agreed. Meanwhile, as this volume bears witness, there is no longer doubt among child psychiatrists or members of our allied professions that problems of illness, of dying, and of bereavement are central to our work nor that research, both empirical and theoretical, is urgently called for.

JOHN BOWLBY, M.D.
Past President of the
International Association of
Child Psychiatry and Allied
Professions

Preface

This second volume in the series *The Child in His Family* continues the tradition of bringing together original contributions from invited international authorities representing different disciplines and cultures who focus their expert attention on some common problem or set of problems besetting the human family. As in the first volume, the approaches are wide ranging in their scientific scope and encompass both the clinician's invaluable impressions and intuitions as well as the researchers more objective methods. Saliently, and refreshingly, the text includes material in which the children are allowed to speak for themselves from the perspective of their own stage of development. In these verbatim accounts, one is able to discern the authentic voice of childhood in situations of stress and distress. The book also makes it abundantly clear that although cultural variations in response to disease and death run a gamut of responses from India to Peru, people from all over the world (parents and children) resonate to the basic human condition in much the same ways inwardly. The repertoire of reaction is extensive since families have had many centuries of exposure to suffering and death in which to elaborate their coping techniques.

This current volume has some claims to originality. It assembles for the first time a large amount of new work coupled with reviews and revisions of the old and has placed them in a spectrum extending from sickness to survival. It is true that there is already in scattered existence a voluminous bibliography on the psychological, social, and cultural adjustments to disease and death, but nowhere else have they been put together for clinicians. Its primary usefulness will be to the large group of professional and paraprofessional personnel who have to deal with seriously ill and dying children and families in which death has occurred. There is also a section on violent death covering suicide, infanticide, homicide, and parricide.

We wish to express our gratitude to the contributors for their cooperation in working with us, to Professor Serge Lebovici for furnishing material for editorial comment in addition to his own excellent contribution, to the publishers for accelerating the process of publication in order to keep the series up-to-date, to Mrs. Martha Kniepkamp for once again helping with the time-consuming and arduous task of preparing the manuscripts for publication, and to Mrs. Laurel Sitek for producing immaculate typewritten pages from those mutilated by indecipherable editorial scrawls.

E. James Anthony, M.D.
Cyrille Koupernik, M.D.

St. Louis, Missouri
Paris, France
September, 1972

Contents

General Aspects   1

A Working Model for Family Studies   3
> *E. James Anthony (U.S.A.)*

A Survey of Family Reactions to Disease and Death in a
Family Member   21
> *Michel Gourevitch (France)*

Disease   29

Editorial Comment   31
> *Cyrille Koupernik (France)*

Psychological Adjustment of Children with Cystic Fibrosis   37
> *Leon Cytryn, Peter Van P. Moore,*
> *and Mary E. Robinson (U.S.A.)*

Psychological Study of Parents of Children with Cystic Fibrosis   49
> *Stanley J. Leiken and Patricia Hassakis (U.S.A.)*

Problems of Emotional Adjustment in Juvenile Diabetes   59
> *A. Zeidel (Israel)*

Psychological Problems in the Chronic Nephropathies of
Childhood   65
> *G. Raimbault (France)*

Psychological Aspects of Congenital Heart Disease in the Child   75
    Nina Rausch de Traubenberg (France)

The Roots of Hypochondriasis in the Child   85
    Cyrille Koupernik (France)

Dying   **97**

Editorial Comment   99
    E. James Anthony (U.S.A.)

Meaningful Communication with the Fatally Ill Child   105
    J. Vernick (U.S.A.)

The Fear of Death in Fatally Ill Children and Their Parents   121
    Joseph M. Natterson (U.S.A.)

Crisis and Adaptation in the Families of Fatally Ill Children   127
    Edward H. Futterman and Irwin Hoffman (U.S.A.)

The Doctor and the Dying Child   145
    N. Alby and J. M. Alby (France)

The Dying Child in Hospital   159
    W. H. G. Wolters (Holland)

Symposium: The Dying Child in an American Hospital   **169**

Jimmy—A Clinical Case Presentation of a
Child with a Fatal Illness   171
    C. M. Binger (U.S.A.)

Death and Mourning   **189**

Editorial Comment   191
    Cyrille Koupernik (France)

Childhood Leukemia—Emotional Impact on Siblings   195
    C. M. Binger (U.S.A.)

The Experience of Death on an Adolescent Pediatric Ward   211
    John E. Schowalter (U.S.A.)

The Need to Mourn   219
    Norman L. Paul (U.S.A.)

A Child's Capacity for Mourning   225
    Robert A. Furman (U.S.A.)

Pathological Mourning   233
    Marilyn Winograd (U.S.A.)

✓ Who Mourns When a Child Dies?   245
    Albert J. Solnit (U.S.A.)

Mourning and Psychic Loss of the Parent   255
    E. James Anthony (U.S.A.)

Suicide, Homicide, and Parricide   **265**

Editorial Comment   267
    E. James Anthony (U.S.A.)

Childhood Parental Loss, Suicidal Ideation, and
   Suicidal Behavior   275
    Kenneth S. Adam (Canada)

The Impact of a Father's Suicide on His Latency Son   299
    Eliezer Ilan (Israel)

Children Who Torture and Kill   307
    S. Lebovici (France)

Children Who Kill Their Mothers   319

    John E. Mack, Donald J. Scherl,
    and Lee B. Macht (U.S.A.)

Adolescent Girls Who Kill or Try to Kill Their Fathers   333

    E. James Anthony and A. Rizzo (U.S.A.)

Survival   **351**

Editorial Comment   353

    E. James Anthony (U.S.A.)

Symposium: Children of the Holocaust   **357**

Introductory Remarks   359

    Judith S. Kestenberg (U.S.A.)

The Analysis of a Child of Survivors   363

    Moses Laufer (England)

Children of Survivors   375

    L. Rosenberger (Israel)

The Impact of the Nazi Concentration Camps on
the Children of Survivors   379

    Erna Furman (U.S.A.)

Children of Concentration Camp Survivors   385

    Dov R. Aleksandrowicz (U.S.A.)

Children of the Holocaust: Mourning and Bereavement   393

    Hilel Klein (Israel)

Hypotheses and Methodology in the Study of Families of
the Holocaust Survivors   411

    John J. Sigal (Canada)

The Transcultural Experience of Death, Dying, and Disability 417

Introduction: Transcultural Approaches to the Experience of
Death 419

    Geoffrey Gorer (England)

Death, Grief, and Mourning in Britain 423

    Geoffrey Gorer (England)

The Child Who Leaves and Returns or the Death of the
Same Child 439

    H. Collomb (Senegal)

Discontinuity in the Female Role Within the Traditional
Family in Modern Society: A Case of Infanticide 453

    Phyllis Palgi (Israel)

Dying and Death: Some Hindu Cultural Rules and Paradigms 465

    R. S. Khare (U.S.A.)

The Reaction of Peruvian Families to the Disablement of
the Father 479

    *Renato Castro de la Mata, Maria A. Silva de Castro,
Alegria Majluf, and Luis Estrada (Peru)*

Symposium: The Dying Child in an African Hospital 489

Death of a Child in Nigeria 491

    T. Asuni (Nigeria)

Epilogue 501

    E. James Anthony (U.S.A.)

Index 507

The Child in His Family

THE IMPACT OF DISEASE AND DEATH

VOLUME 2

GENERAL ASPECTS

A Working Model for Family Studies*

E. James Anthony, M.D. (U.S.A.)

Problems in Family Research

We, who are born in families and, for the most part, live and
die in families, have an unresolvable problem in studying families
and the impact of events upon them, since we can hardly do what
the scientific observers are generally asked to do, that is, stand outside our field of investigation and look at it objectively with proper
emotional detachment. We are so deeply and inextricably inside
the field of study that our observations are inevitably biased and
contaminated. Furthermore, when we attempt to conceptualize our
investigations, it is hardly possible to blot out the echoes arising
within us of our own families of origin and orientation. This is the
scientific predicament of man as a psychosocial investigator. He is
always, whether he knows it or not, prejudiced by his preconceptions which are built into the very fabric of his way of looking at
things.

The second problem of the family researcher stems from his being
a child of his times and thus reflecting the mysterious *Zeitgeist* that
pervades a given field at a given time causing a spawning of ideas
that are similar but that, unfortunately, are labeled differently. Investigators have their share of suggestibility and are as prone to the

*Based on the address given at the plenary session of the 6th International Congress of
Child Psychiatry and Allied Professions in Jerusalem, August, 1970.

contagion of fashionable ideas as are nonscientific members of the community. The assimilation and transformation of concepts deriving from a total contemporary pool are so subtle and universal that the process of unconscious plagiarism remains largely undetected and undetectable. It is therefore difficult to ever be sure that one's notions are a product of one's own experience and not of the collective wisdom of the field. This might place us more frequently than we like between the proverbial horns of a dilemma were it not for the fortunate fact that our scientific narcissism is such that we generally manage to give ourselves the benefit of any doubt regarding our originality.

The third and final problem has to do with the presentation of our findings to others. This is a problem for all clinicians who must translate their living encounter with the patient into the abstraction of words for the purpose of communication. To the student of psychodynamic processes, the family in transaction is a thing of endless wonder as the interactions are bent to serve the many and varied needs of the membership. To reduce this to a formulation is to lose the essence of what is happening. Today one-way screens and audiovisual techniques attempt to preserve the vitality and rhythm of life although their intrusion may add an artificial element to the proceedings.

These three problems are each concerned with the impediments to knowing a family — observationally from the outside, intuitively and empathically from the inside, intellectually from the ideas generated during appraisals, and affectively from counter-feelings provoked by contact. Another mode of knowing is by living-in with the family and participating intimately in their daily lives. Knowing the family in these different ways gives us a better chance to understand their reactions when confronted with internal or external crises. However, to utilize our total knowledge to the best advantage, we must construct a frame of reference or heuristic model that does justice to both the complexity and the range of the child in his family.

A Developmental-Transactional Model

Family theorists today have adopted three separate positions with regard to family process. One position emphasizes the individual in the family and his intrapsychic response. The family is regarded as being made up of various individuals whose internalized disorders may have repercussions on the family life. The second position sees the family transactionally as a communicating and interacting group in which psychology and psychopathology is essentially familiar and the individual is simply a part in relation to the whole. Midway between these two positions are those who focus their attention both on the individual and on the family with each member contributing his idiosyncratic share to the total pathology which, in turn, provokes pathological reactions in the different members.

In the model presented here, the transactional viewpoint (as outlined by Anthony and Benedek [4]) subsumes much more than the existential interchanges on a single level. It includes conscious, preconscious, and unconscious levels of exchange, systematic cross-identifications of personality, conscience, and drive; and inevitable collisions between immature and more mature modes of functioning. The model includes a time axis in the evolution of the family as a group through various stages of development. We are becoming increasingly aware of the mutuality of the psychodevelopmental process and the way in which parents respond to the various developmental stages through which their child passes. The parent finds himself or herself running along the same developmental course, but this time more in retrospect. For this second time around, the parent may react to the child's developmental phase, interact with the child during the phase, and reactivate some of the conflicts left unresolved from the same phase in his own childhood.

The psychology and psychopathology is further complicated by the transference of feelings and attitudes from the family of origin to the family of orientation. Developmental psychopathology in the family, therefore, always has a dual genesis as the family of the past and the family of the present continue to interact. When the psychopathology of the present demands a scapegoat, the family may turn to a transference object, a particular child, or to a particular stage of development. Families, like individuals, may have specific difficulties with certain developmental stages, so that each time a particular child comes up to a particular phase, the family as a whole may become disturbed. In addition to the intrapsychic and interpersonal tensions and conflicts that have to be resolved stage by stage, the family has to learn to cope with repercussions within the wider network of relationships outside of the family, as well as the ambient culture.

As it develops, the family, like the individual, tends to develop its own special identity that is a composite of the system of identifications operating within it. During early family life, the group may present a confused and fluctuating image to the outside world, but sometime after the first five years, the family identity consolidates and a "family likeness" begins to develop. The members display the same basic personality characteristics, the same coping skills, the same defense mechanisms, the same prejudices, the same humor, the same language patterns, and, when they decompensate and become conflicted, the same psychopathology with the same symptom clusters. After ten years, there is altogether less variability within the family and a greater susceptibility to common manifestations. As the children reach adolescence, the special identity problems of this stage interact with any identity problems already latent within the family and diffusion of family identity may result.

In the area of psychopathology, certain abnormal trends serve to give the family its hallmark. For example, there are families that are generally mistrustful and nurse their suspicions against a background of poor communication; there are hypersensitive families who have a hard time managing their interpersonal relationships since everybody is ready to be hurt and everybody is fearful of hurting others; there are aggressive families where aggression is a way of life and the members quickly learn that the best means of defense is attack carried out either actively or passively; and finally, there are sado-masochistic families in which torturers pair off with sufferers in orgies of painful interactions.

Families also evolve idiomorphic ways of dealing with the basic affects of anxiety and depression. In some anxious families, a great deal of free-floating worry pervades the atmosphere, whereas in other families, this may be quickly transformed into phobias, ob-sessions, compulsions, and conversions. Depression is also a particu-larly contagious affect within the family. Developmentally, a de-pressed mother can give rise, in succession, to a depressed infant, to depressive moods in the toddler, to depressive emotionalism in the latency child, and to sad and mournful adolescents. (It is important to realize that these depressive reactions are not simple reflections but an internal development in the child in relation to the with-

drawal and psychic loss of the mother.) A dominant parent can often
set the emotional tone of the family in addition to dictating the
major characteristics of its psychopathology, but it is the system of
crisscross identifications and counter-identifications between the
family members that helps to configure a pattern of family psychopathology.

If one observes a family together, one immediately becomes conscious of the generational and gender differences that govern the
interchanges. Role theory has scrutinized the family with respect
to manifest functions, but developmental roles imposed by psychosexual status have received scant attention. This is because family
theorists have generally not received any intensive training in child
development, while child psychiatrists and child psychologists are
usually woefully untrained in transactional dynamics. The bringing
together of the developmental and transactional within a single
model should certainly provide a fuller understanding of family life.

We can look at the family in several different developmental-
transactional ways. Cognitively, within the framework of Piaget, it
may represent a very heterogeneous group with members at the
sensori-motor, the symbolic, the intuitive-representational, the concrete operational, and the formal operational levels, each one of
which implies a radically different way of thinking and communicating. It should not be surprising, therefore, to find that transactions
are at times confused and that members may fail to get through to
one another. There is no doubt that a great deal of incomprehensibility is taken for granted in family living. The communications that
do penetrate may be grossly distorted by the inadequacies and im-
maturities of the cognitive apparatus. Vocabulary in itself sets
limits to understanding for different members. To some extent,
this inherent problem is overcome by the fabrication of a basic
family language which, like Esperanto, serves the purpose of everyday life by the use of simple concrete expressions and neologisms
that have been manufactured for private family use.

On a psychosexual scale, the oral, the anal, the phallic, and the
genital members may have basic difficulties in understanding or
empathizing with one another. For example, the child who has put
the anal phase for the most part behind him may behave unsympathetically and even punitively with the child still in the throes of
this particular period. Older children may react with repugnance to

the coprophilic interests of the toddler or the gluttonous preoccupations of the infant. A great many children, of course, pass through childhood trailing unresolved conflicts behind, and these are the ones that resonate to all the developmental conflicts occurring within a family at any given time. The adolescent, struggling with the reactivation of early conflicts within him, may display extreme intolerance to all the younger children in the family. To a certain degree, being in a certain developmental phase offers the child some immunity from the stimulations and provocations of other developmental phases, and, for the same reason, he has also some protection from traumata that is not phase-specific.

On a psychosocial scale, while younger members may be struggling to assert their autonomy, to carry out serious and satisfying work, and to achieve clear-cut roles and identities for themselves, the older members of the family may feel themselves in a rut and isolated from each other. So engrossing are these crises that the different members may find it hard to help one another with their own past experience.

The developmental-transactional picture of a family can be highly dramatic. For instance, in a particular household, the baby's six o'clock feeding is due, and right on time he starts to yell vociferously. The other members all respond in their own particular way. The mother's breasts begin to drip with milk; the toddler becomes cranky and messes his pants; the five-year-old girl, like a surrogate mother, runs to the baby to comfort him; the latency child continues to operate his chemistry set industriously and takes no apparent notice; the adolescent complains that the place is like a mad house and that he cannot think clearly in such a setting (this, by the way, while his stereo set is blasting with cacophonous melody); and the father finds himself unexpectedly grouchy and heads for the kitchen to fix himself a sandwich. Family life is like an orchestral performance with instruments of different range and different sounds playing together but not always harmoniously!*

The external family is matched by an internal family that each member carries within himself. This internal representation reflects the developmental stage of the individual allowing him to create a

---

*Adapted from a vignette provided by Brazelton, T., *Infants and Mothers. Differences in Development.* Boston: Belacorte Press, 1969.

more predictable environment for himself. It gives him some indication how members will react and interact and the more experience
he has of family life, the less surprises there are for him. At times,
he may manipulate the external family to have them correspond
more closely to his internal construct and this may occasion angry
and bewildering interchanges.

The model does not function in a vacuum but in a rich social and
cultural milieu which must be taken into account when evaluating
families. Freud was not unaware of the gulf between the lower
classes of Vienna and the middle-class patients whom he treated. In
a letter to his fiancée in 1883 he wrote: "I will not follow these
thoughts further, but one might show how *das volk* judges, believes,
hopes and works quite otherwise than we do. There is a psychology
of the common man which is somewhat different from ours."*
It is only very recently that psychoanalysts have returned to the
question of class differences.

The model described is a complex one to work with in practice
since it attempts to take into account simultaneously several interacting developments and to investigate them biologically, psychody-
namically, and culturally. Most investigations described in this book
confine themselves to one part of the model and therefore to only
one aspect of the problem.

Toward a Developmental-Transactional Epistemology

Although part of everyday life, serious disease and death invariably evoke surprise when they occur at any time but especially
in young families with children where the vital emphasis is on
growth and development. Young families, lacking experience and
well-established homeostatic mechanisms, are likely to react to a
powerful somatic threat against one of their members more catas-
trophically than older families which have suffered and endured
enough to have developed a repertoire of coping capacities.

The family collectively represents an encyclopedia of knowledge
into which the individual members dip according to the needs of their
particular stage of development. Depending on the family, the
amount of knowledge available may be limited, distorted, or trans-

Letters of Sigmund Freud, 1873–1939, edited by Ernst Freud. London: Hogarth
Press, 1961.

lated into more acceptable forms; it is frequently left to the individual members to construct their own theories out of a medley of
facts, fantasies, and fictions that reach them from various sources.
Investigators have attempted to tap this knowledge during different
stages of development in the manner of Piaget. In terms of disease,
the child's concept of his body and its functions and the child's
concept of bodily dysfunctions go hand in hand and both of these
have been described in part by Anthony [1,3] together with naive
dynamic theories and fantasies that develop along with them. It
was demonstrated, for example, that the attitudes toward feces and
bowel action were closely linked to childhood notions of animism.
For the younger children, feces were credited with a life of their
own, whereas with older children, they were alive as long as they
remained inside the body and became lifeless when excreted. With
the development of colitis and constipation, the dynamic notions
altered appreciably. With the loss of control over the bowel mo-
tions, feces became endowed with living and reacting properties and
were not only able to move by themselves but also to attack the
children. The latter concept was especially likely in those who had
received a harsh and punitive toilet training, within the transactional
dyad of what Anthony [1] called "the potting couple." Experience,
together with the stage of development, determined the nature of
the knowledge.

There have been several attempts to outline the development of
the child's conception of death, but they have all lacked a dynamic
and transactional viewpoint and have taken only manifest developmental responses into consideration. An exception would be the
work of Susan Isaacs [13] in which peer group transactions were
considered and dynamic elements explored but, unfortunately, in
no way systematically. Questionnaires and drawings with interroga-
tions have constituted the main approach. Sylvia Anthony [5] found
that the child's notions of death corresponded very closely to his
notions of life as outlined in stages by Piaget. Nagy [19], who was
referred to by her child subjects as "Auntie Death," obtained her
data from essays written by seven- to ten-year-olds in which they
were encouraged to "write down everything that comes into your
mind about death." Death was viewed by those under nine with
"infantile realism" (Piaget) and personified in different stereotyped
ways. The "death man" was sometimes a skeleton, sometimes a

woodcutter, and frequently depicted as a man in a white coat with long legs and arms and eyes as big as sequins. On one hand, the person who is dead cannot move and does not speak; yet if you pass by his grave he knows that you are there and he hears you talking. For the younger children death is a temporary separation that is reversible. When the fact of irreversibility is recognized at about the age of ten, the fears are counteracted by new fantasies and theories of rebirth, reunion, and reincarnation. In the sensitive death-oriented child, the topic can become an intense preoccupation and lead to an existential crisis with phobias and nightmares, as described by Anthony [2]. A child's actual experience of death of sibling or parent may exert a major effect on his notions. Cousinet [7], Schilder and Wechsler [20], and Mitchell [18] have all explored the child's developing attitude toward death, but the results were limited by the inadequacies of method. In Giabicani's study with Heuyer and Lebovici [12], a number of questions relating to the diagnosis and etiology of death were put to 110 French children between the ages of four and fourteen. The findings of the survey were, on the whole, disappointing. There was no evidence of any "innate ideas and the general conclusion was that the child simply replicated the information from parents and teachers and that personal experience played only a peripheral part except for deaths in the immediate family. More productively, the study did attempt to relate the child's notions of death to his aggressive propensities. Weber [22] found that 50 to 60% of children between six and fifteen years of age have seen a dead body, although according to him, the child is unlikely to become preoccupied with death before puberty. Weber believes that there is no reason to doubt the profound and primitive roots of the death experience in the child.

As yet, there are no systematic developmental-transactional studies. Two sets of crises regarding death may occur during childhood in sensitive children living in a family in which free emotional expression is accepted and even encouraged. The first crisis, based on separation anxiety and fear of abandonment, occurs between four and six years of age, and the second crisis, an existential crisis at an age between nine and eleven years, is brought about by the realization of the irreversibility of death, in relation to both the self and loved ones.

Belsley [6], in a personal communication, reported the following reaction in her four-year-old son.

One morning Eric watched a television program on the funeral of General DeGaulle. He sat very intently and then started asking questions about it. When I explained that a very famous man had died, he asked what it meant that he was dead. I told him that it meant he would not be living anymore and would not move. Then he saw the coffin and when he found out a man was in it, he wanted to know how he could get out. I explained that he would not get out and then he asked a whole lot of questions, one after the other, about how he got in there, why he was in there, and why he died. I said that he was an old man and that when people get old their bodies do not work as well and that they sometimes get sick and then they die. He asked whether young people died and I answered that some did but usually people died when they were old. He then asked about his grandparents dying, his parents dying, and him-self dying, and I could see that he was beginning to get very upset about it and rather frightened. He kept on asking questions very nervously, such as could I die. What then would happen to him? Would he die? When would I die? And so on. I said that I was not sure, but that it was pretty likely when I and his father die, he would be a grown-up man which was quite a few years from now. He got more and more upset. When, however, I tried to turn the television off, feeling that things had gone too far by this time, he begged me to leave it on being he was very interested in seeing what happened. You could see that the whole idea was gripping him and hitting him with some force. So I left it on and sat there with him, and held him, and tried to answer his ques-tions as best I could and as honestly as I could without making it sound too frightening. A little later, he began to almost cry, walking around in a kind of daze, keeping on with his questions. He would be quiet for a few minutes after I had answered him, and then he would come back with the same kind of questions: "Why do people die? I don't want you to die. I don't want to die. What will happen if Daddy dies and you die and Karen (his sister) dies and I am left alone?" His father then tried to give him some idea of how many years it would be until he probably died so that he could see it was not an immediate worry. Since Eric knows how to count, he started counting with him saying: "We are going to count all the way to 70 and just see how long it is," and he counted very slowly. After this, Eric seemed to feel a little better. The more Eric talked, the more I realized that although he was very attached to me and very dependent on me that his main fear was that he was going to lose me, he was also very afraid of not being anymore. Since he was quite upset about the whole matter, I tried to give him a lot of physical attention that day. He would feel a little better for a while and then start again. When he went to bed at night, he said to me: "I'm not going to wake up in the morning. I won't be here. I'm going to die during the night," I assured him that that surely would not happen. In the weeks that followed his concern with death remained but it gradually became less disturbing. However, whenever he felt out of sorts, the thoughts came back and he would explain to me earnestly that he was only a little bit sick and not really sick enough to die. When I tried to coax him to eat certain foods and take his vitamins (as I've always done) he began to worry about whether people died if they did not eat well, and would he die. I said that if children did not eat the right kind of foods for a long time, they could get sick and die and that this sometimes happened in very poor countries and I showed him some pictures of children with malnutrition. But I told him although he did not eat well enough as far as I was concerned, and that I wanted him to eat better, he really had nothing to fear and that he certainly got enough food to stay alive. It was just that I thought he might be a little healthier and more comfortable if he could eat a little more regularly. Curiously enough, his sister Karen, at the same age, had the same kind of reaction when we watched the funeral of Martin Luther King on television. She asked the same kind of questions that Eric did, but wanted to know more about what happened to the body after it was buried. Like Eric, she then went on to ask about people that she knew, such as her grandparents and parents, and whether they would die. She said one thing that was omitted by Eric; she was very concerned that I did not die before she did. She wanted everyone that she loved to wait and die after she died. After this, Karen's feelings about death went underground, but lately (she is now nine) she has disclosed a lot of death concerns in her diary, for example, "Eric looks like he is dead when he is asleep"; and "I don't like the way Mommy lies with the back of her head on the pillow"; and other such anxious comments.

It would be an oversimplification to state that the first crisis (four to six years old) has to do with fantasied loss and the second crisis (nine to eleven years old) with actual loss. From a developmental point of view, gleaned retrospectively, the conclusion seems plausible, but a transactional account at the time suggests a much greater complexity. One is struck not only by the intensity of feeling involved and their persistence over time, but also by the ramifications into the child's life and family. The case of Robert (reported by Zeligs [23])bears all this out. Robert's one-year-old baby brother died suddenly and mysteriously in his crib. The mother had left him in the care of her cleaning woman while she went to see the doctor. The shock and pain seemed greater to her because she had not been with the baby when he needed her most. Robert, five years old, and Louise, three years old, had been sent to a neighbors during the crisis of death.

When the children were brought in, Robert ran up and said immediately, "Is David alright? I want to see David." I [the mother] tried to hide my grief and said, "You can't see him now, he is asleep." The children spent the night at a neighbor's. Robert worried about the baby all night and had to be given a sedative to sleep. The parents decided to tell the children the truth.

The father took Robert on his lap and the mother held Louise on hers, and they said: "David is not alright. He got sick suddenly, yesterday. He died and fell asleep, never to awaken. He is with God in heaven, now. His memory will always be in our hearts, but he will not be with us anymore." "He's not dead! I want my baby! Tell God I want David back!" Robert jumped up and down and screamed hysterically, "I want my baby!" His grief was uncontrollable and he wept bitterly. Louise simply repeated the words, "David died, David died." But did not seem to really understand what was going on. Robert had always felt a great responsibility for the younger children. Everytime David cried he would run up and talk to him. The first thing he did when he came home from school was to look for the baby. They would have a lot of fun together. David seemed to love him, would gurgle in delight when Robert played with him. "Why did God take our baby? Will God know how to change the baby's diaper? Are the angels watching him? Will they give him his bottle?" After the funeral Robert was very sad and cried a lot, especially when it was time to go to bed. He seemed afraid to close his eyes. The parents tried to hide their grief in the presence of the children, but they seemed to sense their sorrow. When the father had to return to work, the mother felt very frightened and insecure and the father said to Robert: "If I'm not here and your mother cries, you must help her." When he left a great loneliness swept over the mother and she could not control her grief. Robert clung to her and they cried together. He was very frightened to see her cry. "If I draw horses for you, will it help?" he asked. When she said it would help, his face brightened, and he drew horses for her all morning. He seemed to feel a great responsibility for taking care of her. The mother felt that they had always burdened this willing and serious child with too many responsibilities. Once, when Louise was a baby, she had been left alone in the car with Robert while his parents went into a shop, and Robert was asked to "watch the baby." When they returned, Robert was hysterical. He was afraid something would happen to the baby. After that he refused to be left alone with her because he felt something might happen to her and he would be blamed. The pediatrician suggested that Robert might be jealous of Louise, but the parents remarked that he had always been overly concerned about her, and he acted the same way about David, too. The father had always warned him to look after the younger ones. He was somewhat strict especially with Robert. He himself had been an only child and his mother had been very strict and had spanked him hard. On the other hand, he tended to spoil Louise. At bedtime Mother use to sing lullabys to her children and they would all have fun together, but after David died, this stopped. Robert himself had had a succession of serious illnesses since infancy. At 19 months, he had been hospitalized for a week and it had frightened him very much. Three months after the death of David, he became ill with nephritis and had to stay in bed for two months. One day, while he was in bed watching television, the program showed a grave. He burst into tears and said "What is this—a cemetery? Is David buried in a cemetery like this?" Then we had to tell him that the baby was buried. "I want to go to see him. I want to see David in the cemetery," he demanded. Mother said that he was too sick to do this. Robert wept bitterly and the parents did not know how to comfort him. After the loss of David, the parents decided to have another baby. They tried to feel that it was not a replacement, but, as the mother said, she could hardly wait until she had a baby in her arms again. Robert seemed very concerned about the pregnancy and asked her whether she would have had another baby if David wouldn't have died. He also asked whether the baby was going to be healthy and suggested that it be named David. The parents suspected that he had some idea that David would be returning in the form of the new baby. Mother remarked that he seemed confused about birth and death. He developed two major problems. He seemed to be always on edge and would cry at the slightest thing. Any scolding brought on uncontrollable sobbing. A little frown from the parents would upset him and make him almost hysterical. If his sister cried it also upset him. He also worried that the children would call him a cry-baby. He seemed fearful and insecure and unable to make the slightest decision. It was nine months since David's death and he still has not been able, reported the parents, to get over it. At the suggestion of the teacher, the parents consulted a psychologist and Robert told him, "My problem is that I cry too much and I'm afraid to go to school because the children will call me a cry-baby. I don't know why I started to cry....I have another problem. I don't like to go to sleep. I am afraid to close my eyes." The psychologist told the parents that they should share their sorrow with the children so that they did not feel excluded and also to concentrate more of their love and attention on the living rather than the lost child. She felt they must help Robert understand the facts of David's death, that it was no one's fault. Then they should explain about the funeral and tell him where the body is buried. Take him to visit the cemetery and place flowers at the grave site if he wished to do this. The parents were told not to hide their grief, but rather to share it. They were also told not to tell the children that death meant going to sleep and never waking up, otherwise the two would become inseparable in his mind. The psychologist got Robert to differentiate sleep from death in a very simple pragmatic way. She said to him "You are afraid something will happen while you are asleep. But nothing will really happen. You can hear things and feel things in your sleep. You are breathing. Your body and your heart are working. What happens when an alarm clock rings?" Robert: "It wakes people up." The psychologist continued: "Yes, and they hear it in their sleep, so they wake up. If someone would throw some cold water on your face, you would wake up. It would make you mad, too. Sleep is good because it helps your body rest from the work of the day. If you don't feel well in your sleep, it wakes you up. Your Mommy and Daddy have especially good ears when it comes to hearing if their children are alright while they are asleep. They watch over you. . . .It is not like being dead." And Robert replied: "Yes, I know. I know it is different." He improved dramatically and began to do well at school again. He became a little upset when the new baby was born, and it turned out to be a girl, but he recovered rapidly from this.

There have been no satisfactory developmental-transactional

studies of disease and its effect on the child and his family. The
finding of group differences with a selected number of variables has
constituted the main approach. For example, diabetic children as a
group are rated more pathologically with regard to psychiatric disturbance, self-perception, sexual identification, body image, manifest and latent anxiety, constriction, dysphoria, dependency, and
oral preoccupation (Swift, 1967 [21]). Comparing good and bad
adaptation to the disease has been a method of study by Mattsson
and Gross [17] (1965) with respect to hemophilia. They found
that the crucial factor determining good adaptation was the mother's
ability to master her guilt over having transmitted the illness. They
felt that in the poorly adapted cases, the hemophilic child was
identified with a deceased close relative, usually a bleeder, with the
result that the mothers saw their sons unrealistically as vulnerable
at all times. They felt that this was an important predisposing
factor in the development of the "vulnerable child syndrome," defined by Green and Solnit [11] (1964) as a serious disturbance in
the parent-child relationship following parental reactions to an acute
or chronic life-threatening illness in the child. Such a child senses
his mother's expectation of his vulnerability and premature death
and he may challenge this at the risk of injury, in a counterphobic
manner. Josselyn [14] studied a group of children with rheumatic
heart disease over a period of eight years and came to some tentative conclusions regarding the role that the illness played in their
lives. She felt that there was a tendency for a sick child to regress
to a dependency level, the illness offering a gratifying experience
in the amount of care provided. This could be tempting to a disturbed child. To the child with an unsatisfactory infantile relationship with the mother it compensated for what he had missed, and
for the child with a satisfactory relationship during infancy it reactivated the happy times. For the boy at the oedipal level of development, it gave the opportunity to seek out his mother on an
infantile, helpless level. The child also sought relief from his overpowering anxiety regarding his illness by regressing to a safer level
of development. A notable effect of the illness was on the capacity
to deal with problems aggressively. Aggression becomes dangerous
since it carries the possible punishment of death. One child expressed the wish to grow up and die sooner, because this would
allow him to go to heaven where there were no bad attacking people.

Heaven represented to him the only place where he would be free from the aggression of others. This was important to him since he could not, because of his general physical weakness and because of the danger underlying strenuous activity, defend himself. In Dubo's [8] study of children with pulmonary tuberculosis, the problem of repressed hostility was also in the forefront as well as its unfavorable influence on the course of the disease. She also observed characteristic reactions of anxiety, depression, dependency, and regression. Tuberculosis itself was equated with death and assumed the aspect of "a menacing introjected malignancy." The dreams, fantasies, and drawings of the children were filled with morbid and threatening symbols. The regressive trends were strong and reached "infantilization." Another disturbing threat to the children stemmed from the necessary stress on isolation and precautionary measures so that many of them reacted with a "pariah complex," and felt different, stigmatized, unclean, and ashamed. These feelings at times amounted to almost paranoid proportions. The children generally tended to assume personal responsibility for the illness as a punishment for disobedience or wrongdoing and protected parents from blame by displacing hostility inward. The persistent preoccupations with thoughts of death were related to a world-destruction fantasy and appeared to be an intensive fear of abandonment, in that, for the child, death meant that everyone went off and left him.

It would almost seem as if investigators have concerned themselves with dynamic, transactional, or developmental facets but never together in a comprehensive approach. Anna Freud has attempted to look at the natural history of illness with respect to the child's psychological responses. In the pre-illness phase, he may be bored, listless, and withdrawn. During the illness, he may respond to the love, attention, and indulgence generally shown by parents to sick children; he may object to the restriction in terms of eating, activity, and play; and he may resent or enjoy the regression in the service of the illness.

Following the illness, he may develop typical neurotic disorders or a "convalescent syndrome." Pain is the great problem for the sick child. "The child in pain is a child maltreated, harried, punished, persecuted, and threatened with annihilation." In a more or less whimsical comment, Gardner [9] has epitomized childhood development from one to twelve years in a series of dangerous D's—desertion, dismemberment, death, deprivation, defeat, disfigurement, dissection, disability, and disgrace—all of which may at times be represented in the stress of disease and dying. Another Gardner [10] (1969) has focused not on the child's guilt, but on the inappropriate guilt reaction of parents to the child's illness. He considered the Freudian hypotheses relating this to an excessive amount of unconscious hostility toward the stricken child or to a parental superego that was unduly severe in its tolerance of even normal hostility, and suggested that a third reason might stem from the parent's need to gain control over the uncontrollable and that this guilt could be utilized as a defense mechanism in the handling of existential anxiety.

Conclusion

We have attempted to construct a model with both longitudinal and cross-sectional properties, examining it in the context of clinical observations. The result is a *tableau vivant* rather than a statistical analysis that can be described only by an observer with a fundamental delicacy of perception together with a sensitivity and flair for the nuances of developing transactions. That it remains largely incoherent is a reflection of its detail and complexity. As we watch the picture unfold, we keep an eye on the antecedents since we believe them to play an integral part in the subsequent events. It is not an easy task to disentangle and make sense of the whole and its parts. In this context, comments by two shrewd observers of developing, changing man are highly appropriate. The physician-philosopher, John Locke [16] had this to say: "I see it is easier and more natural for men to build castles in the air on their own, than to survey well those that are to be found standing. Nicely to observe the history of Diseases, in all their changes and circumstances, is a work of time, accurateness, attention and judgment." The second observation derives from the anthropologist-philosopher, Claude Levi-Strauss [15] who adds this to the importance of the "work of time": "Every landscape offers, at first glance, an immense disorder which may be sorted out howsoever be pleased. He may sketch out the history of its cultivation, plot the accidents of geography which have befallen it, and produce the ups and downs of history and prehistory: but the most august of investigations is surely that which reveals what came before, dictated, and in large measure explains all the others."

This deals with the life event seen from the outside by an observer with a fundamental delicacy of perception and flair. The life event, such as disease and death, seen from the inside requires another special faculty, made up on empathy and intuition, to discern the dimensions and dynamics of the representation within. It is with this two-pronged approach over time with which this presentation is concerned.

Bibliography

1. Anthony, E. J., An experimental approach to the psychopathology of childhood: encopresis. *Brit. J. of Medical Psychology*, 30, (1957), 146–175.
2. Anthony, E. J., The Behavior Disorders of Childhood, in *Carmichael's Manual of Child Psychology*, Vol. *II*, (edited by P. Mussen) John Wiley & Sons Pub., New York, 1970.
3. Anthony, E. J., The child's discovery of his body. *J. Amer. Phys. Ther. Assn.*, 48 (1968), 1103–1114.
4. Anthony, E. J. and Benedek, T., *Parenthood—Its Psychology and Psychopathology.* Little, Brown, and Co., Boston, 1970.
5. Anthony, Sylvia, *The Child's Discovery of Death.* Harcourt Brace, New York, 1940.
6. Belsley, J., Personal communication.
7. Cousinet, R., The child's concept of death. *J. Psychol. Norm. Pathol.*, 36 (1939), 65–76.
8. Dubo, Sarah, Psychiatric study of children with pulmonary tuberculosis. *Amer. J. of Orthopsychiatry*, 20 (1950), 520–528.
9. Gardner, G., Quoted by W. S. Langford, in *Amer. J. of Orthopsychiatry*, 31 (1961), 673.
10. Gardner, R., The guilt reaction of parents of children with severe physical disease. *Amer. J. Psychiat.*, 126 (1969), 5.
11. Green, M., and Solnit, A. J., Reactions to the threatened loss of a child: a vulnerable child syndrome, *Pediatrics*, 34 (1964), 58–66.
12. Heuyer, G., Lebovici, S., and Giabicani, A., *Revue de Neuropsychiatric Infantile*, Vols. 5 and 6, (1955).
13. Isaacs, S., *Social Development in Young Children,* Routledge and Kegan Paul Ltd., London, 1930.
14. Josselyn, I., Emotional implications of rheumatic heart disease in children. *Amer. J. of Orthopsychiatry*, Vol. XIX, (1949), 87–100.
15. Levi-Strauss, C., *Tristes Tropiques* (Translated by J. Russell), Criterion Books, New York, 1961.
16. Locke, J., *Essays Concerning Human Understanding,* Oxford, London, 1860.
17. Mattsson, A. and Gross, S., Adaptational and defensive behavior in young

hemophiliacs and their parents. *Amer. J. of Psych.,* Vol. 122 (1966), 1349–1356.

18. Mitchell, M. E., *The Child's Attitude Toward Death,* Schocken Books, New York, 1967.

19. Nagy, M. H., The child's view of death. *J. Genet. Psychol.,* 73 (1968), 3–27.

20. Schilder, P. and Wechsler, D., The attitudes of children towards death. *J. Genet. Psychol.,* 45 (1934), 406–451.

21. Swift, C., Seidman, F. and Stein, H., Adjustment problems in juvenile diabetes. *Psychosomatic Medicine,* Vol. XXIX, (1967), No. 6.

22. Weber, A., Children's experience of death. *Monat. Psychiat. Neurolog.,* 107, (1943).

23. Zeligs, R., Death casts its shadow on a child. *Mental Hygiene,* 51, (1967), 9–20.

A Survey of Family Reactions to Disease and Death in a Family Member

Michel Gourevitch, M.D. (France)

A study of the general literature of this subject confirms the existence of the gap that E. J. Anthony and C. Koupernik emphasized in an Editorial Comment [3]: "What is less fully described and discussed, and may well be a stimulus for further investigation, is the influence of loss on family life and the ways in which the surviving members look to one another for solace, surrogation, and emotional support. The vicissitudes of detachment, searching, and reattachment behavior within a family group surely need to be explored transactionally."

On the other hand, the influence on the individual of bereavement and, more specifically, the death of one of his parents has been well investigated both with regard to immediate effects, that is, mourning [8, 11, 14] as well as remote effects, that is, permanent psychiatric consequences [7, 9], the validity of which has been denied [16].

Chronic illness in parents, like death of parents, has also been held responsible for the development of psychiatric illness in children [19]. There is a difference, however, between considering such effects on individual family members and on the family group as a whole. True, a child's death initiates the work of mourning in each one of his parents but as soon as one considers the couple together and the interactions that take place between them, one is faced with quite a different dynamic picture. More intricate still are the changes brought about by a father's disease or death in the dynamics of the relationship between his wife and their children. To add to the difficulties, the study of such facts can only be of the follow-up type, whereas it was by proceeding from effect to cause, along an anamnestic line consonant with the usual medical inquiry, that Bowlby and Birtchnell traced the probable source of disease in established patients and isolated the factor of an absent parent [7, 9]. The family's reactions can only be examined within the context of ongoing transactional observations that take into account the large number of variables involved, and this probably accounts for the dearth of studies of this type.

As far as reactions to *disease* are concerned, Anthony has undertaken a field study in which he has observed disturbed families in their own homes [4]; he refers in this to Lesage's "Lame Devil" who used to lift the roofs off houses in order to observe what went on underneath, which, etymologically, is detective work. He begins by reviewing his forerunners in the literature, most of them sociologists. Koos, some years ago [13], observed that the better a family's premorbid organization had been, the more efficient was the adjustment of the various members to stress; that disease altered the reciprocal relationships between family members, the sick father, for instance, losing his authority and regaining a permanently impaired one when he recovered. Parsons [17], well known for his inquiries into the sociology of disease, emphasized the inadequacy of the modern family's capacity to cope with illness. Spiegel [22] took a rosier view in postulating the establishment of a new balance within the family as the result of a series of readjustments. Sampson et al. [20] studied the effects of schizophrenia upon the relation between husband and wife and found that the more tolerant the family was to the pathological behavior, the later did therapy get started, a finding amply borne out by clinical observation. Every psychiatrist who has had the experience of diagnosing a case of severe schizophrenia of long duration is not unlikely to have been confronted by a blind disbelief on the part of the family, even those of high intellectual and socioeconomic status.

Finally, Anthony extrapolated from Toynbee's "Challenge and Response" thesis [23] to account for the way in which his families, like societies, responded in three different ways to the dangers that threatened them—namely, by growth and differentiation, by collapse followed by recovery, and by regression and disintegration. In order to see whether this same historical trend held true for families, Anthony set out to "unroof" homes. The family is a microsociety and the psychiatrist here made use of sociology and history in a profitable and convincing demonstration of multidisciplinary cooperation. Having extracted the historic-sociological lesson, he once again reverts to his clinical point of view and concludes with a psychopathological analysis that must be read in toto for a full appreciation of his findings. To summarize briefly, he discovered that in any psychotic patient's family a "genetic premonition," based on nothing but vague behavioral inferences bolstered by suggestion, may generate a pseudopsychotic clinical picture in selected children. On the more positive side, the family may conjointly elaborate a "theory of the disease" that helps to explain deviant behavior, clarify psychotic mystifications and, therefore, enhance the total adjustment of the group. Such theories have primitive foundations beneath the upper level of rationalizations. These mechanisms may also throw light on Sampson's [20] description of the family's coping maneuvers in response to the stresses provoked by psychosis and may represent a significant factor in the genesis of family psychopathology.

Most of these studies, whether conducted through an "open roof" or not, deal with the effects of *mental* illness. Anthony does, in fact, quote one case of tuberculosis that had a positive outcome in terms of growth and differentiation but the home circumstances were so psychologically disturbed that the case might well have been included in the "mental" series. Nevertheless, he emphasizes the need to differentiate between the effects of physical and psychiatric disease. A catatonic mother or a paranoid father, in most cases, have morbid attributes long before they become psychologically ill and, therefore, exert effects of longer duration than, for example, rheumatoid arthritis or multiple sclerosis that overcome a hitherto healthy adult. There are many other "roofs" left to be lifted off including the obsessionalization of life brought about by the need for daily care in certain chronic illnesses as pointed out by Alby [1].

The impact of death on normal family life has been abundantly covered in the literature but mostly in relation to childhood leukemia. Childhood mortality was not inconsiderable in the past and was acknowledged as an event of everyday life. It was evident in Rousseau's statement in *Emile* [18] : "The less one has lived, the less one may expect to live. Of all the children who are born, not more than one-half will reach adolescence."

Nowadays, with the increase in life expectations, childhood and death have become so antithetical that their coincidence invariably promotes a sense of shock and mention of it has become suppressed. "Death seems to have been banished and has replaced sex as our most prohibited biological subject. The Victorian child had death in his prayers and in his precepts; modern children are more likely to be taught about their origin than about their departure from this world," says Yudkin [25].

The fate of the leukemic child has recently prompted several studies on both sides of the Atlantic. Perhaps, as Solnit has suggested, these authors were "confronted with what we expected to avoid in children by electing to become interested in death, chronic physical illness, and the end of a life rather than the beginning of one" [21]. From this current literature (as well as from absence of literature that preceded it and from the silence that still covers many of the problems connected with death), one can perhaps gain some insight not only into the family's reactions but also into this curious reticence of the physicians.

There are children who succumb to chronic illness but they are a minority, at least in developed countries, as compared to the child victims of accidents. About the families of this latter group, little or nothing has been published [15]. It is, therefore, speculative to consider which situation entails a heavier taxation on the family's resources. One would be inclined to feel, with Alby [2] and Friedman [12], that mourning is less intense if prepared for during the slow process of dying from chronic illness. Yet it is difficult for the physician not to identify with the parents as suggested in the opposing view put forward by Yudkin when he says: "Perhaps we are more able to help the parents of a child who has been killed in an accident than those of a child who is dying of an illness: the first is someone else's responsibility; death from disease we think of as ours" [25].

Much of our knowledge of the family's reactions to death, therefore, is derived from studies involving some progressive illness in the
child such as leukemia [6, 10, 24]. "As the victims of an overwhelming assault on their parental identities as protectors and providers . . .," these parents will experience "not only the loss of a
child, but the impact of that loss on family relationships and atmosphere. For many parents, the loss of a child represents a permanent
severing of one line that they have put out to immortality" [24].
To this attack on their parental self-image, they will respond by a
coping strategy based upon certain mechanisms of defense, namely,
isolation of affect, denial, and increased motor activity [10].

But above all they will, antemortem, prepare for the inevitable
loss by an *anticipated mourning*. This is emphasized by all authors.
While still alive, the child is subjected to a progressive withdrawal of
cathexis, a detachment that takes the guise of "philosophic resignation." This is associated with denial, a defense mechanism that appears in the form of stubborn hope, often incompatibly linked with
a clear knowledge of prognosis, accepted at the conscious level.
Speaking of resignation, it is worth noting that the religious factor
is totally absent from the French studies, so deeply secularized is
this country, and the more so in matters of life and death. Anglo-
American authors, on the other hand, make frequent allusions to
the part played by religion [6, 12, 25] but its treatment gives the
impression of superficiality. In the face of death, the deeper psychological mechanisms appear to be the same in both believer and
atheist.

Guilt is a normal component of mourning, whether anticipated
or not, but as an individual response it lies outside the scope of this
review. We cannot, however, refrain from mentioning the part it
occasionally plays in the decompensation of a previously pathological personality with the development of delusional phenomena.
Guilt may be introjected as in the case of Alby's patient [5] who
was convinced that he had become syphilitic as a result of indulging
in one free gesture* with a female workmate and had then contaminated his son. Guilt may also be projected onto the physician
generating intense aggressive feelings, intentions, and plans (Alby,
personal communication).

*Laying his hand on a girl's gluteal region without any "interchange."

What are the effects of a child's death upon the reciprocal system of relationships within his family? The parental tie may get stronger but only insofar as it was strong before; where the link was previously weak, as Binger observes [6], neither parent can do anything to help the other. Alby [2], in fact, goes so far as to state that death may provide an index of the latent precariousness of the parental union. She has observed quite a few divorces and separations as an outcome of a child's death and even in good marriages, the mother may be unable, for a while, to look after her husband and remaining children. Fathers have shown themselves to be particularly vulnerable: The same author quotes the pathetic case of a physician who was unable to visit his son in hospital because the latter's condition signified for him: "You are a bad father as well as a bad doctor."

Siblings suffer very much from feelings of guilt stemming from death wishes, from fears of falling ill in their own turn, from jealousy at the exclusive attention paid to the patient, and from rage at the leniency with which he is treated at home during remissions. As a consequence, they are very apt to develop various psychosomatic disturbances and academic shortcomings as an aftermath of death.

The farther one goes from the family nucleus, the farther one gets from diagnostic realism and from genuine, deep feelings. The influence of the grandparents is almost constantly negative because they constitute the first of the "concentric circles of disbelief" (toward the diagnosis) [12], the diameter of which extends to the perimeter of the extended family group where unrealistic disbelief and indifference go hand in hand. The culture generally adds its own arbitrary demands that expect the parents to comply in stereotyped fashion to the dying process. They are forbidden to lose hope, to amuse themselves, or to leave the child at all, all of which may amount to an unbearable burden when one considers the many years of remission induced by the newly available methods of treatment.

During the weeks following death, Binger [6] has observed quite a few clinically depressive reactions in previously sound parents. They may be quite unable to return to the hospital where their child died [2] or can only do so if they can suppress the process of mourning which mechanism may have begun before the death of the child when they were unable to accept the inevitable [12]. In this connection, Friedman has reported the development of pregnancies in 20% of the mothers of his terminal patients.

Bibliography

1. Alby, N. and Alby, J.M., Le Mèdecin face a la mort de l'enfant. *Mèdecine de l'Homme,* 30 (1970), 30–34.
2. Alby, N., Raimbault, G., and Friedman, H. L., Les parents devant la mort de l'enfant. *Concours médical,* 11 (1971), 1874-1883.
3. Anthony, E. J. and Koupernik, C., Editorial Comment on "Family Vulnerability and Family Crisis," in *The Child in His Family,* Wiley-Interscience, New York, 1970.
4. Anthony, E. J., The Mutative Impact of Serious Mental and Physical Illness in a Parent on Family Life, in *The Child in His Family,* Wiley-Interscience, New York, 1970.
5. Bernard, J. and Alby, J. M., Incidences psychologiques de la leucémie aiguë de l'enfant et de son traitement, *l'Hygiène mentale,* 3 (1956), 241-255.
6. Binger, C.M., et al., Childhood leukemia: emotional impact on patient and family, *New England Journal of Medicine,* 280 (1969), 414-418.
7. Birtchnell, J. Early parent death and mental illness, *Brit. J. Psychiat.,* 116 (1970), 281-288.
8. Bowlby, J., Grief and Mourning in Infancy and Early Childhood, in *The Psychoanalytic Study of the Child, Volume XV,* International Universities Press, New York, 1960.
9. Bowlby, J., Effects on Behaviour of Disruption of an Affectional Bond, in *Genetic and Environmental Influences on Behaviour,* Oliver and Boyd, Edinburgh, 1968.
10. Chodoff, P. et al., Stress, defenses and coping behavior: observations in parents of children with malignant diseases. *Amer. J. Psychiat.,* 120 (1964), 743-749.
11. Freud, S., Mourning and Melancholia, in *The Standard Edition, Volume XIV,* Hogarth Press, London, 1957.
12. Friedman, S. B. et al., Behavioral observations on parents anticipating the death of a child, *Pediatrics,* 32 (1963), 610-625.
13. Koos, E. L., *Families in Trouble,* King's Crown Press, New York, 1946.
14. Lagache, D., Le travail du deuil. *Revue Francaise de Psychanalyse,* 10, (1938), 4.
15. Lindemann, E., Symptomatology and management of acute grief. *Amer. J. Psychiat.,* 101, (1944), 141.
16. Munro, A., Parent-child separation. *Arch. Gen. Psychiat.,* 20, (1969), 598-604.
17. Parsons, T. and Fox, R., Illness, therapy and a modern urban American family. *J. Soc. Issues,* 8, No. 4, (1952), 31-44.
18. Rousseau, Jean-Jacques, *Émile,* 1762.
19. Rutter, M., *Children of Sick Parents,* Oxford University Press, London, 1966.
20. Sampson, H. et al., *Schizophrenic Women; Studies in Marital Crisis,* Atherton Press, New York, 1964.

21.   Solnit, A. J., Who Mourns When a Child Dies? in this volume.
22.   Spiegel, J. P., The Resolution of the Role Conflict Within the Family, in *The Patient and the Mental Hospital,* Free Press of Glencoe, Illinois, 1957.
23.   Toynbee, A. J., *A Study of History* (abridged version), Oxford University Press, London, 1934.
24.   Wallace, J., Family functioning, in "Care of the Child With Cancer." *Pediatrics,* 40, (1967), 487–545.
25.   Yudkin, S., Children and death. *The Lancet,* January 7, (1967), 37–41.

DISEASE

Editorial Comment

A ghost dressed in black has settled in the house. He will not leave unless he can take away with him his chosen prey. The only way for the family to cope with his intolerable presence is to invite at the same time his enemy—the "man in white," the doctor. The disease is in the cell named the family. It introduces a new parameter that will profoundly modify its metabolism.

We will mention only briefly the problem of the sick parent. The topic has already been partially covered by Anthony [2] in the first volume of the International Yearbook. It is also dealt with in the paper by Koupernik in the present volume. One of the main problems involving chronic illness in a parent is that the child, in his naiveté, may come to consider that it is normal for a parent to be sick; only later, when he discovers the outer world, will he be able to conceive that sickness is the exception and that his own family is not like those of other children. He will also begin to realize that he may possibly lose the sick parent. Even worse, he may actually believe that he is guilty of the illness or the death of the parent because, like all children in the ordinary course of development, he may entertain hostile feelings or death wishes toward the mother or father from time to time, and, since he is still under the rule of magical thinking, he may take his omnipotence for granted.

Turning next to the problem of the chronically sick child, we find that guilt still continues to play an important role both with regard to the child himself (punishment for past misdeeds) as well as his parent (retribution for inadequate or bad parenting). This is particularly true for children who eke out their lives in the penumbra between health and death. The advances in medical science have led to the situation, emphasized by Cytryn, that we have to cope now with an increasing number of such "halfway" children who are being kept alive with conditions of cystic fibrosis, nephropathy (Raimbault), diabetes (Zeidel), or congenital heart disease (Rausch de Traubenberg).

The children with such illnesses have certain problems in common. Since the discovery of disease takes place within the normal process of development, the child imperceptibly becomes his illness, but as a result of enhancement of body feeling, the *psyche* and *soma* are not too well integrated, so that, whereas the healthy child *is* his body, the sick child *has* a body that is constantly making its presence felt through pain. It is this suffering appendage that makes him feel acutely different from others.

The young child gradually begins to elaborate magic-phenomenalistic theories of disease that account for his feelings of guilt, his selection as victim, and his projected ideas of hostility from those in his environment. ("I'm sick because I'm bad;" or "I'm sick because others have bad intentions toward me.") These initial hypotheses persist even into adult life. Nevertheless, the older child, at the beginning of latency is undoubtedly becoming more realistic. Rausch de Traubenberg mentions that children with congenital heart disease become aware of the uniqueness of their fate around the age of eight; hemophiliac boys, studied by Mattsson and Gross [5], come to the same realization at about the same age.

The existence of the chronic disease creates important modifications in the intrafamilial balance. The parents in the first case reported by Leiken and Hassakis are overwhelmed by the weight of their caretaking task; they quarrel with each other and resent the doctors. The parents in the second case blame the doctor because he chose to spare them when their first child was born with cystic fibrosis and refrained from telling them the truth. They then decide to replace the dead child with the consequence that the substitute child closely identifies himself with his dead sibling and experiences increased death anxiety at each anniversary of his lost brother's death. The event is for him a dramatic memento mori.

The whole psychic economy of the family is disturbed as the sick child becomes a permanent epicenter of a disequilibrium. He crystallizes the family's feelings of compassion, pity, overprotection, solicitude, sympathy, and helpfulness, a certain amount of which, varying in different cases, represent overcompensations for anger and resentment. The siblings may be frustrated to the point of wishing to be sick themselves in order to attract a part of the parental attention; others, on the contrary, will dedicate themselves to the well-being of the sibling. Finally, there is a third type of situation described by Mattsson and Gross, where the impaired siblings have the same deep feeling of solidarity that characterizes oppressed minorities.

The chronically sick child also learns to live in permanent contact with the "man in white" whom the family has been compelled to invite so that they can get on with the business of everyday life in spite of the sinister presence of the black ghost. The "man in white" fascinates and frightens the child at the same time. A study by the Israels (quoted by Ajuriaguerra [1]) offers us some clues through the medium of drawings as to how the sick child views the doctor. He is seen ambivalently; sometimes he is the one who brings the sickness; sometimes, he is the ideal parental figure, and sometimes, he may even be a rival for maternal love. He relieves pain but at the same time, he inflicts pain through "shots," etc., toward which the child may assume a sadomasochistic existential attitude.

There is also another world that the chronically sick child has to discover, namely, the hospital. Hospital means for him exile in a milieu that is sometimes a prison or a concentration camp and at other times, a community of children linked together by a chain of common distress. This is probably even more so when he is admitted in a highly specialized unit where he meets children of whom some are going to die and others are likely to raise with him the possibility of his own death. A new relational unit comes into being made up of the sick child, his ward mates, the doctors, the nursing staff, the visiting parents, and may even include, in an almost personalized way, the device such as an artificial kidney, that is going to save his life or, at least, prolong it. Doctors and nurses may respond in a wide variety of ways; sometimes they escape into rationalizations; sometimes into detachment and impersonalization; but a certain number find themselves unable to carry their feeling of helplessness in the face of the child's impending death and guiltily quit the case.

In this chapter, because of space limitations, we have been able to present only a few disease entities. Some of them, like diabetes mellitus, because of their chronicity, may interfere with a normal life style, the child being permanently under treatment. In the case of congenital heart disease, especially in cyanotic cases, a drastic limitation is imposed upon the child's activity. This limitation interferes with the discovery of his own body and with the relationship with the peer group. Other chronically disabled children are condemned to a lack of mobility and, in some cases, they may be completely paralyzed. The personal experience of illness depends not only on personality but also on the nature and extent of the handicap. The fate of the polio child, for example, depends upon the extent of the damage but brain activity is unimpaired (with the possible exception of some clinical varieties characterized by respiratory involvement and cerebral anoxia) and the child, therefore, fully appreciates his predicament. The other characteristic of this disease is its nonprogressive nature so that the family needs only to orient itself to the prospect of rehabilitation. Nevertheless, the need for movement in the child is so intense that it gets canalized into compensatory fantasies. At the other end of the scale, we find the cerebral palsy child impaired both in his cognitive abilities as well as his emotional life, and the possibilities for sublimation are much more limited. A study carried out by Graham and Rutter [4] lent some support to the view that those with lesions located above the brain stem have a greater percentage of intellectual and emotional difficulties.

Between these two examples of motor handicap, one finds progressive muscular dystrophy. At one time it was believed that there were no specific mental difficulties in these children, other than those imposed by the limitation of movement but recent work, reviewed by Demos [3] suggests that about one-third of these children have an intellectual deficiency, the reason being a vascular impairment located in the brain as well as in the muscles; some other writers claim that the disease might well be neurogenic, the primary lesion being cerebral. This situation is similar to what is found in some cyanotic cases of congenital heart disease, where the brain suffers from an insufficient blood flow or is perhaps the site of vascular anomalies.

Another trait that is specific to muscular dystrophy, at least in the majority of cases, is the genetic factor. The impact of the genetic factor is discussed by Cytryn as well as by Leiken and Hassakis in connection with cystic fibrosis and the guilt on the part of both parents, if inheritance is of a recessive type, or one of them if it is dominant.

In the majority of the cases, muscular dystrophy becomes progressively worse and this course, in spite of psychotherapy and attempts at rehabilitation, creates a tragic climate in the family.

The problem raised by epilepsy is less striking but nevertheless worrying. Three main mechanisms, singly or in combination, have been described:

1. There are "primary" impairments, in Bleuler's meaning of the term in which the disorder is directly due to organic impairment, such as in psychomotor or temporal lobe epilepsy. In this group are found the greatest proportion of permanent intercritical or nonparoxysmal behavior disorders which contributed to the ill-founded notion of an epileptoid or epileptic type of personality.

2. The second mechanism is iatrogenic. Most of the anticonvulsant drugs have side effects such as mental retardation, impairment of memory, and behavior disturbances.

3. The third is an existential explanation for the difficulties experienced by epileptic children and their families. Epilepsy is still considered a curse, a symptom of the mythical "nervous degeneration" spoken of in the last century by some European psychiatrists. This may induce in parents, influenced by such conceptions, an attitude of rejection and lead to a segregation from normal school life and peer interaction. In addition, the epileptic child is under continuous treatment which becomes for him a way of life as well as evidence of some unalterable badness inside of him. He may, like the hemophiliac and the diabetic, accept this until adolescence, and then, the chances are that he will rebel even to the point of endangering his own life.

In this review, we cannot overlook the impact on families of mentally retarded and autistic children, whose presence inflicts a deep narcissistic wound on parents and siblings alike. The same effect may be obtained with children who have a sensory handicap. The whole life of the family may become geared to such a condition or, in contrast, the child may be hidden from the public eye and brought up in relative isolation.

All these factors help to create a complex situation, the severity of which is determined in part by the degree of impairment, the cultural traditions of the group concerning sickness and handicap, the childhood experiences of the parents (as shown, for instance, in the first case reported by Leiken and Hassakis), and finally by the support systems within the community.

Cyrille Koupernik

Bibliography

1. Ajuriaguerra, J., de, *Manuel de Psychiatrie de l'Enfant,* Masson and Cie Ed., Paris, (1970), 888–889.
2. Anthony, E. J., The Mutative Impact of Serious Mental and Physical Illness in a Parent on Family Life in: *The Child in His Family;* (The International Yearbook for Child Psychiatry and Allied Disciplines) Vol. 1, John Wiley & Sons, 1970.
3. Demos, J., Probleme de l'existence et de la signification des troubles du fonctionnement cerebral dans la myopathie a forme de Duchenne de Boulogne. *Rev. Fr. Neuro-Psychiat. Inf.* 18, (1970), 315–317.
4. Graham, Ph. and Rutter, M., Organic brain dysfunction and child psychiatric disorders. *Brit. Med. J.,* 3 (5620): (1968), 695–700.
5. Mattsson, A. and Gross, S., Adaptational and defensive behavior in young hemophiliacs and their parents. *Am. J. Psychiat.,* 122 (1966), 1349–1356.

Psychological Adjustment of Children with Cystic Fibrosis*

Leon Cytryn, M.D., Peter Van P. Moore, M.D., and
Mary E. Robinson, Ph.D. (U.S.A.)

.

Introduction

Cystic fibrosis (CF) was once considered a very rare disease. Now,
with improved diagnostic methods, the illness is being recognized
in many children throughout the world. It seems to occur in about
one of every 1500 live births, which would amount to over 3000
new cases a year in the United States [1, 2]. The condition varies
in severity and degree of disability. The involvement of the lungs
is the most serious complication and often leads to chronic respiratory infections, bronchiectasis, emphysema, and sometimes to
cor pulmonale [3].

The outlook for patients with CF has improved considerably in
the last ten to fifteen years. This is reflected in a shift in the
average age of patients attending CF clinics as well as by the increased age of survivors [4]. This welcome trend, however, presents some problems to the professionals concerned with the care
of CF patients. The disease constitutes a heavy burden to the
families. There is a constant worry about medical complications
and eventual death of the child as well as financial strain due to the
need for expensive drugs and constant medical supervision. In

*Supported by a Research Grant No. 219 from the U. S. Children's Bureau.

37

addition, the care of a patient with CF is a full-time job for the family.

While it is obvious that CF is not an easy disease for parents to live with, how much more difficult it must be for the child. His body functions in strange, unpredictable, and often frightening ways. He frequently does not feel well and at any time may become quite ill. Doctor's appointments, medical examinations, and hospitalizations are a regular part of his experience. He has to be careful of what he eats and take a variety of pills at all hours of the day. Postural drainage takes time from play and nights must be spent in a mist tent.

Normal peer relationships are difficult because of the need to avoid contagion, limitations on physical energy, and the desire to keep the condition secret. Most difficult of all, in a world which admires physical health and normality, the child must deal with the fact that in truth he is neither healthy nor totally normal. It is almost inevitable that he will have fears of dying. He will sense his parents' anxiety about his condition yet may find them unable or unwilling to help him cope with his own anxiety. Finally, particularly where he has well siblings, he will have to answer the question of "Why did it happen to me?"

It was in an effort to find out what CF children think of themselves as people, what they understand of their condition and how they handle the emotional stress that it engenders, that our research was undertaken.

Demographic Data

In the course of our study we evaluated 29 children with CF. The majority of the patients were being cared for in the Cystic Fibrosis Clinic of The Children's Hospital of Washington, D. C. and the rest in the Cystic Fibrosis Unit of the National Institutes of Health. There were 15 boys and 14 girls, ranging in age from 8 months to 9 years. Ten were under 3 years old, 9 were 3 to 6 years, and 10 were 6 to 9 years. Twenty eight were white and one was black.

Eighteen of the children were the only ones in their family who suffered from cystic fibrosis. Six had one CF sibling, three had two, and two had three. Five children (from two families) had had a sibling die of CF before they were born.

With three exceptions the families studied were intact. In one case the father had died and in two the parents had divorced. All school-aged children were attending regular school and were at grade level, although two were having moderate difficulty.

The socioeconomic status of the entire group was relatively high, as exemplified by the mean yearly income per family of almost $10,000.

Appearance

When observed in the interviews, eleven children looked quite healthy and showed no signs of illness. Nine had mild manifestations of their conditions, such as cough and slight dyspnea on exertion, and eight were judged to be in moderate distress on the basis of pallor, persistent wheezing, clubbing of fingers, and moderate dyspnea on exertion. Only one child, a four-year old girl, was thought to be in severe distress.

While the relative paucity of obvious signs of debilitating illnesses in the children attested to the excellent medical care they were receiving, it might also have reflected a reluctance of the cooperating physicians to refer families where there was a seriously ill child. Of 26 patients who were rated clinically, using a four-point scale (Schwachman and Kulczycki [5]), 19 were rated as good or excellent, seven as mildly affected, and none as severe.

In spite of their generally healthy appearance, half (fifteen) of the children appeared small for their age. Shortness of stature is a common finding in cystic fibrosis.

The overwhelming majority of the children (26) had adequate large and small muscle coordination as evidenced by their agility, ability to manipulate objects and their performance on visual motor tasks. For three children, small muscle coordination was rated as only fair, but none were rated lower.

Intellectual Functioning

Children under three years were routinely seen at home and given the Bayley Mental and Motor Scales and, when necessary, the lower levels of the Stanford-Binet. The mean Development Quotient (D. Q.) for this group was 101, with a standard deviation of 9:49.

Eight of the ten children had D. Q.'s between 90 and 110, while one child had a D. Q. of 131 and one a D. Q. of 80. The latter was an eight-month-old who had been quite sick during the early months of her life, so it is unlikely that her performance reflected her real intellectual potential.

In the three- to nine-year-old group, most children were seen in the office and all were given Form L-M of the Stanford/Binet. The mean I. Q. was 107, with a standard deviation of 5.48. I. Q.'s ranged from 94 to 132, with one-third of the children scoring above 110.

When the results were broken down by sex, the boys in the under-three group did somewhat less well than the girls (mean I.Q. of 95 as opposed to 107 for the girls) but were closely matched with the girls in the three- to six-year group with mean I. Q.'s of 104 and 105, respectively. In the six- to nine-year group the boys did significantly better than the girls, with a mean I. Q. of 119 as compared to 101 for the girls.

It is quite clear that, at least for our group, CF is not related to any impairment in intellectual functioning.

Child's View of Himself

Each child expressed whatever concerns he had about his self-concept and body image in different ways and in different contexts. Some did human figure drawings with clear indications of concerns about body integrity such as disproportionately large, shaded, or excessively detailed chest areas, missing limbs, or small constricted figures. Others gave a large proportion of anatomical, blood, and mutilation responses on the Rorschach, while others produced fantasy material which suggested that they saw themselves as younger than they were, dependent, and inadequate.

As a group, the girls had a more adequate view of themselves than did the boys. Their appearance, bearing, interests, and ambitions for the future were consistently feminine, as was their choice of play material.

Most of the boys seemed to have a positive sexual identification but as a group they were not as aggressive and self-assured as the girls or as other boys their age. Half of the older boys saw themselves, especially on a fantasy level, as younger, dependent, and inadequate. Some were vague about what they wanted to become, or chose occupations requiring exceptional health and physical stamina (astronaut, football player). They were more concerned than the girls about shortness of stature and inability to engage in strenuous activities, which they felt set them off from their peers.

The most important finding was that the majority of our older subjects were functioning effectively in their families, at school, and with their peers. Their general self-confidence and poise suggested that at least at pre-adolescent age levels, their concerns were not interfering significantly with their functioning.

Defenses and Coping Styles

The children made use of a variety of defenses to ward off anxiety and in most cases these were both effective and adaptive, helping the child to maintain reasonably good emotional balance and freeing his energy for constructive purposes, including learning. In the minority of children, defenses were inefficient and broke down under stress or were successful at the expense of restriction and inhibition in total functioning.

Reaction formation was seen in two children who persisted in engaging in strenuous physical activity despite their illness. However, each child seemed aware of his physical limits and there was no indication that either had caused his physical condition to worsen. Unquestionably, both children derived a great deal of satisfaction from their activities which facilitated their peer relationships.

Several of the older children were striving for and achieving academic success which seemed the best available use of aggressive energy and drive when success in competitive physical activity was denied to them.

Many children made use of fantasy in which they expressed aggression, saw themselves as leaders of peers and hoped to grow up to be "superman," yet in every child fantasy seemed to be used only as a respite from the problems of reality. Fantasy was recognized for what it was and reality testing was not impaired.

Most of the older children seemed to have great trust in their doctors and felt that the latter would not let anything terrible happen to them.

As previously noted, none of the children had totally withdrawn from peer relationships; a few had managed to maintain virtually normal social contacts and the remainder continued to desire and reach out for more friends. In view of this, the children's desire to conceal their condition seemed a realistic response to the awareness that children are often uncomfortable with peers who are significantly different from themselves.

Less healthy defenses seemed to be regression, withdrawal, and avoidance. Not surprisingly these defenses were most common in the two- to four-year group, although they were also characteristic of the most disturbed older children. Under stress, they reverted to more primitive behavior patterns or became restricted in the range of their activities, interests, and interpersonal relationships.

Frequently, particularly in the beginning of our study, the research team, as mental health specialists, questioned the use of certain defenses by the children. However, it soon became obvious that CF children, faced with a singular, frightening reality which neither they nor their parents could change, did the best they could to live with this reality. Thus, they employed a degree of denial, compartmentalization, and repression of affect which under other circumstances might be seen as pathological. Although such defenses were not always totally effective and had their cost, they were the only ones left open to these children.

We were constantly surprised at the capacity of the children to deny that they were ill or that their symptoms were in any way different from those experienced occasionally by other children. However, our culture is oriented toward the healthy, average child who is as much like his peers as possible and makes no provision for the ill and different child. Under these circumstances the child has little alternative but to aspire to a well-child role and deny his illness.

We also came to appreciate the children's denial of their feelings about their illness. In almost every case we saw, the child's parents, even when they were aware of and understood his feelings about his condition, were unable or unwilling to talk with him about these feelings. They were reluctant to face their own fears, and were concerned lest they create or increase fears in their child since they felt that no amount of talk could change the reality of their child's condition. Even factual information was reluctantly or partially communicated and only in few cases did the children express a full understanding of their illness.

Emotional Health of the Children

Once all the evaluations of the children were complete, the psychiatrist and psychologist reviewed each case in order to arrive at a more general evaluation of total emotional health, including indications of emotional disturbance, if any. This judgment represented a composite rating for each child in the previously discussed categories. Each child was assigned to one of four groups: no disturbance, mild disturbance, moderate disturbance, and severe disturbance.

No Disturbance. In the interview situation, these children were remarkably zestful and persevering, obviously enjoying the interviews and relating well to the examiners. They were conforming and eager to please, but not overly so, had little or no trouble separating from their mothers, and displayed age appropriate independence. They seemed to see themselves as adequate, competent people and if activity in one area was denied them, they were resourceful about finding alternatives. Peer relationships were good and there was no indication of significant depression. While their fantasy material revealed concern over body damage and expression of aggressive impulses, there was no indication that anxiety interfered with their ability to function. Their major defenses were denial, repression, and isolation of affect, and these defenses seemed to be both successful and adaptive. *Twelve children, 41% of our subjects, were in this group.*

Mild Disturbance. In most respects, children in this group were similar to those in the first group. However, they gave evidence of obvious anxiety about body damage and aggressive impulses, and about their physical condition. There were also indications of intermittent mild depression. While not entirely self-confident, they displayed age appropriate independence. In spite of their concerns they were able to function well intellectually and socially. *Five children, or 17% of our subjects, were in this group.*

Moderate Disturbance. Children in this group related to the examiners in a hesitant and tenuous way. They had limited drive, perseverance, and creativity in play. Behavior was listless and activity level was low. They showed limited or highly variable endurance with the degree of endurance reflecting their emotional state rather than their physical status. Emotionally, they functioned like younger children and related to their mothers in a passive-dependent way. In the interview they presented the extremes of dependent behavior, being either extremely passive/dependent or unable to ask for or accept help appropriately. Their concerns about body damage were expressed in terms of questions about their own adequacy and a passive attitude toward life. They were frequently right and tense and evidenced considerable anxiety and regression under stress. In addition to denial and isolation of affect, they employed less mature defenses including regression, withdrawal, and avoidance. While their anxiety interfered with their functioning, it was intermittent and never totally immobilizing. However, they consistently gave the impression of great vulnerability to stress. *There were eight children or 28% of the sample in this group.*

Severe Disturbance. Children in this group showed an exaggeration of the characteristics of the moderately disturbed group. They were generally uncooperative and hostile toward the examiners, and related to their mothers in an infantile, clinging, and controlling way. They displayed generally inappropriate, regressive behavior and severe, disorganizing anxiety, which led to significant impairment in functioning and very poor social adjustment. *There were four children (14%) in this group.*

Among the 12 children in the two most disturbed group, boys outnumbered the girls two to one, and in the most disturbed group, three of the four children were boys. This finding suggests that CF is potentially more disruptive to the emotional development of boys than girls.

There was no definite relationship between age and degree of disturbance, although all children in the most disturbed group were four or over. In the other three groups were children of all ages.

There was also no obvious relationship between severity of illness, as evaluated independently by the physicians, and the child's overall adjustment. The sickest child, a four-year-old girl, was found to be quite well adjusted, as was a six-year-old who had experienced the most hospitalizations.

While only half of the total group were considered to be under-sized, two-thirds of the most disturbed children came from this group. We considered the possibility that the small size of these children negatively influenced their body image and consequently, their self-concept, contributing to emotional disturbance. While a correlation between body size of boys and their emotional and social maturity was suggested [6] no such correlation was found for girls [7].

Discussion

The finding that 4 of the 29 children were considered to be seriously disturbed and in urgent need of psychiatric help is not out of keeping with estimates of the frequency of serious emotional disturbance in the general population, which clusters around the ten percent level [8].

Of greater concern was the finding of significant, if not totally disabling emotional disturbance in an additional eight children. These children were seen by us as emotionally vulnerable and in danger of either disorganizing under stress or becoming unduly rigid and constricted with a resultant impoverishment of personality and disability to function. Ideally, they should have psychiatric treatment.

The interaction of environmental factors with the stresses of CF was obvious in the most and least disturbed groups. In the most disturbed group, three of the four children came from families where there were situations which could be considered hazardous to the emotional development of any child. In one the mother was severely physically handicapped and presented a picture of helplessness and inability to control her son. In another the father was dead, the mother was consciously aloof from both her sick and her well child, and had turned their care over to others. One family were recent refugees from abroad, struggling to adjust to a new culture in which they suffered considerable loss of prestige and social status. However, the fourth family was one in which there were a reasonably stable marriage and a great deal of warmth and acceptance of both the sick child and his well siblings. They shared with many families the difficulty in discussing the child's illness with him, but they were aware of his feelings and were trying to help him.

In contrast to the families of children in the most disturbed group, those who were seen as best adjusted all came from warm, stable families where there was appreciation of and respect for the needs of individual children. However, even these parents had marked difficulty in talking to their child about his condition, either in communicating specific information or in dealing with his feelings.

Conclusion

Even though well over half of the children studied were judged to be functioning well emotionally, socially, and intellectually, it was obvious that it was at some cost. For the 42% judged to be having significant emotional problems, the cost was considerable.

The relatively high incidence of emotional disturbance in our group is of particular concern when the characteristics of the group are considered. All families seen were volunteers and many who were approached refused to be studied, which brings up the possibility that the most disturbed families were not included. The children in our sample were relatively healthy, with fewer limitations on their activities than is the case for many children with CF. Also, our group was young, with one-third being under three and none over eight. Thus, there is the possibility that a group of older, sicker children, most of whom came from unstable homes would show a greater deal of disturbance.

Unquestionably, the future holds many problems for all the children in the study, even those who are now adjusting well to their life circumstances. The onset of adolescence will bring increased concerns about physical stature and bodily functioning and a greater need to be "just like everyone else." Interest in heterosexual relationships will activate questions about marriage and child bearing. Realistic vocational choices will have to be made. Indications are that these difficulties may be particularly acute for the boys in our study.

All the children in our study were receiving excellent medical care. All the parents had been thoroughly informed about the nature of the child's condition, his current physical status, and the purpose of home medical procedures. Physicians were seen as capable, dedicated people who would be available day or night in a medical emergency. However, in none of the cases had the parents been given special help in looking at their and their child's feelings about CF. The results of our study indicate that such help should be considered essential and made routinely available.

Bibliography

1. Goodman, H. D. and Reed, S. C., Heredity of fibrosis of the pancreas, possible mutation rate of the gene. *Am. J. Hum. Genet.*, 4, (1952), 59.
2. Kulczycki, L. L., MacLeod, K., and Schwachman, H., A survey of school children for cystic fibrosis. *A. M. A. J. Dis. Child.*, 100 (1960), 174.
3. Kulczycki, L., Mucovicidosis or Cystic Fibrosis: Its Pathogenesis, Manifestations and Therapy, in *Mucovicidosis*. H. Bohn, H. Dost and E. Koch (eds.). F. K. Schattauer-Verlag, Stuttgart, 1964.
4. Di Sant'Agnese, P. A. and Anderson, D. H., Cystic fibrosis of the pancreas in young adults. *Ann. Intern. Med.* 50 (1959), 1321.
5. Schwachman, H. and Kulczycki, L. L., A report of one hundred and five patients with cystic fibrosis of the pancreas studied over a five to fourteen year period. *A.M.A. J. Dis. Child.* 96 (1958), 6.
6. Jones, M. C., The late careers of boys who were early or late maturing. *Child Develop.*, 28 (1957), 113–128.
7. Jones, M. C. and Mussen, P. H., Self conceptions, motivations, and interpersonal attitudes of early and late maturing girls. *Child Developm.*, 29 (1958), 491–501é.
8. Witmer, H. L., *The National Picture of Children's Emotional Disturbances*, Child Development Center, New York, 1962.

Psychological Study of Parents of Children with Cystic Fibrosis

Stanley J. Leiken, M.D. and Patricia Hassakis, M.D. (U.S.A.)

Introduction

Some years ago one of the authors (SL) was asked to address a
group of parents of children with cystic fibrosis (CF). During the
discussion period after the talk one parent began to tell the group
how frightened she was each time her child was hospitalized.
Finally, she said, "You know each time I think he might not make
it, but each time he does pull through. I am not relieved, however,
because I know there will be another time and sometime maybe he
won't make it. At times I wish he would die and it would be all
over with." At this point the chairman of the meeting, himself the
father of a CF child, arose and abruptly concluded the meeting. The
fear of allowing this discussion to go any further was too overwhelming.

Since that time we have been most interested in the parents of
these children. The family with the CF child must face a potentially fatal illness; but, in contrast to the family with the child with
leukemia or any other definitely fatal disease, these people do not
know the final outcome for sure. As difficult as it may be for the
family of the fatally ill child, the future is indeed predictable and
what the parent does or does not do can make little difference in
the final outcome of things. In contrast to this, the outcome of CF
is in doubt and the parents may often feel responsible. Leaving the

child at home with a baby-sitter may alter the outcome if the child develops a large mucus plug while the parents are gone and the baby-sitter is unable to handle the situation. The parent's inability to pick up a gradual worsening of the child's respiratory condition may affect the immediate prognosis. Giving in to the child's protests about the various aspects of his medical treatment and backing off from vigorous therapy so as not to have to "fight with him all the time" may also be dangerous. In addition to these factors, the parents must also bear the responsibility of carrying the deadly genetic components of this disease. So a number of factors operate to make this situation unique and a particularly difficult one for the parents of a CF child.

Design of the Study

One author (PH) assists in operating a CF clinic where eighty children are seen regularly. The other author (SL) has attended the CF clinic in order to become more familiar with the problems of these children and their families. The four families presented here were chosen as being quite representative of many of the families seen in the clinic. It was felt that at least one of the families in this project is operating as a well-functioning unit, one is doing fairly well in light of the massive amount of stress with which it is forced to deal, and the remaining two are seen as the most difficult families by the staff of the clinic.

A review of the literature on this subject reveals three articles. Turk [6], points out the deprivation which these families seem to feel in all areas of their life. Lawler et al. [2] focused on the severe pathology that existed in that each of them could benefit from psychological assistance. They were particularly impressed with the need of the parents and children to deal more openly with their preoccupations with death. They felt there was a need to deal more directly with the "smoldering resentments and their not infrequent wish to desert their children and be free of the great burden which they must bear." Tropauer's study [5] revealed that depression and preoccupation with death were present in a large percentage of patients when the obvious signs or complaints of emotional distress were absent.

CASE MATERIAL

Family No. 1. Mr. and Mrs. W. are 26-year-old parents of a two-and-a-half-year-old-normal child and a one-and-a-half-year-old infant with cystic fibrosis. They were unhappy with their second pregnancy which was unwanted for financial and other reasons. The child was born with meconium ileus and underwent surgery within the first 24 hours of life. At the beginning of this child's life the parents already had to deal with their intense ambivalence toward even a normal child let alone a severely damaged and, as they put it "deficiently endowed one" [4]. They both began searching immediately to find the cause of this disturbance." Although they are intelligent, medically oriented people (mother is a nurse), Mrs. W. began to blame herself for some pills she had taken early in her pregnancy and wondered what else she might have done to cause this calamity. They both felt badly about not wanting this baby and, although they did not verbalize it, we suspect they felt this wish in itself may have caused the disorder. Amidst this and the tiredness and fatigue attendant with the termination of any pregnancy, was the anxiety about the life of the child which was further complicated by the child's two-and-a-half-month stay in the hospital, during which time it clearly was perceived as a burden. Their life changed more dramatically when the child came home at two-and-a-half months of age, with an ileostomy. Both parents suffered overwhelming fatigue. The mother reports that a huge percentage of the waking day was devoted to the actual physical care of this baby. They had to deal with that "disgusting" part of the body. They felt unable to show the baby off to friends or to leave her in the care of baby-sitters because of this condition. Although they were overwhelmed at this time, it is clear they began to deal with some of their guilt, depression, and anxiety by "doing" for the baby—an outlet which had been denied them during the baby's stay in the hospital. Although this "doing" provided them some relief, it also took its toll. When Mr. W. came home from school he found a totally exhausted wife who wanted to go to bed immediately and leave the responsibility of the children to him. He was angry about this and felt it was not his duty to do this. On the other hand, during the night he found himself getting up each time the baby coughed because he was afraid it might mean the onset of a serious illness. Mr. and Mrs. W. found they had little time to talk to each other and no time whatsoever to spend alone or to do the things which might interest them. This situation is clearly described in the article by Turk [6]. She talks about the massive deprivation these families feel. They criticized each other endlessly. Mr. W. criticized Mrs. W. when she smoked around the baby. He said she didn't change the sheets frequently enough. We learned later that the merciless criticism directed at each other was a projection of their own overwhelming sense of inadequacy. Mrs. W.'s mother was a hypomanic perfectionist with whom Mrs. W. had always sought to compete. Now the production of a "deficient" child clearly put her out of the running in the competition with her mother who had never had a defective child. Even before the baby was born Mr. W. had felt terribly unsure of his career decision. His uncertainty showed itself clearly in his lack of academic achievement. As a child his mother made it clear to him that he was indeed a genius and the world was awaiting his arrival. Life was proving her to be in error and his feelings of inadequacy were overwhelming. Both of these people displaced these feelings of inadequacy onto the physicians, almost all of whom appeared to them to be incompetent. This pattern has tended to persist in a slightly altered form. They now are quite suspicious of all physicians. After this initial attack on all of the physicians who cared for their child they turned to each other and looked there for the "inadequate one." At that point they were close to divorce and had, in fact, planned a trial separation. A brief course of psychotherapy helped each of them to redirect some of the feelings of inadequacy back onto themselves and foster a somewhat more supportive relationship.

Family No. 2. Mr. and Mrs. C. are the parents of two boys with cystic fibrosis. Bobby is nine and Tommy is fifteen years of age. Both are doing fairly well. Tommy has moderate pulmonary disease. Another boy, Jimmy, who would have been eighteen, died of CF eight years ago. Steve, now twenty, does not have CF. The first CF child was born after they were married about three years. The most difficult time for them (as it was for two of the other families) was just after this first child with CF was born. They met with a physician who had the diagnosis in mind but did not tell them about it for quite sometime. Their anger at this physician is well controlled and "nearly forgotten." They point out somewhat sadly that "maybe if the diagnosis had been made earlier Jimmy's life might have been prolonged." They are both angry and disappointed because the doctor did not tell them because "he didn't want to worry us." They both point out that as soon as they knew about the diagnosis and were told squarely and forthrightly about the prognosis they were able to deal more successfully with it than before. They clearly are the kind of people who can deal with reality much better than a nebulous uncertainty. The time during this child's acute illness and the year before his death was the most difficult period they faced. Yet it was during this same time that Mr. and Mrs. C. also began to deal with the question of having more children. (To plan for a new child as the death of one child becomes more of a reality is not uncommon with these families.) They decided in favor of having a child although they knew the possibility of CF was strong. The knowledge that this new child had a positive sweat test and now they had three children with CF one of them about to die, seems like an almost unbearable stress. It was at this time that the Catholic religion was of the greatest help. They clearly saw death as something which is not final. They also see themselves as not being so crucially involved as determinants in the lives of their children. What they might do or not do does not change the end result in their mind. They see their lives in the hands of God. In a sense this gives them great relief from the over-burdening responsibility that other parents seem to face. On the other hand, it does not decrease their devotion to their children and to each other. This feeling of being "God's helpers" comes out most clearly as they talk about how lucky they are as parents to have children with wonderful personalities. The children's personalities are something that God has done rather than feeling they, in any way, are responsible for the excellent mental health of these children. They convey this relaxed good feeling to the children who seem about as well adjusted as any in the clinic. Mr. and Mrs. C. enjoy an extremely warm marital relationship. In contrast to the W.'s neither feels particularly deprived or cheated by having a child with CF. They do not have a constant desire to get away but when they do have the feeling of the pressures being overwhelming, they have arranged to take vacations from the children and even occasionally from each other. Interestingly, however, although they can deal with the idea of death more directly than any of the other families, they do, at times, sidestep the issue and find it easier to talk of their children's feelings. For example, the oldest child became quite depressed at the time of his sibling's death and since then has been acutely aware and frightened of any bodily illness or injury he might suffer. The youngest child has anxiety on the anniversary of his brother's death, and feels very relieved when that anniversary passes. He obviously feels an identification with this dead brother and fears the same fate for himself. The parents deny they have these anxieties but spend much time helping their children deal with these fears. Mrs. C. also tends to deal with her own feelings about CF by being the one who helps others and she is constantly in touch with the parents of children who have recently been diagnosed. This seems to give her strength and is helpful to others in the clinic. They feel strong and capable of mastering their problems, yet they, too, admit they can take only one day at a time and don't often think of the future. "You can't go around always thinking of tomorrow or next year."

Family No. 3. Mr. and Mrs. B. are the parents of a 22-month-old girl, Tanya. She is the youngest of three children and the only child in the family with CF. She was diagnosed at four months of age. The original course was stormy until seven months. She has done exceedingly well with only occasional episodes of upper respiratory disease since that time. The parents mentioned, as did Mr. and Mrs. C., that the most difficult time was just before the diagnosis was made. They talked of their anger with the physician who cared for the child during the first four months of life and did not give them a diagnosis or clear answers to the origin of their child's illness. They focused on how difficult it is to deal with this kind of stress "when one does not know what to expect." Then they were finally given the diagnosis suddenly, without explanation. The news was given to Mrs. B. in the absence of Mr. B. They talk about the contrast between their previous physician and one of the authors (PH) who has been so helpful because "she would spend time sitting, talking and explaining to us." Mrs. B.'s first reaction was to blame her husband, because "I had two normal kids from my first marriage so it must be his fault." The next feeling was similar to that of Mr. and Mrs. W. They felt their whole life would be curtailed. They felt this way throughout the acute stage of the child's illness, from the age of three months until one year. Since that time things have gone well and since the child usually does well they "forget" to bring her in for her clinic visits. Over the past six months they have "forgotten" half of their scheduled monthly appointments. However, during the brief upper respiratory illnesses, they panic and call the author frequently. This particular brand of denial, although affording them some relief, could seriously interfere with the consistent, ongoing treatment of Tanya.

Family No. 4. Mr. and Mrs. T. have four children. The oldest is a 17-year-old boy who is involved "in the drug scene" and also has a cleft palate for which he has had multiple operations. The twin girls who suffer from CF are twelve years old and the youngest child is a six year old with no signs of physical disease. The twins, Sandra and Sabrina, both suffer from respiratory difficulties now. Sandra has severely compromised pulmonary functions and probably has little more than a year to live. Sabrina is doing better and has a much better prognosis for the immediate future. The parents report that the most difficult time for them was just after they found out about the diagnosis. They were overwhelmed by the prognosis. Mother reports, "it was a shock, then I decided that I would do what I could to change the prognosis. First we talked about it all the time but later we talked about it less and less. There is no sense walking around being bugged." Mrs. T. takes on the entire responsibility for the treatment and care of these children. Mr. T. seems totally overwhelmed by the problems of his twin girls and emotionally disturbed son. When one of the authors (SL) attempted to interview this man in his barber shop (it was impossible to get him to come to the clinic or office), he allowed only a five minute interview and then, as the discussion came closer to his feelings, he insisted he had to take care of his customers and left. Mrs. T. talks of how she feels that everyone in the family is deprived. The parents both feel their life has been extremely limited. They have not spent even one day away from their children since the diagnosis was made. They claim there is no one to leave them with and they "never" use baby-sitters. They do not feel they can take vacations because of all the equipment they would have to take with them. We suggested they might exchange baby-sitting services with another CF family. In response to this Mrs. T. said she would be happy to take care of another CF child but knows she could never leave her child with another parent. They avoid looking at any possibility of getting away from their children and refuse to consider the fact that maybe the restrictions are partially of their own making. There is no question that they resent the imposition placed upon them and the restrictions that plague them but they prolong and intensify the situation as they wear the badge of the martyred, masochistic parents. We suspect they use this position in order to insure they never have any time alone for were they to deal with each other more directly serious marital conflicts probably would result. These people tend to "bury themselves in their work" as a way of defending themselves from the overwhelming pain and anxiety. Until recently, Mrs. T. had a full-time evening job five nights a week while her husband worked six-and-a-half days a week as a barber. This is another example of the "doing" defense, that we saw so clearly with Mrs. C.

Discussion

Each of these parents has developed certain defenses or coping mechanisms which they use to deal with this massive reality stress. To varying degrees with each family these defenses have proven successful in reducing stress for the parents and child while at the same time allowing for optimal medical care. However, there are also defensive mechanisms at work which prove ineffective in reducing anxiety and greatly hinder effective treatment of their disease. It is important for the physician, whether he is a psychiatrist or pediatrician, to know whether a successful or unsuccessful operation is taking place so he may be effective in the management of these difficult family problems.

The most frequently used helpful coping mechanism was the "doing defense" [3]. Three of our four families made frequent use of this method of dealing with anxiety. Mrs. C. gave assistance and advice to many CF families and was the prime organizer of a local CF group. Her careful concern for the anxieties of all her children is a further bit of "doing." Mrs. T. not only cared for her two CF children but held down a full-time job. Mrs. W. felt much less anxiety but much fatigue while caring for her three-month-old CF child with an ileostomy. Only after the acute threat to life was no longer present and there was no longer quite as much to "do" was the severe marital conflict manifest. It is clear that each of these parents was able to relieve much of their anxiety by being able to "do" for their families. Friedman [1] talks of the excessive "motor activity" seen in parents anticipating the death of a child. Other authors discuss how parents of leukemic children in hospitals become somewhat more relaxed when they were allowed to participate strenuously in the care of their child.

On the other hand, both the W.'s and the T.'s demonstrate that this same coping mechanism if used to extreme can also be quite detrimental. The T.'s have such a need to keep busy that they rarely see each other and therefore provide little comfort or support in times of stress. Mrs. W. found herself so exhausted by all of her "activity" in caring for her child that she had little time for her husband who soon came to resent his wife's isolation from him.

This same situation of a mechanism operating both in a healthy and pathological way is seen with our patients' frequent use of suppression which borders, at times, on frank denial of reality. These patients must maintain an ability to suppress freely and frequently. All of the families in our study have made it clear to us that they must think of the death of their child only very rarely. If the thought of the ultimate prognosis was always with them each day would bring dreadful pain and suffering. They must indeed suppress or even deny, at times, that the future is filled with uncertainty. The way the C.'s and the B.'s discuss the future with each other and with their children clearly belies their denial. This mechanism, however, is quite helpful to patient and parents alike. On the other hand, massive suppression or denial can be not only totally ineffective in coping with anxiety but can cause severe interference with medical care. Mr. and Mrs. B. cannot tolerate the fact that Tanya has CF and admit that at times they are sure she has "grown out of it." It is at these times that they "forget" her appointments at the CF clinic. By not coming they can change the reality and continue to maintain their fantasies. However, even the slightest upper respiratory infection produces panic in them, so the use of denial not only endangers Tanya's health but really gives them little relief. Friedman [1] points out "there appears to be an optimal range of defending or buffering one's self from the thought of having a child with a fatal disease. Deviation from this range in one direction, by denying reality, interfered with optimal participation in the care of the child by not allowing the parents to fully meet the responsibilities and demands associated with the situation. On the other hand, when the parent lacks adequate defense patterns applicable to these circumstances, his ability to care effectively for his child is also significantly hampered."

It is clear that the physician caring for these children must be aware of the mechanisms these families use to cope with the ever present anxiety—an anxiety which is intense primarily because of the frustrating reality of this disease. He must be aware of both the type of defense and the way in which it is used. In order to accomplish this, the parents must be seen alone and interviews must be directed at the defenses used. The families in this study were seen only three to six times (with the exception of the one family which was seen for brief psychotherapy), yet many deep feelings were touched upon and much support and relief were given. One suggestion which this study implies is that there should be time, possibly as infrequently as two or three times a year, when parents of children with chronic disease have a chance to talk with the physician about their own feelings—a time, when the physician, and the parents as well, strictly avoid discussing the specific details of medication, etc. Above all, both parents must attend this meeting together. This would convey the message that the physician feels that they, the parents, have needs which must be met as well as those of their children. However, in order to accomplish this end, the physician must come to grips with his own feelings about chronic disease and death. We are all aware that one of the frequent, unconscious motivating factors in the life of the physician is the need to be the one who masters and controls illness and disease rather than suffers from it. When a physician faces a disease he can neither master or control he frequently feels frightened, overwhelmed, and incompetent, and fails in his responsibility of dealing effectively with the patient. None of us totally escapes the wish to hide when serious or life threatening disease confronts us, and we must be constantly aware of our own feelings lest they make us unable to effectively deal with our patients. To the extent that we can successfully deal with our own feelings, we then become able to effectively work with these families and become able to support those defenses which are so necessary for the everyday functioning of these besieged parents, while at the same time being alert and aware when these same defenses begin to interfere with the medical treatment of the child and/or the mental health or happiness of the parents.

Bibliography

1. Friedman, S. D. et al., Behavioral Observations on Parents Anticipating the Death of a Child, *Pediatrics*, 32 (1963), 610–625.
2. Lawler, R. H., Nakielny, W., and Wright, N. A., Psychological implications of cystic fibrosis, *Canadian Medical Association Journal*, 94 (1966) 1043–1046.
3. Schwartz, D. A., The agitated depression, *Psychiatric Quarterly*, 35 (1961), 758–776.
4. Solnit, A. J. and Stark, M. H., Mourning and the birth of a defective child, *Psychoanalytic Study of the Child*, 16 (1961), 523–537.
5. Tropauer, A., Franz, M. N., and Dilgard, V. W., Psychological aspects of the care of children with cystic fibrosis, *American Journal of Diseases of Children*, 119 (1970), 424–432.
6. Turk, J., Impact of cystic fibrosis on family functioning, *Pediatrics*, 34 (1964), 67–71.

Problems of Emotional Adjustment in Juvenile Diabetes

A. Zeidel, M.D. (Israel)

At the Beilinson Hospital in Petach-Tikva, I have had the opportunity of following a number of young diabetics within an age range of six to twenty-five years. Out of a group of 80 patients, about one-third were referred for psychiatric consultation because of gross psychological maladjustment, disturbed family relationships, or because of emotional difficulties in maintaining their diabetic regimen. The remaining two-thirds did not manifest any marked psychological disturbances, but when examined carefully, particularly with regard to their adjustment to the illness, they were found to have many emotional problems. A remark by one of the pediatricians in the Endocrinological Unit, to the effect that the major difficulties in diabetic management lay not in the metabolic but in the psychological sphere, stimulated my interest in the emotional side of juvenile diabetes.

The psychological factors can be roughly categorized:

> Psychosomatic factors
> Somatopsychic factors
> Personal-social adjustment factors

Psychosomatic Factors

Under this heading, I would include emotional circumstances, especially psychic stress, that may either precipitate the illness or influence its course.

CASE 1

A thirteen-year-old, conscientious, and rather capable girl, eager to please her parents, was usually very tense prior to school examinations. At such times, her glycosuria increased in spite of the fact that her diet and insulin requirements remained unchanged.

Somatopsychic Factors

Under this heading, I would include the immediate effect of metabolic changes on the patient's emotional and mental state. The effect may be brought about by an impaired cerebral physiology resulting from hypoglycemia.

CASE 2

An eight-year-old diabetic boy was admitted to a psychiatric hospital because of severe aggressive outbursts and paranoid thinking. He was found to be quite manageable except for occasional severe and short-lived attacks of aggression and destructiveness preceded by irritability without apparent external cause. When his blood was tested for sugar during these attacks, an abnormally low blood sugar level was found. Close supervision of his food intake practically eliminated these outbursts.

Personal-Social Adjustment Factors

In order to assess the impact of diabetes on the child, we must take into consideration some of its properties, namely, its chronicity, its relatively mild course for many years, and the unique dietetic and medical regimen. It is a chronic, incurable condition with a fair prognosis regarding life, and a somewhat poor prognosis regarding health. Complications in the latter years are frequent. It shares certain typical consequences with other chronic illnesses such as the fostering of dependency and the evocation of anxiety not only in the patient himself but also in parents, relatives, and close friends.

The disease often follows a clinically benign course for many years, and the patient (unless his blood sugar levels tend to be extreme) may, subjectively, remain in good health. Some patients may vaguely remember experiencing initial symptoms of diabetes, like thirst or weakness or going through a series of infections or minor illnesses at the onset of the disease. So there is not much physical suffering entailed. However, the general management of the condition is both exacting and frustrating. Moreover, the children become aware quite early that those about them are deeply concerned and, at times, alarmed by mysterious laboratory findings. There is thus a perplexing discrepancy between their own feelings of well-being and the worried feelings of relatives and friends. The children fill the gap in their understanding with fantasies that reflect their illness, their personalities and their stage of development. In its internal representation, diabetes is a mystery, a threat, or a punishment for misbehavior.

CASE 3

An adolescent, whose illness had started at the age of 14, firmly believed that it was caused by his masturbation.

CASE 4

A nine-year-old boy is sure that he developed diabetes at the age of seven because he had failed to prevent his older brother from riding a motorcycle on which he subsequently met his death in an accident.

No matter how well informed most children nowadays are with regard to the pathogenesis of their illness (many of them have some knowledge of the role of the pancreas in diabetes), they may still entertain the fanciful notion, that it is caused by eating bad or "forbidden" food or by their disobedience in refusing food offered to them by their parents. The prominence given to harmful foods and poisons in many myths and fairy tales may help to nurture some of these "paranoid" theories.

The diet restrictions and the daily injections and urinary examinations can provoke deep resentments at the unfairness of it all in making them "different" from other children and the accumulation of such feelings may end in rebellion or massive denial. Again, because of the discrepancy between what they feel and how others regard them, they may attribute everything to a capricious whim on the part of their parents and accuse them of hostility and aggression. Later, they may extend this accusation to include a concept of themselves as victims of society in general.

CASE 5

In an essay written by an adolescent girl aged fourteen, she complained about society's attitude toward diabetics in general and toward her in particular. She vehemently protested against being branded as "sick" and imagined that people avoided her because of her illness which they ignorantly regarded as contagious. Underlying this attitude were intense feelings of inadequacy, fear, suspicion, and hostility that she projected onto her environment.

The nature and quality of the diabetic child's adjustment depends on the premorbid personality characteristics, previous and current life experiences, the patient's age and state of development, and the parent's attitudes and behavior. The management of the diabetes frequently interferes with the forward movement toward maturation and essentially reinforces regressive tendencies that are counteracted by an open defiance of the rules and regulations governing their care.

The understandable preoccupation with the workings of the body also impedes the progress from egocentric to more social and altruistic interests. The separation from parents and the transfer of emotional attachments to friends and contemporaries, are also delayed or indefinitely postponed. The anxious and protective mother may maintain her close supervision of the child's food intake and excretory output and may also restrict his activity because of mistaken notions regarding muscular strain and fatigue. As a consequence, autonomy and self-care are difficult to achieve and difficult to maintain. Social embarrassments are frequent and may lead to withdrawal and further turning to the mother. For example, meets and outings with peers help in the process of socialization and emotional emancipation from the family, but diabetic children who often have to bring their own food, eat when others do not, and refrain from eating when others do, may seldom experience the exciting feelings of independence that stem from such ventures. They end up feeling "different" and inferior, or may try pathetically to hide their condition.

Bowel and urinary products and functions are a matter of great importance in the psychology of the preschool child, but soon they become devalued and disgusting to him and he sets them aside forever after as infantile interests that are incompatible with maturity and normal society. In diabetes, however, urine cannot be disregarded and retains its early significance as a measure of the child's cooperation with his parents and other authority figures such as the physician. The child may also see his well-being reflected in its array of colors. Some diabetic children, on the other hand, reject it forcibly as a symbol of regression, some are repelled by it as a distasteful reminder of disease, and for some it is disliked for both reasons.

At adolescence, the difficulties of adjustment usually increase. At this stage the struggle centers around extrafamilial relationships in association with sexual maturation, and instability, ambivalence, and anxiety appear to be an inherent part of normal development. Nevertheless, this stage is harder for the diabetic, especially in regard to the new social obligations. The shame of being "different," of being "handicapped" leads to concealment of infections, diet restrictions, urine testing, and so on. The "normal" rebellion against the mother's care leads to a rejection of "her" diet. The parents may be blamed for the diabetes and even hated for the misery it has brought about for the child. Depression is frequent, alternating with rebelliousness.

In late adolescence things may improve and the child may become biochemically and psychologically more stable. Patients who have learned to accept the reality of the situation are now able to cope with the task imposed upon them. They are able to take over their own care, and the ambivalent ties with the parents are no longer as close or as disturbing. The outlook largely depends on the pre-adolescent history of dealing with emotional and interpersonal problems. Prognosis is poor in at least two instances: when parental overprotection and dependency combined with hostility dominate the picture, and second, in cases of neglect and rejection from early life. With the approach of adulthood and the need to make decisions on his own (and possibly to face the prospect of a poor prognosis), the diabetic may understandably begin to feel unfairly treated and deprived, and depression may become a predominant affect. It is at this stage of late adolescence that the diabetic often shows a marked self-destructive tendency as manifested by overeating or undereating and a deliberate disregard of the medical routine. Hypoglycemia attacks may become frequent. The formation of a satisfying object relationship may help to obvert such developments.

CASE 6

A boy in his late adolescence interrupted his studies, withdrew from all recreational and social life, and became preoccupied with thoughts of suicide because of the fact, he complained, that no complete cure had as yet been discovered. He felt ashamed at not having been inducted into the Israeli army, and was not amenable to any logical argument based on the fact of his physical condition.

The personalities of the parents, and their attitudes and behavior toward the child and his illness are significant factors in his emotional adjustment. Their stereotyped views about illness, together with their basic psychopathology may reinforce regressive tendencies, or precipitate and aggravate the conflict between them and the resentful diabetic child. The following attitudes were fairly common in our sample:

1. Severe anxiety and fear regarding the disease and its outcome resulting in a crippling overprotection or sacrifice of the whole family to the well-being of the diabetic child. (Everyone, for example, being put on a restricted diet so that the patient's feelings would not be hurt.)

2. Severe mourning reactions, lasting sometimes for long periods. (For example, one mother had refrained from all recreation and entertainment since her six-year-old daughter had become ill many years previously.)

3. Guilt feelings (especially provoked by the idea that diabetes was an hereditary disease leading to much mutual recrimination between the parents as to the genetic source.)

4. Authoritarian reactions (as, for example, in the case of the father of a twelve-year-old girl, who took over every detail of her diabetic management, including her injections. He was very much annoyed and disappointed when his daughter refused to permit him to examine her infected vulva.)

The normal struggle of the adolescent with his parents thus becomes intensified by the diabetic condition and each side may use the illness as a weapon against the other.

Psychological Problems in the Chronic Nephropathies of Childhood

G. Raimbault, Maitre de Recherches I.N.S.E.R.M. (France)

As in any chronic disease, nephropathies, in addition to somatic problems, raise some very important psychological questions not only for the patient himself but also for his familial and medical entourage. Because of its chronicity, and particularly when it strikes in childhood, a complex relationship gets established between the medical team and the "sick" group (made up of the child and his family), an understanding of which is necessary and sometimes even essential if the pediatrician is to achieve his medical goal to keep the patient alive and at the same time assure him of an acceptable way of life.

In this study* of the doctor-child alliance in the chronic nephropathies, there has been a collaboration between pediatricians, nursing personnel, psychologists, psychoanalysts, parents, and children.

The Nature of the Stresses Involved

Chronic nephropathies in childhood are characterized by an early diagnosis, a prolonged course interrupted by remissions and relapses and giving rise, at times, to wavering convictions of recovery or death and, at times, to similar uncertainties regarding the interventions made.

*At the Children's Hospital in Paris under the direction of Professor Royer. Translated by E. James Anthony, M. D.

With the development of chronic dialysis and transplantation, a new universe of possibilities has opened up when renal insufficiency worsens but paradoxically the terminal phase is curtailed and the immediate prognosis becomes again uncertain. These treatments are carried out with the approval of the parents who, at least at first, see in them nothing more than a desperate hope for the survival of their child. The proposed procedures stimulate unrealistic expectations as well as real fears and fantasies. The everyday life of the family is measured out in a series of hoped-for interventions that intensify the uncertainties produced by the nature of the illness. The dialysis offers a sort of moratorium during which a great many questions haunt the minds of the people involved. What will happen tomorrow? When will the transplantation take place? How long will it last? Will the child ever reach adult life?, etc., etc.

During this waiting period, a bond of dependency is established between the nursing team and the artificial kidney machine of such intensity that any severance from it becomes unthinkable since it would mean the death of the child.

We will make an arbitrary separation of the different points of view contained in this situation—the child's, the family's, and the physician's—always keeping in mind the fact that the disease creates a field of converging and interacting psychological problems stemming from each and every one of the participants in the therapeutic relationship.

The Child

A disease presents itself to the child as an indivisible ensemble made up of physical sensations localized internally coupled with external aggressions mediated through medical investigations and treatments to which he must submit himself. A chronic development of the illness signifies an irreversible transition from a relatively normal state in which he is "like others" to the abnormal state of being "not like others." In this sense, a chronic nephropathy implies temporary physical modifications (oedema), permanent limitations (growth retardation) affecting physical and academic performance (particularly with repeated hospitalization), constant restrictions and constraints (as with the use of special diets and drugs), and, at conscious and unconscious levels, anxious preoccupation regarding the changes in the kidney and its consequence for life.

While the child, during normal development, is constantly attempting to acquire control over the functioning of his body at the same time as he is consolidating his ego controls, with the onset of illness he is, in many ways, depossessed of his body which becomes instead a supervised object for others who exercise absolute rights over it observing it constantly and influencing its responses.

In a parallel development to this, the adults who normally would support his autonomy and self-esteem demonstrate contradictory attitudes in driving him, in the service of his illness, in the direction of submission, dependence, and passivity. The reactive attitudes of the child toward the illness are extremely varied. Nonacceptance of it can be explicit: it is the business of others and he wants to know nothing about it. This sets up a kind of dissociation between him and what is sick inside him—the kidney, the albuminuria, and the hypertension. The disorder can also be repudiated or even denied, the children in such cases being apparently unable to recognize the reality of the illness and the threat that it poses for them.

Other children, in contrast, may accept and resign themselves to it at the risk of becoming psychological invalids or pseudodefective. The best adjusted, however, are those who integrate it into the self-system and familiarize themselves with its effects, its course, and its treatment.

In a number of cases, the picture is of an identification with the aggressor—the ministering attendant who needs to inflict pain—that may lead to a passive-into-active reversal with the child gradually becoming his own physician-cum-nurse.

This diversity of reactive attitudes is heavily imbued with anxiety. Some of this can be displaced into spheres other than concern with health such as intellectual rivalry, emotional relationships, or psychosexual striving where they manifest themselves in an elaboration of fantasies and dreams around themes of persecution, abandonment, mutilation, amputation, and destruction indicating the impact of the disease on the child's inter- and intra-personal life and body image. Caught in this senseless entanglement of destructive and ruinous relationships, the child may try to make sense of it all by constructing explanations most often based on wrongdoing, guilt, and punishment. The "harmfulness" of the disease is interpreted in the sense of the "harm" that he had done to others or that others had done to him. In some cases, the psychological "aftereffects" take the form of phobias, of aggression directed toward others or turned against the self or of partial or massive regression.

What happens to the child when the treatment by hemodialysis becomes his daily ordeal? On the level of general adjustment, the physical recuperation—progressive and sometimes spectacular— and the possibility of resuming scholastic and social activities amount almost to a rebirth.

However, besides these real gains, recuperation creates a problem that is, if not specific, at least crucial: the integration of novel life elements into his development and into his world. The artificial kidney that modifies all other relationships, as a psychological fact, is not easily absorbed into ordinary, everyday life and exerts a general influence on all functions and activities. The youngest ones clearly show their inability to integrate this powerful man-machine relationship to which they are linked by a veritable umbilical cord. They may demand a human presence at their side during the dialysis so as not to feel utterly alienated and abandoned.

The same demand may come from the older children although disguised as anger, aggressiveness, negativism, and indifference to a host of people in a variety of settings at home, hospital, and school. There is a real risk of dismissing such manifestations as linked with their personality without searching for its meaning—an appeal to help them to integrate a nonsymbolizable situation.

The Parents

When a child becomes ill, his parents ask the doctor for a diagnosis, a treatment, and a prognosis. In the case of chronic nephropathy, the answer to these questions is neither immediate nor satisfactory. The doctor who has followed a logical course in establishing the diagnosis would like the parents to accept and maintain the same logical approach in their contact with him. In fact, the word "chronic" and the uncertainty of the prognosis are regarded by the parents as a verdict toward which they react in anything but a logical way. A delay in making the diagnosis may give them time to "metabolize" it but quite often the announcement comes too rapidly and leads either to a paralysis of effort or to a frantic "shopping around" for a more optimistic evaluation. Denial becomes the first bastion of defense. The physicians are exposed to an incessant barrage of questions and requests to the point of exhaustion.

As with the child, so with the parents, the illness may be viewed as an attack that reactivates personal problems and leads to continuous efforts at formulating a sensible reason for the "non-sense" of the disease and its absurd intrusion into their lives.

To justify this "unjust" illness, a search for causative factors first investigates possible psychological determinants: the presence of psychological symptoms in the child, psychological elements in mother and child, the relationship between the mother and her own mother, and the relationship between the mother and her husband.

The numerous questions regarding nosology can be symbolically understood as an attempt to discharge anxiety and free the individual from guilt. The guilt feelings, which are stronger the more ambivalent the parents are toward the sick child, may appear sometimes in a depressive guise as self-accusations and sometimes as projections of the fault onto others—the sick child, another member of the family, the medical profession, the family as a whole, destiny, God, and so on.

It is as if the parent were identifying himself with the child whose body can support the physical disease while the parent carries the load of mental suffering. This identification, which forms the basis of the projection of the parent's problems into the setting of the disease, leads them to present their own problems to the doctor at the same time as they report the problems of the child. This constitutes the background to the relationship between physician and parents and it is against such a background, varying with remissions and relapses, that emotional conflicts arise. The physician must be constantly on the alert with regard to these if he is to reach a diagnosis.

Although the physical diagnosis can be established once and for all, the psychological diagnosis and the problems besetting the doctor-patient relationship are continually undergoing change.

Beginning with the chronic hemodialysis (in addition to the important socioeconomic problems attached to it), there comes a crystallization of psychological problems associated with the integration by the parents of a new type of relationship with their child. The presence of this machine (this "wire mother" in Harlow's terms) that seemingly restores their child to life and upon which they remain essentially dependent has the effect of modifying their own status of "parent."

This modification is never expressed or recognized as such but can be inferred from their attitude toward the machine, the dialysis session, and the attending doctors, or less directly toward insurance or Social Security, or, very indirectly, toward such abstractions as medical sciences, civilization, and so on.

Behind every occasion when these different instances are incriminated, there is generally some attempt to work out a relationship with their child impeded by some authority whose influence it is difficult to identify and upon whom it is impossible to project anything definite.

The Physician

The pediatricians who have the clinical responsibility for the management of childhood nephropathies asked for a study to be made of the psychological problems involved. They also agreed to be included in the study. It seemed essential to us to ask them to specify, during the team sessions and during individual conferences, the problems with which they were confronted in practice. After hearing the child and his family, we tried to bring out certain aspects of the doctor's problems.

This guidance is possible at different levels of diagnosis, particularly where the doctor-patient relationship and the doctor's language itself are concerned.

The Doctor-Patient Relationship

In some rare instances, the doctor may deny any psychological interest in the case or turn a blind eye to the psychological aspects of it. A common denominator appears in all other cases: whether explicitly or implicitly, there is a feeling of guilt that activates, at different times, different states of tension in the relationship, three of which are particularly clear, having to do with accusation, recovery, and justification.

The accusation is sometimes conscious and directed against the doctor himself or implicit against a third party, another doctor, laboratory, parent, or even the patient. It seems to correspond to a need to locate the responsibility and to make manifest the inevitable. Once the accusation is made, the doctor determines his own function as one of "recuperator" to restore the sick individual not to his original level of function (i.e., "cure" him) but to a level at which he is functioning pathologically but sufficiently. The medical enterprise as a whole is then justified in its reparative aim in spite of the difficulties entailed, the anxieties and reproaches that the doctor, as a person, directs toward himself and the nature of therapeutic measures that might seem draconian in comparison with the tentative result.

The medical activity may then take the form of a challenge in which the doctor is trying to prove that one can do something against all expectation, against all hope and, in spite the suffering entailed, take a lost cause and restore it, never admitting defeat. Against the objective reality of the ailing body, the doctor, with the help of medical knowledge and its advances, struggles untiringly. He has difficulties in maintaining a continuous relationship with the sick child and his family, especially where the broad areas of technical and psychological responsibility overlap. The disruptive moments are significant in this respect. In some cases, the breaking point coincides with the termination of the technical action: a dialogue that was accepted and pursued during the course of the action, in terms of facilitating it, may come abruptly to a halt with its conclusion. The technical procedure covers up, sometimes quite obviously to all parties concerned, the doctor's difficulties in maintaining a "therapeutic alliance" with the patient. The problem may resolve itself when another member of the team takes over the responsibility.

Sometimes the technician cannot combine the empathic attitude necessary to establish the therapeutic relationship with the unavoidable aggressiveness involved in a technical procedure that requires a withdrawal from identification. This means that the therapeutic attitude is interpersonal, both parties being on an equal level, but when the technician does his job, the patient becomes a mere object. Either he will not be able to pass from action to words when he finds himself confronted, for instance, with the need to speak the truth or he will withdraw from the relationship after the action when this implies the involvement of new members of the therapeutic team.

In other cases, the rupture may be due to the limitation of medical knowledge so that the doctor can no longer have recourse to science nor use it as a protective screen—as a result, being completely bereft of all resources he is unable to sustain the relationship any further. On other occasions, the defense mechanisms of the doctor against his own anxieties are such that the patient is no longer seen as a suffering child but as an object of practice and research: the doctor-patient relationship then comes to an end.

The Problem of Communication

Psychological problems are also found in what we have called the "failures" of medical discourse. Thus, when a problematic fact in the doctor's personal history is reflected in the history of the patient and his family, a peculiar repetitiveness appears in the case record at points when the explicit needs of the family are intermingled with the implicit needs of the physician. From this confrontation, or rather collusion, the doctor's "therapeutic style" takes shape determined by the personal theme at the base of his guilty feelings and his restitution fantasies, the latter a product of the history of each pediatrician as of each individual.

Another pathognomonic sign of difficulties in the doctor's relationship is in the occurrence of certain "blanks" in his communications. Sometimes he does not talk of the problem in question or does so tangentially, briefly or brusquely. Sometimes there is a dissociation between the words spoken and the feelings they express.

Finally, in addition to these momentary "blanks," more substantial "blanks" may appear with the shifting of the problem, just described, onto another person and into another sector.

Chronic Hemodialysis

In the context of the chronic nephropathies of children, with their frequently fatal outcome, the physicians are becoming aware of their identifications with patients, of the impact of their personalities, and of the psychological value of their medical actions and are thereby recognizing the need to think out their own defense mechanism against death—the death anxieties of the patient revealing or concealing their own.

Setting up the treatment of chronic hemodialysis which, to some extent, covers up the reality of death constantly mobilizes, in an almost daily struggle, forces engaged in the apparent denial of fundamental, psychological problems. Putting this aside, partly consciously and deliberately, partly unconsciously, they rationalize, justify and judge the behavior of the children and their families and respond to it with the same rationalization, the same justification and the same judgments without trying to understand anything beyond what is said, how it is said or why it is said. This appears very clearly in the group discussions which are often centered on the daily behavior of patients treated by dialysis.

When these mechanisms of defense are no longer effective, ruptures take place in the relationship, very obviously, for instance, at the level of the nurse who asks to be transferred to another service.

These problems, in the therapeutic team, seem to us to originate from the same difficulty as the one experienced by the patients and their families in the emergence of a new type of therapeutic relationship involving a machine that plays a vital part in keeping the patient alive and thus abolishing, for the time being, the reality of death.

Conclusion

To analyze psychological problems in any disease implies, among other things, the analysis of the following given facts: the disease itself (its nature, length, seriousness, symptomatology), the diagnosis and technical care, the child's personality, the conscious and unconscious network of relationships within the family, and the child's place within this network. From these elements, the enumeration of which is by no means exhaustive, one can attempt, first, a definition of the patient's problems; second, an analysis of the therapeutic team which, whether good or bad, can in no way be considered equivalent to a perfect robot technician in the service of the medical profession but is constantly called in question by the sick child and the child undergoing hemodialysis, in terms of his survival, and the quality of this survival.

To study, in this way, the problems from the patient's point of view on the one hand and from the doctor's and nurse's points of view on the other hand is an artificial process which can give only an imperfect account of the problems of doctor-patient relationship, of those composing it and of those who must be taken into consideration if this relationship is to remain therapeutic.

Making a diagnosis of these problems may not be possible, but from an understanding of its nature and its ramifications, one might deduce from them a possible therapeutic mode of behavior deriving, on the one side, from an analysis of the communications involving the chronic illness considered as a field of convergence and projection for the psychological problems of each one rather than the cause of these problems.

As for prognosis on the psychological level, only observations made over a long period of time and into adult life will permit us to draw valid conclusions. It is always when an event is over that it begins to make sense.

Psychological Aspects of Congenital Heart Disease in the Child*

N. Rausch de Traubenberg, Ph.D. (France)

Introduction

The singling out of one aspect from a composite situation is always an artificial procedure, and this is especially the case when a child's development is seriously hampered by some major physical handicap with dramatic implications. In fact, at the different stages in the life of a sick child, we may find ourselves confronted with a variety of different aspects, some emerging at a given time and others receding and reappearing later—all this against the constant background of a threat to life and a fear of death.

In the face of such threat, an adult usually responds by attaching lesser significance to all other concerns so that to him they become secondary. Apparently, unaware of any danger, the child continues to satisfy his own needs to the best of his ability. It is this difference in attitude that characterizes the pattern of life in a family with a child afflicted with congenital heart disease. It goes without saying that the development of any child has to be viewed within the context of the family's life and this is even more so in the case of a sick child.

Assuming that he is not immediately affected by a threat to life, what then does a child in this predicament experience? We shall

*Translated by E. James Anthony, M. D.

attempt to answer this question by examining the results of a
neuropsychological investigation of open-heart surgery in children.
The psychological tolerance to surgical situations was studied.
Ostensibly, the problem seemed to be clear-cut but it was soon
apparent that it could not be adequately covered without the help
of a multifactorial approach that took into account the numerous
social, psychological, and medical factors involved. Thus, the initial objective underwent expansion when the investigation focused
on *the patient as an individual* with all his resources, failings, aspirations, and sufferings.

Experimental Conditions

Do all children respond in the same way to a cardiac disability? If
not, what are the factors that account for individual differences?
Do such differences lie in the medical diagnosis, or in such factors
as age, the socioeconomic status of the family, the parent-child relationship, or in the specifics of hospitalization with its promise of
the anxiously waited improvement? Last, but not least, there is the
major factor of the child's personality.

To provide a satisfactory answer to all these questions we examined the psychological records of 114 children between the ages of
five and fourteen before and after surgery in the context of the
above-mentioned variables, comparing them to control groups.

Psychological Data

Two psychological methods were used: group comparisons of psychosomatic findings and individual comparisons of personality tests
and interview material. The latter threw more light on subtle individual responses and revealed how the child coped with his disability,
compensated for it or denied its consequences.

Cognitive Effects

The psychometric data made evident a deficiency in perceptual and
motor functioning particularly in the cyanotic cases, the conspicuous disturbances tending to corroborate the hypothesis of an
organic susceptibility produced by an inadequate cerebral flow.

Our finding also indicated a high incidence of low I. Q.'s raising the fundamental question of difference in the mental potential of cyanotic and noncyanotic children. The finding itself is of secondary importance. What matters more are the implications of this deficiency; that is, whether it is a basic defect in the intellectual apparatus or a simple retardation brought about by inadequate schooling, irregular school attendance, insufficient socializing, a poor cultural background, or a lack of stimulation that eventually reduces the child to a state of passive withdrawal thereby further diminishing his interests and motivations. The exposure to a subcultural background or to an overprotective mother can have the same detrimental result as stimulus deficiency because the resources available to the child are not drawn upon or because his needs are disregarded on the grounds of protecting his health. Fatigue and listlessness do the rest and the child is relegated to a state of indolent resignation.

The above observations show that, in his daily life, the child experiences a restriction with regard to his activities, his intellectual and social experience, and his innate curiosity and drive for self-expression. This state of mind can be attributed both to factors influencing his maturation and to the lack of stimulation of his environment.

Emotional Effects

Observations, drawings, and projective tests were analyzed in terms of the child's self-concept, his response to frustration and deprivation, his fantasies (especially of mutilation and dismemberment), his attempts at handling his often precarious balance, his security-providing images and, finally, his progress following surgery. Our findings proved invaluable in offering some explanation of how the child learns to live with his disability, how he compensates for his handicap, and how he reacts to chronic illness and to the stress of surgery.

FROM AGES FIVE TO EIGHT YEARS

Between the ages of five and eight, the physically most vulnerable group displays a range of reactions reflecting strong needs for power and self-esteem in the face of equally strong feelings of inadequacy, insecurity, and inferiority. These reactions represent an attempt to come to terms both with the medical situation and with the outside world, and stem from the child's conception of a dangerous and disorganized world rather than from his reaction to his heart condition per se. He seems to seek relief in images signifying security and reassurance that are not usually observed at this age. The undeniable suffering is associated with generalized fears of abandonment rather than with any particular concerns regarding mutilation or physical disability. The body image as shown in drawings and in symbolic associations is that of a manipulated, incapacitated and disjointed object. The quest for identification images appears to be intense and there is clearly a projection of suppressed wishes manifested in the rather naive forms of activity attributed to human images. Seriously ill children (such as those with the tetralogy of Fallot, most of whom did not live long after surgery) talked freely about their illness, referring to their "heart," their "veins," and insisting that it is "good to talk about it," that their "auricles hurt," etc. However, these somatic concepts are not part of a fantasy system, whereas the unexpressable aggressivity is intensely immersed in fantasy and projected onto the outside world.

The pre-surgical mental state is usually characterized by a robust attitude and a dynamism that undergo recession after the operation and are superseded by depressive or persecutory tendencies and, not infrequently, by a rather pronounced feeling of "emptiness" of being "a broken, dismembered thing." Subsequently, a restructuration takes place either along the lines of a traumatic neurosis and/or of an hysterical or obsessional state.

FROM NINE YEARS ONWARD

After the age of eight the child is often greatly affected by the thought of being different from others and the feelings connected with this are externalized as serious inhibitions or states of anxious hyperactivity. Passivity or inertia are not only due to the lack of energy and considerable fatigability but also to the many taboos imposed by the parents that the child internalizes and which explain his neurotic withdrawal. The latter is much appreciated by the parents for whom it provides a certain measure of security. This "mummification" of the child, who becomes the parents' "object" or "doll," is an induced state since some children, after the operation, may inverse this behavior and become explosive, disjointedly driven, and dynamically reactive. Obviously, the imposed inhibition has an adverse effect on the subsequent development of the children. Some develop a state of excitation, instability, and exaggerated restlessness; they have to be in constant contact with adults and manifest a great deal of anguish without being able to internalize it. These children are wary and alert in the medical environment, continually attempting to unravel the technical mysteries and to become a part of the nursing staff. They respond to the "conspiracy of silence" that frequently surrounds them by an exacerbation of anxiety because more often than not they have no idea why they have been hospitalized. This explains the frequent diminution in excitement after the child is told about the pending operation. Regressive attitudes are often manifest in games and in interactions with the parents.

The closer they are to *the adolescent stage,* the less do the children seem affected, having apparently put a certain amount of coping experience behind them. As a rule, the child at this stage tends to exaggerate the "normality" of his life and to become excessively sociable, obedient, and conventional but inhibited in an adultomorphic way. He is often markedly dependent on the parents and bent on pleasing them with his "normality" and does in fact succeed in this since it is easier and less anxiety provoking for the parents to adjust to a healthy child. Immaturity is the basic characteristic. The emotional needs find no expression other than in social contact, and individual and dynamic manifestations are stifled.

From our observations it would appear that all motor and cognitive restrictions imposed upon the child are usually accompanied by an inhibition of the emotional life. The restrictions, supposedly serving to protect the child, are often replacements for warm reciprocal relationships. It is as if a contract is made that relegates the patient to a state of sickness and deprives him of all initiative. The child may react to this by developing internal feelings of opposition that further impede his psychological development.

Interactional Effects

THE MOTHER-CHILD RELATIONSHIP

There is a continuous and dramatized interaction with the mother starting at birth or at the time when she learns of the heart condition; the depressive responses usually appear very early and profoundly influence the mother-child relationship. There is a constant state of anxiety in the face of a situation that is not liable to improve suddenly but which, on the contrary, becomes profoundly embedded and may at any given time come to a fatal end. Some mothers assume the responsibility for the malformation and experience guilt feelings, the latter being nurtured by the child's condition; the child is told: "You will get a new heart, a lovely heart after the operation" for there is always the element of wishful thinking. There is no doubt as to the variety of contradictory feelings experienced by the mothers who project their own fantasies onto the diseased organ and the sick child and then take it out on the outside world or on themselves in an attempt to defend themselves against the deep-seated anxiety. This may result in quite unreasonable behavior. The tendency to be overprotective reflects not only the fear of possible disaster but also a reaction to the unconscious hostility toward the child and the situation in general. These attitudes soon turn into possessiveness and an exclusion of all other influences that might interfere with the passive depending of the child on the mother.

There is every reason to believe that the latter (and the family in general) may communicate an uneasy sense of worry to the child, particularly when they try to conceal the facts and refrain from discussing the operation. The child, in turn, may not share his feelings with them since he may have developed a confused notion that the topic was explosive and prohibited. Thus, the mother-child contact is punctuated by uncomfortable silences determined by underlying taboos, with neither side daring to discuss the feelings of the other so as to avoid any overpowering emotional response. A status quo is established and the contact during the hospitalization period is frequently reduced to admonitions to be good and to lie still. The child adjusts readily to the parental behavior as if he senses that this is what they imperatively need. Although there are some advantages in trying to preserve the child's equanimity, there is also a real danger that the emotional tension may reach a breaking point, or that unconscious disturbing fantasies may flood the child's mind. A psychodiagnostic interview may sometimes help to externalize the conflict.

The Effects of Paradoxical Parental Attitudes

These attitudes are appreciably marked by the family pattern and do not directly depend on the state of the patient. Between the two extremes, i.e., rejection and overprotection, the latter is more frequent and leads to restraints imposed upon the child. This is particularly true when the illness is considered hereditary. More often than not, the adults manage to convey a double-bind communication with an atmosphere of permissiveness around the child infiltrated with constant warnings and restrictions about what he can do. As a result he may have a difficult time understanding this paradoxical situation in which, on the one hand, everything seems to be allowed and, on the other, not even the slightest effort can be made. This may interfere radically with the development of autonomy and self-reliance. "Your heart won't allow it," is what the parents say making use of the somatic excuse to exercise their restrictive attitude and to divert the child's aggressive response and resentment away from themselves. These difficulties are aggravated by the presence of healthy siblings. The child's belief that he is *different* is then confirmed. He experiences this difference on several levels and more acutely at certain ages, but invariably on the assumption that he is an *object* rather than a subject. It is hard for him to disengage himself from this idea and he adjusts to it as best as he can.

Responding to the family's expectations, the child may assume a dependent, submissive role and obtain a vicarious satisfaction in becoming the focus of parental attention. Conversely , he may belligerently challenge the adults and the restrictive world that they represent. The latter attitude, being more self-assertive, is also more conducive to a healthier personality development although the parents usually find it much more difficult to accept.

It goes without saying that such parental attitudes stem from a concern over the somatic condition rather than a wish for a satisfactory psychological outcome; the fear of a disaster and the specter of a fatal seizure are always present, overshadowing every other consideration. Maturer and better-balanced parents learn how to cope with the situation and accept its inherent risks to the ultimate benefit of the child in terms of satisfaction and personality development. On this level of educational interaction the family should receive competent and clearly oriented help so as to avoid their fears getting the better of them, leading them to exaggerate or ritualize medical advice. We have found, time and again, that medical advice was insufficient to meet the needs of the parents who may actually regard the child as more fragile after surgery than before it.

We are led to assume that the mother-child relationship contains a specific structural element in the case of children with a congenital heart disease because of the constant fear of death, a factor that is absent when children suffer from motor or sensory disabilities alone.

Conclusion

A child suffering from a congenital heart disease seems to "ignore" the illness per se; the experience he undergoes and the way in which he handles the situation depend on his capacity for psychological integration and on the response of his parents (his mother, in particular) to his condition.

We would assume, on the basis of our findings, that the young child is less affected by his physical disability than he is by the concomitant undifferentiated distress which he tries to overcome by a recourse to images that represent stability and security. The body image is incoherent and disjointed, and as such readily conceived as an object of manipulation by the adults.

An older child will internalize the restraints imposed by the parents. Seeing his activities curtailed and his energy thwarted, he will either compensate for it by seeking relief in images that replace life experience or withdraw into a neurotic state of inertia and dependence.

Whatever the child's psychological state, it undergoes an evolution after surgery. Both the parents and the child greatly benefit from effective and consistent help during the post-operational period in as much as it establishes a link between the intensified stress of surgery and the readjustment to everyday life.

It should be emphasized, however, that these conclusions hold only within the framework of our particular investigation and it would not be appropriate to generalize from it. It was carried out during the hospitalization period and our approach was not therapeutic but investigative.

Bibliography

Bret, J. and Kohler, C., Incidences neuropsychiatriques des cardiopathies congenitales chez l'enfant. *Pediatrie,* 11, (1956), 59.

Cooper, H., Psychological aspects of congenital heart disease. *South African Med. J.,* 33, (1959), 349–352.

Delay, J., Deniker, P., Ginestet, D., Verdeaux, G. et J., Rausch de Traubenberg, N., Effets neuro-physiqués des interventions avec arrêt circulatoire prolongé en hypothermie profounde. *Presse Med.,* 69, (1961), 2539–2542.

Egerton, N. and Kay, J. H., Psychological disturbances associated with open heart surgery. *Brit. J. Psych.,* 110 (1964), 433–439.

Glaser, H. H., Harrison, G. S., and Lynn, D. F., Emotional implications of congenital heart disease in children. *Pediatries,* 33 (1964), 367–379.

Green, M. and Levitt, E. E., Constriction of body image in children with congenital heart disease. *Pediatrics,* 29 (1962), 438–441.

Landtman, B., Valanne, E., Pentti, R., and Aukee, M., Psychosomatic behaviour of children with congenital heart disease. *Ann. Paediat. Fenn.,* 6 Suppl. (1960), 15.

Rausch de Traubenberg, N., Implications psychologiques des cardiopathies congenitales. Effets des interventions correctrices. *These de Doctorat de Psychologie.,* Paris, 1965.

Schlangee, H., Die korperliche und geistige entwicklung bei kindern mit angeborenen herz und gefassmissbildungen. *Arch. Kinderhlk.,* 47 (1962).

The Roots of Hypochondriasis in the Child

Cyrille Koupernik, M.D. (France)

> *"La théorie c'est bon, mais
> ça n'empeche pas d'éxister"*
> *(Charcot [14]).*

The classical attempts to understand hypochondriasis, as Charcot attempted to understand hysteria, came to very little in the end, and physicians continued to apply rigorous medical investigations to expose its somatic pretensions. The final diagnosis, delivered with authority, branded the ailment as "imaginary" and stigmatized its complainant as an imposter. On a more benign level, its intention may have been to reassure the patient, which it seldom did. The "psychic reality" was generally more potent than the reality produced by the doctor. The hypochondriac continued to resist evaluation and treatment and remained proudly "incurable."

Three major attempts have been made in this century to explain the mystery of an "imaginary malady" that apparently caused so much suffering. These can be labeled the neurophysiological, the psychodynamic (including in its orbit, in some instances, the sociodynamic), and the developmental. Each attempt has contrived "models" elaborating mechanisms in the production of the disorder. The quintessence of each model lies in a system of oppositional forces supposedly at work.

The Neurophysiological Model

In this first model, older archaic structures of the brain are brought into opposition with more recent ones. This corresponds to the Jacksonian or to the neo-Jacksonian (Ey [3]) concepts of levels with different somatotopic representations at each level. For example, Penfield's classical parieto-frontal homunculus is represented on the neo-cortical level, but there is no doubt, judging from the recent work of McLean and others that a more nebulous representation of the body and its sensations operate at the level of the limbic system, or "visceral brain." It has been suggested, simplistically perhaps, that a lesion of the limbic system might give rise to the complex manifestations of hypochondriasis. In Ey's [3] formulation, a partial dissolution of consciousness with regression to an inferior level (normally under the control of the superior level) could unleash primary symptoms (directly from the lesion) and secondary symptoms (from the lifting of cortical inhibition). This viewpoint would suggest, therefore, that hypochondriasis is a real, somatically based entity but so deeply located as to defy any efforts at physical demonstration.

A second oppositional system has involved the two sides of the brain, the body being represented differently in the two hemispheres; the representation in the dominant hemisphere would be more "epicritic" or exactly localizable, and the representation in the subdominant hemisphere being more "protopathic" or diffuse. Hypochondriasis, in this context, might relate to a disorder of the minor hemisphere.

Within this model, the child would be regarded as less "corticalized" than the adult, and therefore further away from the ability to interpret bodily sensations more precisely. This could lay the groundwork for future hypochondriacal developments when the adult undergoes an organic regression to a more archaic interpretation of body feelings. The concurrent affective disturbances could be ascribed to the fact that the limbic system has been regarded as an essential link in the circuit of emotions.

One should add, as a corrective, that these are all in the nature of speculations rather than proven fact.

The Psychodynamic and Sociodynamic Models

The psychodynamic model also includes the opposing wishes to keep well and to become sick, where sickness is unconsciously understood as being helpless, passive, protected, pampered, significant and loved. A passive-regressive illness experience in early childhood can bring about a "convalescent" persistently ready to relapse when things prove stressful in the outside world. The quality of the mothering (nursing) may conduce to the patient posture. It may be the only type of relationship open to the child. Loss of mothering at a critical period may force the child to mother itself, worry about itself, and cater to its own special needs. Identification with a sick parent or sick sibling and the need to draw attention away from the sick family member may force the child to develop somatic symptoms and thus to become the recipient of loving physical ministrations. He may also enjoy the stimulation involved and crave the sensations aroused. In a household where the patient is king and the mother a devoted nurse, the developmental thrust to be active and strong may be unequal to the regressive pull. All these considerations would support the view that hypochondriacs are created in childhood although the illness may show itself later.

The sociodynamic model is based on the body language employed by the hypochondriacal patient. Illness becomes one of the games that people play in order to achieve certain interpersonal aims. Szasz [16] refers to them as "play games" and speaks of the myth of mental illness; the hypochondriacal state could be termed the mental aspect of a mythical illness whose antecedents might be steeped in witchcraft. The opposing forces in this model are magical and logical thought; primitives and children would show a proclivity toward understanding somatic experience in a magical rather than a logical context, and projecting this on to the social environment.

In the psychodynamic model, individuals become ill because people need them to be ill or because they need themselves to be ill. In the sociodynamic model, people in society malevolently conspire to make them ill.

The Developmental Model

During development, the individual normally progresses from a cared-after to a caring-for-self person. If the first experience is not overdone, the second experience will not range beyond a normal amount of narcissistic self-concern and body concern.

Two aspects in the formation of the model need to be considered: (a) the development of the body concept and (b) the development of the notion of illness in the child.

THE GENESIS OF THE BODY CONCEPT

There is an aspect of the body concept that is easy to discern and has been well studied. It is the image of himself that the child recognizes as his own, from mirror or photograph, from the second year and is a primordial element in his individuation. It is through this reflected image that this outer body concept not only becomes recognizable to him but also to others. It serves as a vehicle for description and self-description and displays to the outside world his emotional life.

It is the inner body concept or the "space within," that is essential in the understanding of hypochondriasis. This internal body is partly proprioceptive and partly visceroceptive. The child can easily identify himself with the proprioceptive part since they are the manifest vehicles of voluntary motility. The ideas concerning the visceral structures are much more vague, and the same holds true for the uneducated adult. The unseen, intangible nerves and blood vessels are invested with a magical quality; they permit the transport of the "bodily humors," and can be incorporated into obsessional and delusional systems. The uterus may float around and cause disorders, and the spleen and liver become responsible for temperamental reactions.

We will next consider what the child makes of the interior of his body. Schilder [14] interviewed forty children, aged four to thirteen years (the majority of borderline intelligence) and found them to be singularly disinterested in the internal structure of their bodies. The majority were content with the idea that the inside was full of food. Others included blood and bones. This type of answer is on a par with the concrete nature of reasoning in a child of this age. The question is, did these children confabulate? When a child is confronted with the internal epistemology of the "black box," he has to fall back on fantasy and speculation. He knows what happens at the input end (ingestion) and at the outlet (excretion), but in-between, there is a mysterious gap that can only be imaginatively bridged. In a later, more sophisticated study with the Inside-the-Body Test, a developmental sequence was shown regarding knowledge of "inner space," and the space itself was "richer" because the children were more intelligent. The culture may determine the level of sophistication of such knowledge.

This speculation is frequently and directly linked to the primitive health-illness concept of the individual. The ideas may persist past childhood. A great many uneducated adults think that in the absence of ingestion of food, there is no excretion or that if the digestive apparatus does not function, food is eliminated unprocessed.

The problem is further complicated when the functions of ingestion and excretion are given emotional significance. Ingestion is regarded with positive emotion because it appeases hunger and/or thirst, is associated with good taste sensations, and because it is also linked with pleasing the parent.

Ingestion can also be linked with negative feelings because what he eats may be regarded by him as forbidden, bad, or dangerous, or because during the negativistic phase, to eat may mean to concede or to lose face.

Excretion, similarly, has ambivalent meanings and feelings attached to it. It is pleasant because it stimulates anal and urethral sensations and because evacuation puts an end to a state of tension; and because the act of excretion is like the act of ingestion, a pleasing conformity to the demands of the mother. On the other hand, from very early on, the products of excretion become synonymous with what is shameful, dirty, dangerous, and threatening, and according to Klein [7], children can have fantasies regarding the poisonous and explosive nature of their excreta. These persist into adult life and are the basis of powerful insults.

Finally, in many cultures, a concept of the undivided cloaca appears in the child and persists in the adult, mixing the excretory and sexual functions and consequently confusing the younger child's reproductive and gastro-intestinal concepts during the period of pre-operational thinking.

According to Schilder [14] again, the adult has the idea of a full internal body (comparable to the embryological stage of the morula), while the child feels it as essentially empty (stage of the gastrula).

This notion of the empty body was put forward by a child during an interview with Anthony [1] when comparing his body to a house in which it would be boring to live forever.

The interior of the body is generally silent; it makes itself heard only when something goes wrong. Pain is one of the features that helps to awaken consciousness, to localize parts of the body and to differentiate self from nonself.

GENESIS OF THE CONCEPT OF SICKNESS IN THE CHILD

It would seem that this concept is acquired through the cognitive and affective processes of acculturation at the center of which is the type of relationship that Schilder (cited by Anthony [1]), refers to as "appersonization." This implies an unconscious imitation of someone else's emotions, experiences, actions, and body image. This operates mainly during childhood but continues, more or less, throughout life. During childhood, the sick role together with the behavior and expectations related to it are learned from the family, and illness becomes intimately associated with the dynamics of family life. In primitive societies, individual sickness is experienced as an event linked to the group and its dynamics.

In the preschool-aged child, illness is chiefly registered within the framework of the mother-child dyad. From the neonatal period onward, disagreeable and painful sensations are brought to the attention of the mother by means of vocalizations. Lewis [11] has stated that vocalizations, from the beginning of life, invariably have a negative message, the state of contentment being silent. It is the mother's task to decode the nature and location of the unpleasant sensation, and to assuage the discomfort. Thus, from the very start, there are *emotional* elements that from the essence of illness, namely, the distressing internal sensation, the call to the other, and the amelioration gratification in return. The less competent the mother is in diagnosing and relieving discomfort, the less confidence will the infant develop in the reality of "cure." The attitude of the mother (or substitute mother) is critical in determining later attitudes toward illness. The illness of the infant is felt as her illness and the way in which she treats it corresponds to the way in which she treats herself—with loving care or disregard. As distance develops between her and the child, she falls back on the culturally-approved sense of duty and responsibility and, under certain circumstances, this may become exaggerated. When the mother, for example, has unconscious feelings of hostility and rejection toward the child, she may compensate for them with an increased concern for his health. The child, in his turn, quickly learns that the most effective way to mobilize her attention is to be ill or pretend to be ill or pretend to be more ill than one is. Since the pretense is not too conscious in the first place, he soon manages to convince even himself that he is not well. Since both mother and child are deriving satisfaction from this particular functioning of the dyadic relationship, it is easily perpetrated and becomes a way of life for both parties. This provides another key to our understanding of hypochondriasis.

As the child grows, he undergoes the process described by Mahler [12], of separation-individuation. However, in order to "learn" his role as an individual, he must still identify himself with significant people in his environment. If these are sick, or worse hypochondriacal, he is liable to develop a patient identity. Anthony considers that this process can eventuate in a physical folie a deux in which the child identifies with the sick one. Kanner [6] has given some striking examples of this in his well-known textbook.

We began by presenting illness as a central component of the dyad, and next in terms of identification with a sick or hypochondriacal parent. A third, or phenomenological, aspect is concerned with the coming into consciousness of the concept of illness which undergoes an evolution similar to the concept of death, emerging from magic and animism into an understanding of the biological reality.

An accelerated realization occurs on the occasion of the illness within the family when the dramatic paraphernalia of medicine surrounds the patient and stamps itself indelibly on the impressionable mind of a susceptible child. Shaw and Lucas [15] make the following comment on this point:

> The hypochondriacal child, the neurotic child complaining of somatic symptoms, has probably been overprotected. Often, he (or she) has learned the somatic orientation in imitating a parent who is sick or believes himself to be sick (complaining). Thus, an eleven-year-old girl begins to experience thoracic pains and a fear of dying after her father died of a heart attack. She lies on the bed where he had lain, professes an intense pain, and refuses to go upstairs to sleep for fear of not waking up again.

The authors here have perhaps put too much weight on the more simplistic notion of overprotection (without offering too much evidence for it) and somewhat underplayed the effect of the resounding impact, deep and perhaps lasting, that the death of the father may have had on a sensitive child. Until then, she was probably hardly aware of the beating of her heart, and then suddenly, she is made to realize that it can stop. What did she "learn" from this event? Did she "imitate" her father to keep him "alive" inside her, or had she become him through the process of loss, or was she authentically frightened by the prospect it opened up for some effect on her own heart, for which she might have been prepared by overprotection?

The possibility has been raised that hypochondriasis, in its genesis, may be linked to the presence of what has vaguely been termed "neuro-vegetative" disorders in the child. Freud [5] had considered these among the "actual" neuroses without psychogenesis, and it may be that hypochondriasis belongs originally to this group and is later "psychologized" by the mechanisms that have already been described under such labels as somatic acculturation, appersonization, body language, etc.

The notion of illness, according to Canguilhem [2] is based in the popular mind, on two models, an ontological and a dynamic one. The first attempts to explain illness by the intrusion of noxious material ranging from demons and potions to worms, viruses, and bacteria. (This is basically the Pasteurian model.)

The second model, in contrast, sees illness as the result of some disruption in the state of "universal harmony." (An example would be the Chinese doctrine of Tao.)

In the first model, the responsibility for illness is attributed, along with the guilt, to the outside world (the paranoid attitude). An important part of the education given to children aims at putting them on guard against the aggressions from the external environment. Within this framework, the child may develop two submodels, one of paranoia (that includes several states of obsessive nosophobia, such as fear of microbes or poisoning), and the other of retribution for noncompliance. (The child is convinced that he has fallen ill because of disobedience: "You did not cover up," "You don't eat enough," "You go to sleep too late," etc.) This latter explanation corresponds better to the child's mode of concrete reasoning.

The second model is generally applied to phenomena with cyclical recurrence, such as menstruation, the popular concept of which is largely mythological and includes a variety of superstitions and superstitious practices. The girl is supposed to feel unwell at this stage, to be more disturbed, accident prone, and erratic, and to be more susceptible to infection. (Curiously enough, some recent research has tended to lend support to such popular ideas.)

Masturbation exercises its effect through both models. In one, the consequence is castration, directly or indirectly threatened by the outside world; in the other, the consequence is insanity as a result of a "softening of the brain." (Once again, one should not disdain the popular concepts, as they sometimes turn out to be right; the earlier Freud found masturbation an important etiological factor in the genesis of neurosis, although later it was the guilt associated with fantasy that he felt was crucial.)

CASE ILLUSTRATION

L. B., nine years old, is referred "because she has every illness." In fact, she is markedly hypochondriacal, intensely anxious, and constantly preoccupied with her internal organs—liver, spleen, stomach, kidneys, intestine, heart, lungs—that she believes are diseased. She is the only daughter of an elderly Jewish couple. The father suffers from multiple sclerosis, and between him and his daughter there is almost a competition as to who has more symptoms. The mother is a profoundly nervous person, not strongly maternal and yet overprotective. The maternal grandmother's contribution to this disease melange in the family has been to create a state bordering on panic in the child by threatening to "have her 'zizi' (clitoris) cut off" by the surgeon (who was due to operate on her for chronic appendicitis) if she continued to masturbate.[8]

In this case, therefore, we find summarized all aspects of the popular models of disease: a parent attacked by a serious neurological disease (and very nervous besides); a mother who is overprotective and tense; and a grandmother with a propensity for rousing fear and guilt feelings in relation to the body. Can one, from this case, or even from an aggregate of many such cases, elicit generalized profiles of the parent who generates hypochondriasis or the child fated to become hypochondriacal?

Conclusion

At the present state of our clinical art, this would seem unlikely.

The literature is extraordinarily confused. Nothing clear-cut follows from the considerable work done by Ladee [9] and there is in Laughlin's [10] work, a confusion between actual case history and the theoretical conceptions of Freud and Klein [7] that are never resolved. Pilowsky [13] has found a statistical correlation between the fact of having a hypochondriac father and the presence of what he terms "primary hypochondriasis" (that is, monosymptomatic) in the male progeny.

There is therefore, at the present time, no certain correlation between physical illness and hypochondriasis, nor is it evident either that a child afflicted with a chronic illness is more likely to develop hypochondriacal attitudes. The opposite is as likely.

The question of whether a preceding hypochondriacal disposition may lead to the development of hypochondriasis when actual physical illness intervenes also remains to be demonstrated. The general climate of disease fearfulness generated by organized medicine will also help to determine the reactions of society, families, and individuals to physical illness and the threat of physical illness. The evolution of social institutions (medical aid from the state, public health insurance, workman's compensation, etc.) may afford such substantial secondary gratifications to the sick person that one can envisage a time when entire communities are precipitated into a massive hypochondriasis unless, as in Erewhon, disease becomes regarded as a punishable crime. The physician in the future may be as much occupied with preventing or curing illness as with preventing or curing the fear of illness, or the inclination to fall into illness as the line of least resistance.

The first line of defense against this travesty of disease, this mythical illness of hypochondriasis, must be set up in childhood where it all begins. Kanner [6] gives a convincing example of such preventive measures.

Gregory, a young boy, has developed marked hypochondriasis to the point of no longer leaving his bed. The therapist first of all establishes his influence by creating a positive relationship with the child, and then gradually helping him to relinquish the role of invalid that the boy has chosen for himself. His efforts are successful (by steady persuasion rather than deep-going interpretation), and ten years later, the boy has become active, well-adjusted and ready to enter military service.

It is within this framework of continuity, of the child of today becoming the adult of tomorrow, that the problem of hypochondriasis must be tackled. The function of children's clinicians is to combat the disease myths that pervade the culture by engaging in a constant clarifying dialogue with the individual and the community after we have gained their confidence.

Bibliography

1. Anthony, E. J., The child's discovery of his body, *J. Amer. Phys. Ther. Assn.,* 48 (1968), 1103–1114.
2. Canguilhem, G., *Le Normal et le Pathologique,* Presses Universitaires de France, Paris, 1966.
3. Ey, H., Discussion of F. E. Kenyon's paper, *International Journal of Psychiatry,* 2 (1966), 332-334.
4. Freud, S., *Charcot (1893),* in Standard Ed., The Hogarth Press, London, 3 (1962), 11-23.
5. Freud, S., *Contributions To a Discussion on Masturbation* (1912), in Standard Ed., The Hogarth Press, London, Vol. XII (1958), 239-254.
6. Kanner, L., *Child Psychiatry,* Second Ed., C. C. Thomas Press, Springfield, Ill., 1950.
7. Klein, M., *Developments in Psychoanalysis,* Hogarth Press Ltd., London, 1936.
8. Koupernik, C., and Dailly, R., *Developpment Neuro-Psychique Du Nourrisson,* Presses Universitaires de France (Collection sup) (1968), 378.
9. Ladee, G. A., *Hypochondriacal Syndrome,* Elevier, Amsterdam, (1966) 424.
10. Laughlin, H. P., *The Neuroses,* Butterworth, Washington, 1967.
11. Lewis, M., *Infant Speech, A Study of the Beginnings of Language,* The Humanities Press, New York; Routledge & Kegan Paul, London, 1951.
12. Mahler, M., Child psychosis and schizophrenia: autistic and symbiotic psychosis, *Psychoanalytic Study of the Child,* Vol. VII, International Univ. Press Inc., New York, (1952), 286–305.
13. Pilowsky, I., Primary and secondary hypochondriasis, *Acta Psychiatrica Scandinavia,* 46 (1970), 273–285.
14. Schilder, P., Studies in the constructive allegories in the psyche, *The Image and Appearance of the Human Body,* International University's Press, New York, (1950), 353.
15. Shaw, Ch. R. and Lucas, A. R., *The Psychiatric Disorders of Childhood,* Second Ed., Appleton-Century Crofts, New York, 1970.
16. Szasz, T. S., Foundations of a theory of personal conduct, *The Myth of Mental Illness,* Paul B. Hoeber, New York, 1961.

DYING

Editorial Comment (Section III)

Dying, as a Dickens character once remarked, is a very funny business, and by "funny" he meant "funny peculiar" rather than "funny ha ha" although a certain type of gallows humor may help to relieve the more peculiar side of it. Dying is not only a funny business but, even under the best management, it is an awkward business and none of the participants seem quite to know what to say or what to do. When the child is still labeled sick, those about him can function reasonably well in their professional or caretaking roles, but once he is reclassified as dying, everyone seems suddenly to become an amateur and strangely at a loss. Moreover, they learn very little from experience so that each occasion of dying is treated like a first in history to be approached with adamite naivete. In spite of a growing literature (Vernick has collected a bibliography of 1494 references dealing with the subject of death and dying), it still remains a very awkward business for all concerned, as illustrated so fully in this section

Dying is like adolescence, a transitional period that, unless ritualized and routinized within a cultural setting, is liable to generate anxiety and maladjustment not only in the individuals undergoing the experience but equally in those connected with it. Like adolescents, the dying are in-between people who are in the process of change and, therefore, not easily categorized. They are marginal individuals belonging neither to life nor to death but occupying a psychological limbo where they are imbued with group attributes devoid of idiosyncrasies. They are on the way to join the characterless dead. There is a gap, similar to the generation gap, between the living and the dying, and communication across this gap is not easy. Those within the transitional group are nearer one another than they often are to relatives and friends. The group behavior in a ward of leukemic children has a peculiar dynamism of its own. The children are not intensely attached to one another, but they are extremely sensitive to absences. They get to know the other child in a stark and different way. They learn about his disease characteristics, symptoms, his medication, and even his life expectancy. All this creates a curious adhesiveness that Vernick describes so vividly.

When the dying children are seen in these groups, it becomes clear that they deal with death and dying in as wide a variety of ways as dying adults, exhibiting fear, denial, resentment, puzzlement, and even humor. For children, however, dying is more quintessentially a separation. It is not that *they* are going away but that people are leaving them. They are being deserted and what they feel is loneliness, isolation, and separation anxiety; what they suffer from is the neurosis of abandonment. This is based not simply on interpretation but on the undeniable fact that people around them who love them and care for them are beginning to detach themselves and institute the mourning process. It would seem that at this time more than at any other closeness would be the order of the day with attachments strengthened rather than weakened, and "anticipatory mourning" put into cold storage for the postmortem period. If a trend can be observed at all in this confused field, it is toward maintaining contact to the limits of consciousness and even beyond, humanizing and personalizing the dying phase, and allowing the dying to die in comfort and dignity in familiar surroundings, attended by loving, familiar people. The "flogging" of the dying creature, whether child, adult, or horse, is disgraceful.

One of the questions raised in this section is whether a specialized facility, having to deal at times with dying children, should appoint an individual to convoy the dying children through this oftentimes disturbing and distressing period. Once the child dies, the administration takes over, and the procedures are clear—the undertaker, the mourner, and the minister have assigned roles and relationships. It is before death that everyone, the child, his parents, the nurses and physicians, and the hospital authorities are at sea. What sort of person should this be and what should he do? Vernick suggests someone doing what he himself has done so well—making life-space interventions, clarifying mysteries, abreacting feelings, supporting sagging egos, and altogether acting as an honest reliable resource person for the children. The children responded to him because he had time to be with them and talk to them openly and candidly.

He clearly identified strongly with them and shared emotionally in all their ups and downs. This requires a very special and dedicated individual with no other commitments. The Albys come up with a different suggestion requiring less psychological involvement in the dying child himself but more concern with the relationships between the child, his parents, his physicians, and his nurses that are particularly prone to suffer at this time. The Albys feel that the individual emotional needs of all participants are well-nigh insatiable and that it would be impossible for any one person to meet them all. They also think that in a specialist unit of this kind, carrying out psychological interviews in depth could easily interfere with the smooth working of the treatment program. For them, therefore, the "Psy" person is more a catalyst of relationships than an analyst who helps to make manifest the latent demands of the patient.

One gets the impression that a cultural factor must be at work here and that the organization of a hospital in France would make it difficult for a person like Vernick to operate as freely and as flexibly as he apparently does in Washington. This is probably one aspect of the general hypothesis that it is easier to die in some cultures than in others.

The same is true of Vernick's insistence on dealing with death and dying so directly and authentically with the children. There is an element of "permissiveness" here and freedom—the way liberal Americans want to treat their children. In France it is different, and the Albys recognize the difference. Nevertheless, they see more to the problem than just whether it is good or bad for the child. They feel, like Vernick, that one is often only telling the child what he already knows and has picked up from a thousand cues around him. On the other hand, they wonder about the "counter-transference" problem. Why does the teller need to tell? Is it to relieve the feelings of the child or his own feelings? What are *his* motivations? Would he take into account the age of the child, his personality, his degree of distress and disturbance, and his wish to know or not to know? The Albys, like Solnit, would treat each case on its merits bringing it into line with other "telling" problems, such as whether to tell the child that he is adopted, whether to give him the "facts of life," or whether to disclose marital problems. (Again, he probably knows already.)

The Futterman article is an American (as compared with European) approach in that the field is systematically explored, and concepts are carefully defined within a general frame of reference containing such working ideas as anticipatory mourning, resignation to the inevitable, detachment from the present, reconciliation to the future, and memoralization. As seen in this context, the parents keep themselves psychologically busy mastering, adapting, searching, and participating, leaving them little time to ruminate on the emptiness and nothingness confronting them. The American way of dying, in fact, does include a great deal of "organizational comfort" to deal with existential anguish, and "botanizing on a mother's grave" can be a highly effective defense.

The physician probably comes off the worst in the dread encounter since nothing in his training prepares him for the task of coping with the demands. He receives no help from any medical "last rites." Under the circumstances he may become omnipotent or impotent. The parents may look to him as the last word on this side of the grave but may then gradually lose faith in him as their hopes diminish. Yet, as one parent put it, who else do they have to trust?

Not only is the physician frequently a rank amateur in the psychological care of the dying, but he may be further incapacitated by his own neurotic anxieties. Lewin (1946) pointed to the role that fantasies play in the development of the physician's attitude toward his sick patients and suggested that because of the doctor's aggressive impulses directed against the patient and his fear of the latter's retaliation, the passive helpless patient was also his ideal patient, an attitude buttressed by the experience which every medical student has with his first "patient"—the cadaver. Neurotic disturbances in this area may not only interfere with the medical care he gives but also with his psychological management of parents and relatives.

In spite of the theorizing, one cannot read this section without a feeling of intense involvement in the predicament of these pathetic youngsters. We are left in the end with an overall picture of children, under sentence of death, talking, grumbling, laughing, quarreling and demanding,lonely, and "whistling in the dark." Death at the end of the human life cycle seems almost logical; a child's death never makes sense and leaves the environment with a feeling of outrage. Jimmy's death, poignant though it is, seems almost an exercise in futility. His therapist has also to live through this "absurd-ity" along with his patient, and he does it as well as it can be done. He does not structure the situation, interpret the latent anxieties, or analyze the dreams. He just seems to make himself available to his young patient and to anticipate some of his emotional needs.

If adults themselves cannot deal with children dying, it is left with the children to show how it can be done. In one of Vernick's unpublished "conversations" with leukemic children, he demon-strates very beautifully the way in which children make use of a sort of gallows humor to detoxicate their situation. A few examples will suffice:

The children were going out and one of them said with a half smile, "I can't go, I am going to die." Vernick says to her, "Well, you're not going to die in the next few minutes. You have time to come out to lunch with us." She immediately looked up with a smile and said, "Yes, I'm coming."

Henry was going on a tour, and Vernick asked where his roommate was. He replied quickly, "Oh, he's dead. He's not going."

One of the boys had tried to get in a certain motion picture. He said to the ticket girl, "Don't I get in for a special price?" She wanted to know why, and he said, "I have cancer." Then she replied, "I don't care if you have leukemia," and they both burst out laughing. He went on to talk about how people in the community acted when they saw him. Many were surprised to find him still alive. Some of his friends said, "Hey, what are you doing alive. I thought you were dead."

The children were going on a trip to a local park, and one of the boys was smoking. A twelve-year-old girl commented on the smoke getting into her nose. She said to him, "What are you trying to do, give me lung cancer?" The boy replied, "Well, what difference does it make; if one doesn't get us, the other will."

As the children were turning into the hospital grounds, a hearse passed them on the way out. The conversation was cut off suddenly, and for a few seconds there was silence. Then one of the girls remarked, "Well, somebody got to go home!," and the group all laughed.

One of the boys related a TV program which included a lady standing at the entrance of a morgue saying to another lady who was knocking on the door: "Room for one more."

One of the boys picked up a tape recorder and assumed the role of a radio announcer. He stated that people were dying from leukemia and that here were some of the sounds of people dying. He went on to make such sounds, and two others joined in. Another boy announced that it was his turn to die. By chance one of the mothers happened to be at the doorway as he made this statement, and it was obvious from the look on her face that she was extremely shocked.

One of the girls said, "I washed my hair last night." After a moment's pause, she said, "I mean I washed my head," and the entire group broke into laughter. (At this point she was almost completely bald from treatment and was wearing a wig.)

If one is at a loss in dealing with these dying children, it is because of not listening. If one is to do the right thing by them, one must listen to what they have to tell us.

E. James Anthony, M. D.

Meaningful Communication with the Fatally Ill Child

J. Vernick, M.S.W. (U.S.A.)

Introduction

The suspicion or actual diagnosis of a fatal illness in a child produces one of the most overwhelming and pervasive stress situations imaginable. Not only the child, but also his parents, siblings, other relatives, friends, neighbors, and even his physician find themselves in a state of extreme emotional tension and discomfort.

Even very young children, as a result of the extensive and perhaps sudden exposure to medical personnel and procedures, and/or hospitalization, quickly become acutely aware that they are in a serious and life-threatening situation. The parents are generally in a quandary as to what, if anything, they should say to the child regarding his illness. Even if they feel that they should talk with the child, they are uncertain about how to proceed. Furthermore, the physicians themselves tend to complicate the issue since many doctors still advise the parents to join them in saying nothing about the illness until the child asks questions regarding it and then to give information which, hopefully, will avoid getting the child unduly upset. It is not only unfair to the child and parent, but psychologically and humanly impossible for the parents to avoid communicating, directly and indirectly, their concern for their child. Clement Smith [1] commented, "Anything you do under such a situation hurts. I think we should get away from the idea that, with children, we must somehow soften blows in a special way. Blows cannot be always softened, but by explanation and sharing, their impact may be made somewhat less concentrated and acute." Although this was written over sixteen years ago, it is amazing how little progress we have made in following his recommendation. At the present time, unfortunately, we all still find it extremely difficult to relate helpfully to fatally ill adults and it is almost impossible to motivate most adults to communicate meaningfully with the fatally ill child. The emotional impact upon each person associated with the child is so great that almost everyone either seeks to avoid such involvement entirely or becomes so "protective" that honest interchange with the child becomes impossible. Frequently, the writer has heard such comments as: "He doesn't want to talk about such things because he hasn't asked questions about what he has"; "If I talk with him about such and such it will only get him upset"; or "He wouldn't understand what I told him."

On the whole we tend to decide for ourselves what the child needs to talk about purely on the basis of what we feel would be most comfortable for us to discuss with him. On the contrary, however, in order to help a child (or any patient, for that matter) develop additional machinery for coping with the many problems which relate to his serious or fatal illness, it is essential to establish an environment in which he feels perfectly safe to ask any and all questions. We must also communicate clearly to the child that all answers to his questions will be honest and couched in terms that he can understand.

Indeed, there is nothing that the child sees, hears, imagines, or wonders about in the hospital environment that cannot or should not be discussed with him. Constant, meaningful communication on all such subjects will free much of his emotional energy from its struggle with these many unknowns, so that it can be more productively directed toward appropriate adjustment to his day-to-day contact with his environment and all the people in it. We must face the fact that the child has many questions, fears, and anxieties about his illness, the medical procedures he undergoes, fellow patients, death, and particularly the process of dying. It is up to the adults around him to help him sift and sort the impacts of these stressful experiences.

It has been the writer's experience that the initial staff contact with the newly hospitalized patient (regardless of the length of his stay) establishes a pattern of relationship between them which changes very little, if at all, during protracted exposure to each other, unless, of course, the approach of staff is later markedly altered. On admission, the child very quickly puts feelers out so he can determine the "worth" of each staff member to him, particularly in terms of whom he can trust. He very promptly learns, through direct and indirect means, which subjects are entirely taboo for discussion and which questions will be answered with half-truths or distortions. He also rapidly determines how far each adult will go in communicating with him.

The child becomes torn between his need to know what is going on in his own treatment program, and in those of the other patients around him, and his desire not to antagonize staff by asking them questions which he senses, or learns, create tension within them. He feels that if he does antagonize staff, they will reject him and thus will not try as hard to help him get better. This would be an intolerable situation for him to be in so, at all costs, he tries to avoid getting into it. He desperately needs every friend and ally he can get at this particular time and will forfeit the satisfaction of his own needs in order to meet the requirements of the environment.

Method of Approach

The major technique utilized in these interviews has been called the "life-space interview [2]," since it allows the staff member to focus on the actual events which are of concern to the children as individuals or as a group. The most effective aspect of this method is the opportunity offered the staff member to deal spontaneously and effectively with significant material whenever and wherever it arises. The goals of the "life-space interview" are the "clinical exploitation of life events" and the "providing of emotional first aid on the spot." To accomplish the first goal, the worker, who may be any person who is part of the child's environment, uses an appropriate experience of the day, or moment, to help the child work on specific problems of adjustment. In order to attain the second goal, the adult offers the child immediate help in coping with situations that provoke an overload of hostility, anxiety guilt, or frustration.

The Problem of the Younger Child

During the initial stages of the author's work with the leukemia patients, all children, from about the age of three years up, were included in the program. The clear awareness of events occurring on the ward, on the part of children even this young, was dramatically illustrated by the following incident.

Prior to becoming seriously ill, Charles, aged five, was a very popular member of the group of youngsters, age three to six years, who romped around the ward playing together. It was obvious that Charles was the most popular member of the group for his name could be heard more than any other. Then Charles was confined to his bed, suddenly became seriously ill and died late one evening. The morning following Charles' death the writer was in the playroom with the group. It was apparent to him that these children knew their friend had died even though they had not asked about him nor been given any information about his death by the staff or their parents. From the time of Charles' death his name was never again mentioned by any of his close friends during their entire hospitalization. It was as if Charles had never existed. The silence of the adults indicated to the children that the former could not discuss this frightening unhappy event with them. The children had correctly interpreted the adult silence to mean that they should keep their questions, thoughts, and feelings concerning such matters to themselves.

It is, therefore, especially useful to be able to refer to the work of two French pediatricians, Raimbault and Royer [3], who have done some work with the very young fatally ill child. While carrying out their first interviews with young patients (1967) concerning their ideas about their illnesses, these authors were struck by the great frequency with which the young children spontaneously approached the death theme. In a more recent paper [4] describing their interviews with and observations on ten children aged five through nineteen, who were hospitalized with chronic diseases of serious prognosis, they reported that these patients too were seriously preoccupied with the idea of death. In all the interviews, the children, either directly through questions and comments, or indirectly through picture drawing, or by both means, themselves brought up the subject of death. After having discussed such matters with the children, Raimbault and Royer concluded that chronically ill and seriously ill children readily and realistically can and wish to speak about their fears, concerns, and ideas about death and dying. Specifically they state, "When the sick child has the possibility to freely express himself with an adult he will approach the subject of death without restraint." They found that it was rare to find a young patient who fled from the opportunity and chose to remain silent.

It should be pointed out that in the interviews held by Raimbault and Royer, even with their youngest patients, straightforward simple communication techniques were used. They found no need to become involved in complicated symbolic and interpretive techniques. This latter approach, according to the writer's experience, is used because of the interviewer's anxiety about dealing directly with the grim subject matter rather than because of the inability or lack of desire of the patient to do so.

Dealing with Treatment Reactions

All patients in this program indicated, at one time or another, that one of the most important things adults could do for them was to let them know continuously what is going on and what might happen in the future.

One of the children, age seven, spoke of some medication he was supposed to get that morning but hadn't gotten yet. During a discussion on this subject, the boy stated that he'd like it much better if the staff would let him know exactly when he was to get it. "I'm scared anyway, but at least I'd know then what's going to happen." He added, with anger in his voice, "Once I got a bone marrow and nobody told me about it before I got it. I get very mad when I don't know what is going to happen. At first I get very scared, and when I feel that way I get mad at the people who make me scared."

The preparation for medical and surgical manipulations cannot be global or nebulous. The anxiety focuses on details and details need to be carefully and clearly rehearsed if the child is to be spared unnecessary anxiety.

A nine-year-old girl was scheduled for a liver biopsy. The author had conferences with nursing staff, the physician and the surgeon. All the steps of the procedure as well as her reactions to them were discussed with the patient. On the morning of the operation, time was spent with the child again going over all the pertinent information and talking with her as she was "prepped" for the procedure. Later in the day, when the anesthetic had worn off, the author went into speak with her and found her very anxious to inform him that he had left something out. She said: "You didn't tell me that they would lift me from the cart onto the operating table!"

As soon as a child enters a hospital, he immediately becomes aware of the other patients and their conditions. On a Leukemia

Service there are many adverse side effects of chemotherapy for the new admission to observe. Thus he may, for example, soon see a patient with loss of hair or even complete alopecia and may become acutely concerned about the same thing happening to him.

Patient-Staff Communication

Saul, age 11, and the author were in a room when a member of clergy entered the room and engaged in a short verbal interchange with the boy. No sooner had he departed than Saul said, shaking his head, "Gee, I wish he wouldn't come in here to see me. I have enough to worry about without carrying him along too."

It was sometimes possible to discuss with certain staff members how they felt they had handled a particular interview. These discussions were aimed at decreasing the communications gap between the adult and child. After giving the child's point of view and his evaluation of the matter, as well as the writer's observations, the staff member was generally able to take a new look at the situation and attempt to rectify it by returning to the patient's room and clearing the air between himself and the child. Each time such a discussion was held with a staff member, the patient or patients concerned were so advised. Both patients and staff were often reminded that part of the author's job was to maintain appropriate communication channels at all times.

The following excerpt from a recorded interview shows a nurse involved in meaningful communication with her patients on a matter of great interest and importance to them. By her words and actions she indicates her willingness to discuss any subject of import to the child in a much more than cursory manner. In fact, not only is the direct question dealt with by the nurse, but she goes on to do a most skillful job of giving further information which is completely understood by the children.

"Sally and Doreen, aged 12 and 13, were lying in their beds talking to me during rest period. Sally saw some patients (a set of twins) being wheeled down the hall and immediately asked, "Hey, what are they going to do to the twins?" I said that they were going to do a bone-marrow transplant. I asked if they knew what that was. Sally said that she didn't, and Doreen said, "I heard something about it, but I want to know more." I asked for a piece of paper and said that I would explain it to them. Sally laughed and said, "Miss L. always needs a paper to draw things on whenever she explains anything." I then went on to illustrate and explain the procedure and purpose of the bone-marrow transplant. When I was through Sally said, "Hey, that's neat!" Sally then asked, "Miss L., what exactly causes leukemia?" I went on to speak about the virus theory. We talked about the common viruses, which they knew about, and I related this information to current ideas about leukemia being caused by a virus. I mentioned that acute leukemia is said to happen to one child out of 10,000 in your age group. "And I had to be one of them!" I said that it was too bad that it had to be this way and added that there were lots of people working to find new ways to treat leukemia and that, hopefully, someday there would be a cure. I said that her doctor was doing just that when he spent time working in the labs . . ."

Patients are not only interested in the details of their own treatment plans, but also in those of their fellow patients. They see and hear many things and attempt to relate the observed progress or lack of progress, and specific treatment plans of their fellow patients, to their own situation. The patients not only discuss their "medical" observations among themselves, compare notes, and seek answers to questions from each other, but they also evaluate staff members in terms of their professional skills as well as their ability to communicate meaningfully with the children. Staff members who can get across to small patients are a minority in any hospital.

Communication with the children is of great importance at all times, but particularly when they are extremely ill. At these crucial periods, much of their apprehension relates to the fears of dying (greatly exacerbated by pain) and being abandoned. Absent or decreased staff contact is then interpreted by the child as an indication that he is getting worse and is going to die NOW.

The writer's experience with many terminally ill children, as well as with some adults, does not lead him to the same conclusions reached by Ross [5] who described five phases in the course of fatal illness once it has been diagnosed. These were denial and isolation, anger, bargaining, depression and acceptance. The last phase was a time when the patient was tired and in most cases very weak and she cautioned against misinterpreting this for a happy state. The patient was actually almost devoid of feelings and oblivious to attention and it was his family that stood in need of help and support. The patient himself preferred to be left alone or at least untroubled by reports and problems from the outside world. Ross concluded that there were "few patients who fight to the end."

Unless a patient is actually completely out of touch with reality, there is a continuing need for those around him to keep up an appropriate level of association with him. We place our needs before those of the sick child if we automatically assume that, when he is very critically ill, all we can do is give him medication. On many occasions the writer, while spending time with a dying child, would ask him if he wanted to play a game, something they had done together all through the child's hospitalization. Even if the child could only nod his head, some familiar games would be adapted to the existing situation. Often the child was so ill that he could neither talk nor move, and the author would then play both parts. This, of course, necessitated working out some method for allowing the patient to communicate with him so that the child's moves could be made as instructed. Of course, not every contact of this kind resulted in the child wanting to play a game or talk. When the patient indicated that he simply wanted someone sitting there with him, this is what was done.

The author was at first uncertain what to do when a very ill child appeared to be completely out of touch with reality. He decided to try holding the child's hand and talking directly into his ear. The first three children with whom this approach was tried died without regaining real consciousness so there was no way of learning if anything had gone through to them. However, the fourth occasion proved to be a very different experience.

Keith, an eighteen-year-old boy, became critically ill, and most of the time lay with his eyes closed giving only vague indications that he might be aware of his surroundings. No two-way communication was possible. However, whenever the writer was in the room he repeated over and over into the patient's ear such brief statements as, "This is Joel," or "The sun is out." At the same time he would hold and squeeze Keith's hand. The boy responded to medication and this particular crisis ended. Later, Keith was asked what he could remember of the time when he was so sick. He had difficulty in recalling any specific verbal communication but said, "I remember your holding my hand. I could recognize your voice, I couldn't answer you. I could feel your voice. All this made me sure I was still alive." Similar responses were obtained from younger children.

We should not, therefore, interpret the silence and withdrawal of the terminally ill patient as evidence that he was resigned to the inevitable nor that this attitude indicated that he was protecting himself against anxiety by denying reality. We need always to consider the possibility that the withdrawal of those around him offered no other alternative. This compelled the patient to turn inwardly to his own psychological resources, limited though they might be. Thus, it often happens that we have given up on a patient and reacted as if he were already dead when, in fact, he was still very much alive.

The Child's Self-Diagnosis from Minimal Cues

Most staff tenaciously hold on to the belief that hospitalized children have little, if any, awareness of what takes place on a ward and that there is therefore no need to talk with them about such matters. There are staff, on the other side, who talk in the presence of children about their illness as if they were deaf or defective, without troubling to explain the technical jargon often translated into anxious information by the child. In fact, very little escapes the sick (and consequently sensitive) child even in the preschool years. The author frequently observed young patients wandering around the ward in what appeared to be random fashion. He later found, however, that they were doing this largely to keep abreast of what was going on in the other rooms. They would either look directly into the other children's rooms or cast side glances inside while going by. In the large dormitory each child could more easily hear and observe what was going on between the other patients and their physicians. As a matter of fact, the staff and parents used the same procedures, particularly when a child was seriously ill. The direct or side glances into the room as they passed by were very common. Furthermore, it was usual practice for the children to stroll through the ward in the morning to check the name plates on each doorway to see if anybody had died during the night. The children quickly came to know what the presence of certain equipment indicated, and that things were really serious when a patient was moved into a private room or to a special section of the ward where more staff were available.

Such events on the ward aroused much anxiety in the patients who immediately identified with the very sick child. This, however, was intermingled with a certain amount of relief that it was someone else whose condition was worsening and this, in turn, caused them to feel bad and guilty. When these complex and conflicting feelings invaded them, it was especially necessary for them to have the opportunity to talk it all out with a sympathetic and understanding adult. Lacking this, they became prey to disruptive anxieties that seriously interfered with their own adjustment to day-to-day experiences on the ward.

Ross [6] found, in her work with adults, that "all terminally ill patients know the seriousness of their condition." In his work with children, the present author would confirm this observation. The children invariably knew their diagnosis, either because they were among the few who had been so informed by their physician or parents or because they had figured it out on their own. Some were aware that they had a life-threatening illness related to the blood without knowing the particular diagnosis. Regardless of age, they all appeared to realize the fact that they could die from their illness.

The process by which they reached a diagnosis may be highly circuitous but most of them are able to recall the confluence of telltale cues that first led them to identify their illness. Here are a set of typical responses from a child who had been consciously kept in the dark about the diagnosis and prognosis..

"All of a sudden I got my room redecorated, and all new clothes for school. . . . When we came back from the doctor's office, things were all different at home. I started getting lots of things I never could have before. I never could have a big machine gun that shoots BB's, but the next day my father comes home and he has this gun for me. . . .Relatives who never used to visit started coming around and bringing me all kinds of things. . . . Sometimes, when I would walk into the room, my mother and father would stop talking and look at me."

By the time a child has undergone some of the procedures used to diagnose and, later, to treat leukemia, he has already completed most of the puzzle for himself. The shock, guilt, anger, fear, and frustration that overcome the parents are transmitted to the child in various ways. He clearly understands that their distress is related to his own situation, and on this basis alone, he is able to conclude that he is in serious trouble. This is when he most needs to have the question discussed with him openly and honestly.

The following are excerpts from interviews indicating what the children had been told about their illness, how much they figured out for themselves, and the feelings that accompanied all this:

A boy aged nine: "Even before I was told that I had leukemia, I figured that was what I had." When asked to explain this statement, he went on to say that he knew that he had a problem with his blood, and then, "One day I was watching TV and saw this thing about leukemia—it's serious—kids die from it—and this was when I figured that I had leukemia.". . .*A girl, aged 12:* "I think I kinda knew. The doctor at home said that I had a blood problem. What kind of blood problem can you have?" She followed this by stating, "Leukemia. I had that kind of feeling. Until the doctor here talked to me it meant that I had to be worried a little longer. I think it is rotten that anybody should keep it from you. My doctor at home didn't want my mother to tell me. I think she would have told me if he had said it was O. K. The doctor told me that I was going on a trip to Maryland, and when I asked why, he said that I had a blood disease. He still didn't say what it was but only that they would know more about it down here. My mother and father started crying, and my father patted me on the head. After the doctor at home told me that I had a blood disease, I already figured that it was leukemia." . . . *A boy, aged eight:* "A boy in the 4th grade at my school died last year, and he had leukemia. When my parents told me that I had some blood problem, I thought of that boy." . . . *A boy, aged 14:* "I was told that I had anemia. Hell, I know some people who have anemia and they aren't in the hospital. I knew that it must be something real serious as soon as I was told that I would have to go into the hospital." . . . *A girl, aged 16:* "I knew that something was up when nobody at home would tell me what was wrong with me and also I thought that it might be leukemia when they had to send me way out here. I had some idea from watching Dr. Kildare—there was a program about leukemia where a patient was getting steroids and since I'm also getting steroids I though that this was what I might have." Laughing, she said, "I doubted the stuff on such programs as really being real, but this one surely seemed to fit me!"

The following answer, on the other hand, is a typical reply from children whose parents and physicians were among the minority not involved in "the conspiracy of silence."

A girl, aged 11, explained, "I knew that something was up after the first few visits to the doctor. My parents talked it over and decided not to say anything to me until they were sure, and when they found out for sure, my mother told me. I know that there is no cure for leukemia, but I feel better knowing what I have." She later explained, "I still have a lot to worry about, but I was even more worried before because I was thinking a mile a minute about what I had."

The child, who is informed by his physician or parents that he has leukemia, often has this act drastically negated by the attempts of other adults to lessen the impact of the news on him. The following are excerpts from interviews on this point:

"My doctor told me that I have a slight case of leukemia." . . . "My doctor told me that it wasn't too bad because they caught it in time". . ."Why is it that my doctor told me that I have the easiest kind to treat? Why do they call it the easiest kind if there is no cure?''

Reaction to Overconcern and Indulgence

Not only does the leukemic child have to deal with the greatly altered behavior patterns within his family, but his difficulties are compounded by the actions and attitudes of all the "do-gooders' and "avoiders" in his life sphere. In many interviews, the children referred to their wish to be dealt with like normal people and not to be given the overindulgent, "Christmas in July" treatment. The following are some excerpts from interviews relating to this:

"There is this lady on the block who always hated me. I used to run on her lawn, climb her trees, and once I broke her window. She would chase me off. She would always holler at me. When I got older and had a car, I used to park it in front of her house which she didn't like, and she used to yell at me for that. Now that she found out I have leukemia, she is very nice to me and even sent me a card and doesn't say anything when I park my car in front of her house. I wish she would be her rotten old self. A guilty conscience—that's what it is. . . . My math teacher in school knew that I had leukemia. He made me so mad. He knew what I had and it was just pity all over the place and I just couldn't stand it. Really, he gave me grades I didn't deserve, and it wasn't fair, you know. The other kids didn't all know, and they knew that Mr. S., you know, was giving me the benefit all the time and they didn't like it." . . .
" . . . but I would want to be treated a little differently." When asked about this the boy explained, "I would like to have extra attention and privileges, but not too much". . . "We should be treated like everybody else. We shouldn't get anything extra just because we have leukemia."

Helen (aged 12), Ned (aged 21), and the author were on the way back to the hospital after a trip to the airport to see Carmen off for home. At one point during the conversation the author wondered aloud about how they handled the situation when their friends asked them about what they had? Ned jokingly replied," I have leukemia. Feel sorry for me." He acted this out and went on to say that his friends probably knew but hadn't asked him yet. Helen wondered whether her friends at school knew she had leukemia. She said, "I'm sure that the teachers know. They try to be so nice to me, and this makes me upset." Both felt that they wanted to be treated as they were before they became ill. "Mostly they don't let you live your life as usual. It's "don't do this" and "don't do that" continued Helen. Ned went on to say that at least he was old enough to say to his parents, "Yeah, yeah," and then go ahead and do what he felt was right. He was indignant that people didn't think that he could handle himself within the limitations imposed by his disease. He guessed that Helen, being younger, couldn't get away with using this approach. She agreed. The author expressed the opinion that parents very often don't give youngsters enough credit for being able to do things right. Helen immediately exclaimed, "Joel, you said it just right!" She went on to describe how her mother did all kinds of things to get her to eat, like heaping her breakfast plate with two eggs when she wanted only one, and so forth.

"When I play baseball my friends say that they will run for me, but I tell them that I will run for myself." . . . "I don't like it at all. My mother gives me everything, even things I don't want. I don't mind being spoiled once in a while, but all the time, WHEW!!!"

The children made it clear that they generally equate the degree of overindulgence and overprotection shown them with the degree of discomfort people feel in relating to them because they have a fatal disease. It is crucial for us to realize that such behavior on our part makes it more difficult than ever for the child to attempt to refocus, as effectively as possible, his own emotional energies toward a reasonable day-to-day adjustment to the stresses of his situation.

Reaction to Death and Dying

A girl, aged nine, saw the author enter the ward one morning and as he approached her, she came close to him and in a low tone of voice said, "I want to tell you something." From her manner, he realized that she was upset and as they walked along together, he put his arm on her shoulder. She immediately said, in a quavering voice, "Nancy (her roommate) died last night." She followed this by saying, "I'm very scared about this." The author stayed with her and talked about her fear of getting that sick and dying. . . A boy, aged 19 was in bed when the author entered his room. He was breathing very hard and several times closed his eyes as if to get a few moments of sleep. The author asked if he was having trouble sleeping at night, and he admitted that he was. He said, "I want to get out of here." The author indicated that his doctor was doing everything possible to get him back home. He pointed out that he had already been hospitalized and sent home in remission several times and then brought up his concern about how many remissions were possible. The author indicated that this was one of the many things that all patients worried about and then returned to the difficulty in getting to sleep at night. The boy said, "I think a lot about the other kids, like Terry" (a boy who had recently died). He went on to add, with much feeling, "Nobody wants to know that they are going to die. Nobody wants to know that it is the end. . ."

Some of the most challenging questions the writer was asked by the children related to the actual process of dying; how this felt, if there was a lot of pain associated with it, and what happened after one died. These questions inevitably led to a discussion of the patient's own ideas on these matters, some of which are reported below:

A boy, aged nine: "One of the things that worries me most about being dead is that I don't know when it will happen."

When the writer asked *a boy, aged nine,* what worried him most about dying, he replied, after thinking for a few seconds, "I guess the fact that I wouldn't see my friends anymore." He then added, "I would be missed."

A boy, aged 12, said, "I wouldn't like to all of a sudden stop breathing." He went on: "I'm worried about the fact that there is no coming back, once I'm dead. Whatever happens, it would mean that I would be dead for millions of years."

A girl, aged 11: "When I'm dead my parents will miss me and so will my dog."

A girl, aged 20: "If I wasn't here, I probably would be floating around up there oblivious of everything."

A girl, aged eight: "The thing that worries me most about being dead is that I would not be here anymore. I would miss my mother and family. When somebody dies, they aren't around anymore." When the writer asked what she thought happened to people when they died, she said, "They get buried and they rot."

On the whole, the children seemed to be particularly worried because they had no control over the time at which death would take place, because they could die suddenly, because they would no longer be on this earth in their customary surroundings, and because death would be accompanied by much pain. The outstanding fear concerned the unknown hereafter verbalized dramatically by a ten-year-old boy who said, "I don't know anything about that up there (pointing upwards) but I do know a lot about here (pointing to the floor) and so I don't want to die."

Conclusions

When lecturing on the subject of communication with the fatally ill child, the author has often found great resistance to the idea that this communication should be completely unrestricted. Even those who find this approach reasonable for older children regard it as unacceptable for younger ones.

They generally attempt to explain the resistance on the grounds that there are many devastating experiences in life that should be kept from immature and therefore vulnerable individuals, and they will cite many instances when society at large sets limits to what might be properly communicated or shown to children.

The author has never recommended or even suggested that a child be told he is going to die. Such an interpretation is usually made by the adult who needs to protect himself from discussing, meaningfully, the subject of death and dying with the child. Certainly one would not emphasize to a patient the fact that he is going to die or that he will probably die soon, but at the same time, one can be fairly certain that the fatally ill child has, on his own, become only too well aware of such a possibility. The reason for noncommunication seems to have little, indeed, to do with the needs and desires of the child but with the fears and frustrations of the adult. The child with a serious illness, at any stage and in any setting, must constantly be offered the opportunity to talk about anything and everything that will benefit him no matter how difficult this might be for the adult.

There is no better way to make the point of this paper than to quote a paragraph from the work of Raimbault and Royer [4], which, while referring specifically to the pediatrician, applies equally well to parents and hospital staff and, in fact, to everyone who comes into contact with a fatally ill child:

> Even when the pediatrician is deprived of his medical treatment, he can nevertheless bring the child support by following advice given by the children themselves, keeping up the relationship, and listening and responding to questions about life and death. On the other hand, to break off the contacts, to stop interchanges, would leave the child with his anguish in a premature solitude that prefigures death.

Bibliography

1. Smith, Clement, Help for the hopeless, *Rhode Island Med. J.*, 39 (1956), 491–9.
2. Redl, Fritz, The life space interview workshop, 1957, 1. Strategy and techniques of the life space interview, *Amer. J. Orthopsychiat.*, 29 (1959), 1–18.
3. Raimbault, G. and Royer, P., L'enfant et son image de la maladie, *Arch. Fran. Pediat.*, 24 (1967), 445–462.
4. Raimbault, G. and Royer, P., Thematique de la mort chez l'enfant attient de maladie chronique, *Arch. Fran. Pediat.*, 26 (1969), 1041–1053.
5. Kubler-Ross, Elisabeth, *On Death and Dying*, Macmillan, New York (1969), 260.
6. Kubler-Ross, Elisabeth, The dying patient's point of view, in *The Dying Patient*, Orville Brim, et al., Eds., Russel Sage Foundation, New York (1970), 156–70.

The Fear of Death in Fatally Ill Children and Their Parents

Joseph M. Natterson, M.D. (U.S.A.)

This chapter will include the following: a detailed review of work on the psychological reactions of fatally ill children and their mothers published by Alfred G. Knudson, Jr. and the author in 1960 [1, 2]; a critique of the 1960 conclusions; and some additional ideas regarding the death problem and the clinician.

Review of Previous Work by Knudson and Natterson

We noted the crude animism of early man and the closely reasoned theological approaches to the death issue of more recent and current history, and we stated that these essentially reflected efforts to relieve man's fear of dying by assuming man's immortality. Modern psychological ideas, eschewing the immortality concept, cast some light on the evolutionary significance of death anxiety. For example, Freud [3] suggested that the fundaments of social collaboration among men were created by prehistoric rivals who agreed to put aside their homicidal rivalry (after killing their leader) on the basis of fear of death by the others. Also, Freud [4] believed that repression of the death instinct is a crucial factor in the structure and function of modern society. We also noted clinical studies by Freud [5], Lindemann [6] and others concerning the effects of death upon the intimately involved survivors. We also gleaned from the literature that important, but unclear, connections obviously exist among separation anxiety, castration anxiety, and death anxiety. We intended to provide basic clinical information about the impact of fatal illness on the children themselves, their mothers, and the clinically involved persons, and we attempted to add some knowledge to the general issue of death in relation to mankind.

Thirty-three children were studied at the City of Hope Medical Center over a 26-month period. They ranged in age from infants to 13 year olds. There were 19 boys and 14 girls. They were a typical group, as regards ethnic background, religious affiliation, intelligence, and behavioral adaptation. The diagnoses were leukemia, cancer, and blood disease—all fatal. In addition to the distress caused by the disease, all the children were exposed to three environmental stresses: separation from mother, traumatic procedures, and the deaths of other children. It was observed that reactions to separation from mother were most severe in the age group of infant to five-year-old; the reactions to traumatic procedures were greatest in the age group five to ten years; and reactions to death were most intense in the age group ten years and older. We felt that these findings were in concordance with the generally accepted view that separation anxiety is the key problem of pre-oedipal years and that castration anxiety dominates in the oedipal and latency periods, and we concluded that existential or death anxiety becomes a prominent problem only for the children in the oldest age group.

The 33 mothers in the study ranged in age from 24 to 45 years. Involvement of the mothers in the parent participation program provided opportunities for significant observations and judgments to be made by nurses, social workers, teachers, occupational therapists, and physicians.

The following conclusions were reached about the mothers. When a child survived more than four months from the time of fatal prognosis, the mother showed a triphasic response—initial, intermediate, and terminal. In the initial phase denial and guilt were predominant, and unrealistic hopes and blames were frequent. In the intermediate phase reality testing improved, and the mothers tended to direct their interest toward realistic measures that gave hope of saving their child. In the terminal phase the mothers' energies moved away from their respective children, and there was acceptance of the child's death. It seemed obvious to us that the initial phase was the most regressed and dangerous period; it was the period when psychosis was suspected in a few mothers. Ego regression was associated with intensification of the mother's identification with the child, and psychologically primitive defenses were impressively evident. After experiencing the initial traumatically induced regression, the mothers moved into the second phase, concentrating on the realistically available resources to possibly prolong or preserve their children's lives, abandoning the sometimes wildly unrealistic fantasies or actions of the initial phase. We inferred that the mothers were now beginning to decathect their children, that anticipatory mourning, as described by Richmond and Waisman [7], had begun. The final phase was rarely observed unless the mother had at least four months in which to do her grief work, to achieve emotional separation from the child before his death. We noted greatest ego strength and maturity in this third phase at which time the mothers became relatively accepting of impending death and could openly express wishes for the death of the child—suggesting that separation from the child, through death, was no longer an adaptive problem for the mothers.

In general, the findings reported above have weathered a decade well. However, three issues do merit further elaboration.

First is the matter of whether and how the children were informed about death. We stated in 1960, "When a child died in the hospital, most of the other children knew only that the child was no longer there. Minimal explanation for such absence was offered, this usually being a statement that the child had gone home. In some instances this explanation did not entirely suffice, either because the questioning child had fairly direct evidence to the contrary or because he was unusually suspicious. The death was not denied in such instances. Interestingly, however, children who probably knew about the deaths of other children seldom asked questions of the staff [2]." There has been justified criticism of our conclusion that children under nine or ten years of age are not significantly troubled by the death issue and of our avoidance of discussing death with the children. Waechter [8], for example, in a recent study, found evidence that death anxiety is intense in younger children. There seems to be no valid basis for any categorical recommendation that children in a particular age group should or should not be talked with about the fatal nature of their illnesses. Rather, each child should be handled as an individual whose emotional conflicts and needs will shift and change in the course of the disease. This would optimally require that, as part of the total management, effort should be made to help the child establish a relationship with a clinician who is equipped to recognize, elicit, and respond therapeutically to the psychological problems and preoccupations of the child throughout his illness. A child psychiatrist with experience in the area of catastrophic illness would be ideal for this role.

A second point requiring amplification concerns the variety of expectable reactions in the parents of fatally ill children. Chodoff et al. [9] found in their group of parents that isolation of affect, denial, and motor activity were the most common defenses. The isolation of affect has a diurnal pattern, becoming less intense at night. They noted that these defenses diminished as the period of illness grew longer thus enabling the parents to achieve less defensive modes of coping with the problem.

Third is the question of the degree of grief work accomplished by even those mothers whose children remained alive four or more months after the mothers were informed of the prognosis. The findings of Chodoff et al. [9] in this regard are in conformity with ours. However, my subsequent clinical experience definitely indicates that grief work is far from complete at this time and that significant depression usually exists for a much longer period. Women who suffer the loss of a young child need psychotherapy, even if the illness lasts more than four months. My psychoanalytic observations indicate that for months, even years, after the child's death, the mother continues depressed, as evident in symptoms, dreams, and fantasies. Gradually, the traumatic loss becomes less like a foreign body and is, in a sense, absorbed into the ego, becoming like other momentous memories, albeit a particularly painful one, slowly receding in intensity. This process requires a very extended period of time, even with intensive analytic therapy. On the other hand, if the mother does have the opportunity to do some grief work while the child is still alive, the emotional havoc wreaked upon her and the family by the catastrophe may be much reduced.

The Death Problem and the Clinician

Many psychiatrists are phobic about working with fatally ill patients and their families. Thereby they neglect an important area of clinical need, and they lose for themselves an opportunity for further conflict resolution and enhancement of their own ego identity.

Kübler-Ross [10] indicates that the psychotherapist can resolve the death problem with the fatally ill patient and engender a genuine acceptance of death in him. Her psychotherapeutic accomplishments are impressive, but she errs in her conclusions. The psychotherapist trades in life, not death. He teaches the patient to live more fully and creatively. He attempts to reduce those ego defenses which impair creative living, and he attempts to help rebuild those defenses essential to effective living. This applies to the victims of fatal illness and their families just as it applies to those for whom death is not an immediate problem. Perhaps it can be said that the psychiatrist working with fatally ill patients and their intimates is not helping them accept death but groping with them to find a way to live with meaning in the shadow of death.

Bibliography

1. Knudson, A. G., Jr., and Natterson, J. M., Participation of parents in the hospital care of fatally ill children, *Pediatrics*, 26 (1960), 482–490.
2. Natterson, J. M. and Knudson, A. G., Jr., Observations concerning fear of death in fatally ill children and their mothers, *Psychosomatic Medicine*, 22 (1960), 456–465.
3. Freud, Sigmund, Totem and Taboo (1912–1913), in Strachey, J., Ed., *The Complete Psychological Works of Sigmund Freud*, Vol. 13, Hogarth Press, London, 1955.
4. Freud, Sigmund, *Civilization and Its Discontents*, (1930), Hogarth Press, London, 1949.
5. Freud, Sigmund, Mourning and Melancholia (1917), in *Collected Papers*, Vol. 4, Hogarth Press, London, 1950.
6. Lindemann, E., Symptomatology and management of acute grief, *Am. J. Psychiat.*, 101 (1944), 141–149.
7. Richmond, J. B., and Waisman, H. A., Psychological aspects of management of children with malignant diseases, *A. M. A. Am. J. Dis. Child*, 89 (1955), 42–47.
8. Waechter, E. H., Children's awareness of fatal illness, *Am. J. Nursing*, 71 (1971), 1168–1172.
9. Chodoff, P., Friedman, S. B., and Hamburg, D. A., Stress, defenses and coping behavior: observations in parents of children with malignant disease, *Am. J. Psychiat.*, 120 (1964), 743–749.
10. Kübler-Ross, Elisabeth, *On Death and Dying*, The Macmillan Company, New York, 1969.

Crisis and Adaptation in the Families of Fatally Ill Children

**Edward H. Futterman, M.D. and
Irwin Hoffman (U.S.A.)**

Coping with the fatal illness of a child has been considered one of the most poignant and stressful events encountered by families in our society [1]. The crisis [2] precipitated by such an unexpected and harsh threat profoundly affects the immediate and long-range adaptation of family members. Family equilibrium is endangered. Coping strategies and adaptive mechanisms which were useful in dealing with previous developmental and adaptive tasks are challenged, and resources are tapped that may not have been formerly apparent.

In order to better understand the nature of the crisis confronting parents and the process of their adaptation over time, we extensively interviewed parents of leukemic children and maintained ongoing informal contact with them and with families of children suffering from other malignancies. In observing parental adaptation during the child's illness and after his death, we have identified some of the major adaptive dilemmas, tasks, and processes that are highlighted by this particular crisis. We have attempted to develop a language which emphasizes the coping rather than the defensive aspects of adaptation [3]. This paper includes a review of our approach to adaptation and of our earlier work describing the task of parental anticipatory mourning [4]. In addition, we will outline the adaptive processes involved in another major task confronting each parent, that of "maintaining confidence" despite the threat which the situation poses to his sense of mastery, worth, and trust.

Sample and Method

During the past six years, extensive open-ended interviews with 23 sets of parents of leukemic children were recorded at various points during the course of the child's illness and after his death. Of a total of 45 interviews, 13 were conducted after the death of the child and 8 were obtained while the child was in medical relapse. Informal contact with these families and with more than 100 additional families with children suffering from other malignancies contributed to the empirical base of the study. This report is based on clinical evaluation of the data obtained from the interviews as well as from observations in the waiting room of the Tumor Clinic, in the hospital during periods of the child's confinement, in the Clinic examining rooms, and in a preventive group therapy program for parents which has been developed in the past two years.

Most of the families in our sample were middle- or lower-middle-class, Catholic, suburban residents of Illinois. Parents ranged in age from their early twenties to their late fifties. In general, systematic effects of socioeconomic variables on the course of adaptation, although not detected, could not be reliably assessed due to the small size and relative homogeneity of the sample.

The Nature of the Crisis

Klein and Lindemann [2] define an *emotionally hazardous situation* as "any sudden alteration in the field of social forces within which the individual exists, such that the individual's expectations of himself and his relationships with others undergo change," The first major category of hazards described is "a loss or threatened loss of a significant relationship." The authors state that the term *crisis* is "reserved for the acute and often prolonged disturbance that may occur in an individual or social orbit as the result of an emotional hazard."

The fatal illness of a child leads to an emotional crisis for parents characterized by marked internal turmoil, temporary interpersonal disequilibrium, and the triggering of coping as well as defensive measures to deal with the danger. When the illness is leukemia, the duration of the crisis may be prolonged and the intensity of the threat varies over time in relation to the course of the disease. With advances in medical treatment, the average life expectancy of the leukemic child has been extended beyond two years and there are growing numbers of children with long-term survivals. Extended symptom-free periods of remission are quite common although episodic relapses and ultimate fatality are still the norm. At the time of this study, the prospects of anything but a fatal prognosis were negligible and the parents were so informed by their physician.

Erikson [5] uses the term "accidental crisis" to differentiate crises arising from environmental resources from those more closely related to development. We prefer the term "situational" to avoid the connotations of spuriousness, infrequency, and lack of universality implied by "accidental." Although the crisis of leukemia is situational, it also resonates with developmental issues. For example, in an earlier paper [6], we dealt with a case of interaction between the situational crisis engendered by the fatal illness and unresolved issues from the separation-individuation phase of development.

Binger et al. report that, in 11 of 20 families of children with leukemia, "one or more members had emotional disturbances that were severe enough to interfere with adequate functioning and required psychiatric help. None had required such help before. . . In other families milder disturbances occurred in both the adults and the children." [7, p. (417)]. On the other hand, along with other authors [8, 9], we have observed few instances of severe psychopathology, severe maladaptive behavior, prolonged turmoil, or permanent family disruption [4]. Discrepancies among findings may be due to differences in the nature of the samples, in the medical and psychosocial care provided, or in definitions of disturbances. The possibility that such a crisis might lead to emotional growth, family cohesiveness, positive redefinition of values, and potential immunization against other threats has been minimally explored [4, 9 (p. 461)].

The Process of Adaptation

Much attention has been paid to the reactive and defensive aspects of adaptation to stress. Hamburg and Adams speculate, "Is it possible that such mechanisms represent only one important class of responses to threatening elements of experience? Or are there other major ways in which the human organism copes with stressful experience?" [10 (p. 277)]. We have been interested in viewing the synthetic and coping aspects of adaptation as well as its reactive and defensive aspects. In addition, we have found Sabshin's emphasis on the temporal context of adaptation useful [11]. Through observing parental responses to the crisis over time, we have been able to characterize their adaptation from a process point of view.

From our observations, we have formulated a number of dilemmas confronting parents in their adaptation to the fatal illness of their child. For each adaptive dilemma, parents need to work out a balance between apparently conflicting adaptive tasks; for example, between acknowledging the ultimate loss of the child and maintaining hope; between attending to immediate needs and plans for the future; between cherishing the child and allowing him to separate; between maintaining day-to-day functioning and expressing disturbing feelings; between active personal care of the child and delegation of care to medical personnel; between trusting the physician and recognizing his limitations; between caring for the child and preparing for his death through gradual emotional detachment.

In this chapter, we will summarize our previous work in describing the adaptive processes involved in the task of parental anticipatory mourning and then discuss the parents' task of maintaining confidence in the face of a profound threat to their sense of trust, worth, and mastery.

Parental Anticipatory Mourning

We have defined anticipatory mourning as "a set of processes that are directly related to the awareness of the impending loss, to its emotional impact and to the adaptive mechanisms whereby emotional attachment to the dying child is relinquished over time" [4]. We were able to identify a series of interwoven and interdependent processes emerging and reaching prominence at different points in time.

Acknowledgment. This entails the progressive realization by the parents that the child's death is inevitable. It involves the continual struggle between hope and despair with progressive deepening of parental awareness and narrowing of hope. Despite parental wishes and defenses as well as fluctuations in the course of the child's illness, parental awareness intensifies as the time of death nears.

Grieving. This includes the experience and expression of the emotional impact of the expected loss along with the physical, psychological, and interpersonal turmoil associated with it. Initial undifferentiated reactions gradually give way to more stable and controlled patterns. Active regulation of grieving occurs so that the process can be delayed, limited, channeled into particular relationships or concealed. Grieving fluctuates with life contingencies and with the course of the illness but gradually mellows in quality and diminishes in intensity.

Reconciliation. This refers to the process of developing a perspective about the child's anticipated death which preserves the parents' sense of confidence in the worth of the child's life and of life in general. Among the adaptive responses included in reconciliation are redefining the implications of the child's death, seeking consolation from the past or present life of the child, and counting blessings.

Detachment. This denotes the process by which parents withdraw emotional investment from the child as a growing being with a real future. The process often involves intermittent clinging as well as distancing and redirection of energies toward other relationships which will continue after the child dies. The timing of detachment is related to the parents' evolving concepts of the child's life expectancy.

Memorialization. This is the process whereby parents develop a relatively fixed mental representation of the dying child which will endure beyond his death. This process includes progressive abstraction by which parents increasingly think of the child in global terms rather than in relation to specific behaviors and progressive idealization (eulogization). Idealization sometimes takes the extreme form of enshrinement whereby the child is conceived of as possessing other-worldly characteristics.

The course of anticipatory mourning was adaptive in the overwhelming majority of parents in our study. In general, the evolving processes of anticipatory mourning were integrated with each other and with other adaptive tasks and served to prepare parents for the tasks of post-bereavement mourning.

Maintenance of Confidence

Maintenance of confidence is defined as the set of processes which facilitates parents' sense of worth, trust, and mastery in the face of potential guilt, rage, and helplessness. We are extending the concept of confidence as elaborated by Benedek [12]. Confidence is manifest throughout the life cycle in the quality of a person's sense of trust in himself, in other persons, and in his surroundings. The threat of a child's death confronts parents with the reality that their control over their own and their family's destiny is limited, and that even the physician may be ultimately unsuccessful in thwarting the relentless course of the disease. Nevertheless, most parents adapt to the child's illness and death with their sense of confidence essentially maintained and, in some instances, enhanced.

Like anticipatory mourning, maintenance of confidence involves a series of processes which evolve and interact throughout the course of the illness and after the death of the child. They are listed below in the order in which they seem to reach prominence.

1. Mastery operations
   a. Search
   b. Participation in care
2. Maintenance of equilibrium
3. Affirmation of Life
4. Reorganization

Mastery Operations

The onset of leukemia in a child represents an assault on a parent's sense of adequacy as guardian of his child and, more generally, as a person with a meaningful control over his own and his family's destinies. In response to this threat, most parents do everything possible to master the disease. During the child's illness, mastery operations are buttressed by hope for prolongation of life and for total cure. After his death, activities may broaden to encompass afflictions in others within and beyond the family. Included in mastery operations are the search for knowledge and resources, and participation in the medical care of the child.

SEARCH

Searching activity encompasses parents' efforts to obtain information about everything pertaining to the child's illness and its ramifications. Parents often begin to develop a cognitive appraisal of the burgeoning threat prior to the physician's pronouncement of the diagnosis. Whether in the form of questioning, seeking information, self-examination or , shopping for other resources, search helps parents to reduce their anxiety about the unknown.

Parents use intellectual mastery to gain some sense of control as though knowledge were actually power. Several authors [10, 13, 14] have emphasized the importance of information-seeking in the process of coping in general. In particular, most authors working with fatally ill children and their families [8, 9, 15, 16] describe intensive questioning of medical personnel and exhaustive reading about leukemia as typical of most parents. In our experience, information provided comfort if it made the course of events more predictable, even at the expense of hope, whereas good news could be upsetting if it undermined expectations arrived at through prior search. For instance, one father stated that he had "built up through reading, hope and an approximate idea as to what would happen". When the doctor told him that the luekemia was of a chronic type (with, in fact, a better prognosis) he "felt like the bottom was out again" because his knowledge was no longer relevant. By means of intellectual mastery, most parents prepared themselves and their families for the future, thus restoring a sense of control over their lives. Nevertheless, some parents insisted that they wanted to know as little as possible. One mother said she preferred "the element of surprise" and another stated, "there is no use studying about it and worrying yourself about it." Even these parents, however, complained at times of not being told enough about their children's condition and medical care.

Search operations can also be used in an attempt to cognitively reverse the diagnosis and prognosis or, as Bozeman et al, put it, to "find loopholes" [15]. Every magazine article, every television announcement of a new treatment, every long-term survival becomes a potential "escape clause" fostering hope. Parents looked for mistakes in the diagnosis and suggested other possibilities such as anemia. Expecially if the child had a prolonged first remission, parents and sometimes ever medical personnel began to question the original diagnosis. "I can't believe she has it. Maybe she had it but not any more. Doesn't the length of her remission surprise you?" one mother inquired adding later, "Could it be that a child's blood changes?" Another family took their child to a famous malignant disease center after a first remission of a year. They were convinced that the diagnosis must have been wrong in the light of their own timetable which predicted that a first remission should not last beyond nine months.

Locating and testing potential resources is another objective of search activity. Parents searched diligently for the best care. They looked over different hospitals, different therapies, and different doctors. Nevertheless, while they might have wished to discredit the physician as a diagnostician, they also needed to trust him as a healer. Therefore, many of their excursions and questions served more to check his competence and to seek reassurance in their choice than to transfer to another source of medical treatment.

Exoneration is another function served by search. Most parents question themselves and raise the possibility of their own responsibility for the illness [8, 9]. Some find solace in religion but several authors [7, 15, 16] report that religious outlets do not play a major adaptive role for most families faced with a dying child. In our sample, parents did seem to be reassured when told that they were not to blame for the illness or its prognosis. Mothers and fathers wanted to know whether the child's illness was caused by radiation from the television set, by tonsil surgery, by poor hygiene, by maternal irradiation during pregnancy, by contagion, and by other factors. They also examined their own responses to the illness to see whether they behaved appropriately, promptly, and effectively. Information about an impersonal etiology helped parents absolve themselves from personal responsibility or guilt. By leaving no possibility unexplored, by leaving no question unanswered, by leaving no stone unturned, parents bolstered their sense of mastery.

After the death of the child, search continued through information gathering about the autopsy findings, about details of the child's illness, about the competence of the medical care and about the state of knowledge in leukemia research. Such operations assured parents that they acted rationally and in the best interests of their child.

PARTICIPATION IN CARE

In the face of impending death, efforts at mastery are vividly manifest in thoughts and action which are life-oriented. The need of parents to participate in the physical and emotional care of their sick children has been recognized by several authors who have encouraged such involvement [8, 9, 16, 17]. Hamovitch found parent participation to be helpful to more than two-thirds of the families he studied [16]. Immediately after diagnosis and at times of relapse or complications, parents in our sample often became very active and invested in the medical care of the child. They involved themselves in helping with procedures, feeding, and the like, sometimes to the point of being seen as interfering and controlling by hospital staff. "Doing everything possible," with approval from medical personnel, allowed parents to feel less helpless and contributed greatly to their sense of continued importance in the well-being of their child. As one mother stated, "When I was giving him medication daily, I felt more useful than when the dose was cut down." Another mother reported being reassured after the death of her child by her own mother's reminder that "Jackie always got his medicine and always got to the doctor when he was sick." Rage against death and helplessness often accompanied and fostered parental involvement in care. One mother exclaimed furiously, "Look! Don't tell me that there is no cure or that there is no hope, because you are not God. You are only a doctor."

As the course of the illness progressed and as hope waned, parental efforts often became less spirited. However, we have observed instances in the terminal phase of last ditch efforts to save the child and of a resurgence of the need to exercise control over the child's medical care. This revival of mastery activity, in a few cases, took an extreme form such as sudden withdrawal of the child from treatment, refusal to allow particular medications to be given, usurping of nursing responsibilities or general rebellion against hospital staff. Such desperate maneuvers to overcome feelings of helplessness, lack of control, guilt, and rage seemed to occur in parents whose confidence was not well-maintained throughout the course of the illness, who also did not show much evidence of anticipatory mourning and whose post-bereavement adaptation was tumultuous. Our observations are consistent with Hamovitch's finding that parent participation that was either very high or very low was correlated with greater adaptive difficulties than was moderate participation [16].

It may be difficult to separate the magical aspects of some caregiving activities with realistic efforts. Parental renunciation of pleasures as sacrifices designed to save the child, while guilt reducing, can clearly be seen as magical in nature. Close and careful observation of the child, however, may have magical overtones but may also serve medically realistic purposes. For instance, a mother stated, "I don't worry about her in school, but I check her every minute when she is outside and never allow her off the block." Such behavior combines partially functional vigilance with an overreaction to separation anxiety. Surveillance is one of the few active caretaking responsibilities afforded parents of a leukemic child and helps him maintain his self-image as a good parent.

Most parents strive to prolong life until the last moment. On the other hand, the parents' longing to be relieved of their burdens and their wish to see the child spared from further suffering make caring for him particularly conflict-ridden toward the end. When asked how she felt when her child cried in pain, one mother admitted, "I just would like to take a shotgun and get it over with."

Extension of caretaking activities after the death of the child is expressed in parents' involvement in funeral preparations and in their concern about proper interment.

Maintenance of Equilibrium

While crisis generates change, it also stimulates development of strategies for maintaining emotional and interpersonal equilibrium. Maintenance includes adherence to familiar routines, continuation of usual patterns of family interactions, and reaching out for emotional supports. All the parents we interviewed worked hard to maintain familiar ways of doing things, especially in essential areas such as work, care of family members, and meeting of basic needs. Other authors have touched upon this aspect of adaptation primarily in describing parental efforts to control their temptation to overindulge and overprotect the sick child [8,9,15,17,18]. In regard to school attendance, we have reported, "children do attend school during remission without excessive difficulties; they may stay home for a few days a week when they have physical symptoms or are found to be in relapse; rarely do they become school phobic" [6 (p.492)]. In other areas as well, parents largely succeeded in preserving the customary pattern of family life.

Stabilizing efforts reached prominence after the initial impact of the illness had subsided and during periods of remission. Relapses, especially when they required hospitalization, tended to tax the ability of parents to maintain equilibrium. Even during prolonged remissions, return to normalcy was never complete. Parents reported changes in their work habits, social lives, friendship patterns, sexual activities, relationships within the family, and expression of feelings. For instance, a couple who insisted that they were simply "making the best of what we've got," "carrying on," and "still able to enjoy ourselves," reported incidents which indicated that new roles and responsibilities had been assigned to their children. The children, in turn, described changes in their parents' moods and sociability. These parents also discussed a common dilemma in wanting to keep things going as before while "feeling guilty that we're hardhearted" in being able to maintain stability. However, this ability to keep things going on an even keel was a source of pride for many parents which bolstered their sense of mastery and self-esteem.

Another maintenance operation involves regulating expression of feelings. By this we are referring not to the use of unconscious defenses such as denial, isolation, and intellectualization as described by other authors [8, 17], but to conscious regulatory operations whereby parents choose their behaviors in accord with appraisal of the life situation confronting them. An example of such regulation, which we have discussed in relation to anticipatory mourning [4], is the timing of parental grieving whereby mothers and fathers actively inhibit, channel, and delay their grieving behavior in coordination with other adaptive tasks. We found that feelings, in general, were monitored, regulated, and modified by parents in the service of maintaining equilibrium. Erecting a facade of calm acceptance was used for concealing anguish, protecting others, protecting themselves, and preserving functioning. Parents usually avoided crying in front of the children, minimized displaying anxiety in the presence of neighbors and relatives, shielded the physician from their rage, and underplayed their fears and doubts before each other.

Reliability of social supports is important to families in maintaining their equilibrium and in the overall task of maintaining confidence. Bozeman et al. describe the need for "tangible services, temporary escape...and emotional support" [15]. Parents report being unable to satisfy these needs through reliance upon their own parents [8, 15], religious affiliations [7, 8, 16], or friendships [8, 15]. In our experience, parents often found that family members and helping professionals such as ministers, nurses, and mental health workers were more likely to advocate either unrelenting cheerful hope for survival or resigned acceptance of the child's anticipated death than to recognize the legitimacy of the parents' rage and grief and to foster expression of these feelings. The child's physician, on the other hand, often served as a major source of support [8, 9, 16, 17]. He is the agent to whom they delegated care of the child. They upheld an image of him as competent and caring. They trusted him, sought his advice and approval, and, ordinarily, found few other persons with whom they felt free to express their anxieties and concerns.* As one mother said, "he treats not only the patient but he takes in the family." His activities support their feelings of mastery. His reliability supports their sense of trust.

Parents frequently insisted that they unswervingly trusted the physician without reservations. As one mother stated, "He is the doctor. If I can't trust him, who am I going to trust?" Although the physician's ultimate helplessness matched their own, parents usually spared the physician from their rage and desperation. Such feelings were sometimes displaced onto others, especially members of the medical team. For instance, one mother spoke glowingly about her child's doctor but complained bitterly about an intern who asked her in the child's presence, "Does anyone else in your family have leukemia?" Even a father who became exceptionally bitter after the death of his son complaining of "neglect, incompetence, and misdiagnosis" verbally attacked everybody who had anything to do with the care of the child except the primary physician.

---

*At the University of Illinois Hospital, this has changed with the introduction by mental health workers of a parental group counseling program and waiting room intervention program designed to broaden the range of resources available to families [20].

When the intensity of participation in the child's care decreased, particularly during long remissions, parents redirected their energies toward relationships and interests that may have been interrupted. These activities, while inhibited during relapses and hospitalizations by concern about potential neglect of the sick child, were generally facilitated by the progressive detachment of anticipatory mourning. Parents branched out to new endeavors which provided feedback supporting their sense of confidence in a broader arena than that encompassed in mastery operations related to the child's illness. They talked more about caring for other members of the family, became more involved in community activities, returned to work, and made plans for the future of the family. These activities continued after the death of the child with the recognition that, although a painful loss had occurred, there were still important areas of continuity, stability, and potential growth in the lives of the family members.

Affirmation of Life

The seeming injustice of a child's death threatens parents' characteristic level of optimism about the meaning and value of life. Nevertheless, parents generally reject bitterness, nihilism, and cynicism in favor of continued affirmation of life. This process asserts itself during the child's illness and after his death. It is manifest in the prevalent devotion by parents to making the most of the child's life in the face of full acknowledgment of his fatal prognosis. It was apparent in our sample in the many statements parents made, along with their expressions of grief and anger, about the richness of their lives, about the gratifying nature of their relationships with family and friends, about their fortune in having found good medical care for their child, and about other things for which they felt grateful. Much of their affirmation took the form of counting their blessings whereby they asserted that emotional investment in living was worth the risks despite the loss they were enduring.

Maintaining an orientation to the child as a living and growing person was often difficult for parents to accomplish. Recently, writers have expressed growing concern about dying adult patients with emphasis on the value of maintaining openness of communication channels [21, 22]. Few authors have dealt with this issue in regard to children [23, 24]. In general, parents try to shield the sick child from full awareness of the nature of his illness and the possibility of a fatal outcome [7, 8, 23]. Glaser and Straus have elaborated on the consequences of lack of awareness in dying adults which tend to create a dehumanized, isolated situation with little opportunity for communication [22]. Our findings suggest that children, no less than adults, are placed in a dehumanized and isolated position when excluded from discussion of their illness and treatment. Parents, however, strongly asserted their convictions that knowledge might be destructive and that shielding maintains a life orientation. Most parents compromised by encouraging communication of feelings so long as the subject of death was avoided.

In the context of anticipatory mourning, affirmation of life took the form of *reconciliation* which, as noted earlier, is defined as "the parents' development of a perspective which preserves their sense of confidence in the worth of the child's life and in the worth of life in general in spite of acknowledgment of the child's fatal condition" [4]. *Affirmation of life* was also expressed in parental *memorialization* of the child and through the continuing impact of his memory on family life. These processes continued after bereavement. In addition to asserting the meaningfulness of the child's life in spite of its brevity, most parents struggled against their feelings of guilt and bitterness by reaffirming their own assets, the worth of cherished others, and the rewards of living.

Reorganization

Reorganization entails a revision of values, goals, and philosophy of life in the light of the sickness and death of the child. Natterson and Knudson described greater "ego strength" of mothers in later phases of the child's illness than in the initial period following diagnosis [9]. Other investigators working with the families of fatally ill children have not dealt directly with the issue of reorganization. We observed adaptive integration of the crisis resulting in some meaningful reorganization prevailing in most of the parents we encountered. While reorganization sometimes began during the child's illness, the process usually reached its fullest articulation after the acute post-bereavement period.

Awareness of personal growth was described by mothers and

fathers. They indicated increased capacity for empathy and intimacy as a direct result of having mastered their own loss. They talked about becoming more compassionate, warmer, more tolerant, closer to their families, more aware of their own and other's feelings. As one mother said, "It really makes you grow up fast." A father noted, "I think we both overlook each other's faults more than we used to" and "appreciate each other more." The growth of warmth and understanding often extended beyond the family. "I'm being more tolerant and patient of people whereas I never had this before." Such maturation may be expressed in branching out to new social roles and care-giving functions such as working for the health and happiness of others. This process is exemplified in the activities of a well-known comedian who has devoted extensive energies to care and research efforts related to leukemia as a consequence of the loss of his own child.

Another form of reorganization involves a change in orientation toward time. Parents developed a heightened sense of immediacy and a tendency to savor the present during the course of the child's illness and dying which frequently persisted after his death. As one mother stated, "Life itself means much more to me. I can't look forward to tomorrow and yesterday's gone so today is the day I worry about and appreciate." A father remarked, "Appreciate what you've got instead of worrying about what you want to have!" In further elaboration of the impact of the death of his son, he added, "If something is determined to happen, it's going to happen and you can't change the future for you. You might be able to help along a little bit but there's no sense in worrying about it and working yourself silly trying to accomplish something that you can't. So I do the best I can and I don't worry about what I can't do."

As their self-concepts underwent reorganization in the light of the prolonged crisis, the confidence of most parents was maintained, and even enhanced, by recognition that they were able to survive the crisis, not only without despair and disintegration but also with new insights, new outlooks and new strengths.

Conclusion

As we have previously indicated [4], a maladaptive outcome was quite rare for parents in our study. Those who were able to accomplish the task of anticipatory mourning were also able to deal with the dilemmas related to the threat to their sense of mastery, worth and trust and to maintain confidence during the child's illness and after his death. To the degree that reorganization occurred, parents responded to the crisis not only with adaptive measures which maintained equilibrium or restored coping and defensive operations, but also with liberation of latent potentialities resulting in further maturation and new adaptive capacities. Successful resolution of developmental crises is generally considered to facilitate further growth and development [5]. Successful resolution of a situational crisis such as described here appears to have similar positive developmental consequences.

Acknowledgments

We would like to thank Dr. G. Honig and Dr. H. Maurer of the Department of Pediatrics for their enthusiastic cooperation with our clinical research program; Miss A. Klein, Dr. I. Borstein, and Miss G. Holverson for their ongoing clinical contribution; Miss J. Ireland and Mrs. A. Hoffman for their assistance in reviewing and classifying data; and Dr. M. Sabshin for his immeasurable contribution to the theoretical aspects of our work.

Bibliography

1.   Paykel, E. S., "Life Events and Acute Depression," Paper presented at Annual Meeting of the American Association for the Advancement of Science, Chicago, December, 1970.
2.   Klein, D. C. and Lindemann, E., Preventive Intervention in Individual and Family Crisis Situations, in G. Caplan, Ed., *Prevention of Mental Disorders in Children; Initial Explorations*, Basic Books, New York, 1961.
3.   Murphy, L. B., Coping devices and defense mechanisms in relation to autonomous ego functions, *Bull. Menning. Clinic*, 24 (1960), 144–153.
4.   Futterman, E. H., Hoffman, I. and Sabshin, M., Parental Anticipatory Mourning, in A. Kutscher, Ed., *Psychosocial Aspects of Terminal Care*, Columbia University Press, New York, in press.
5.   Erikson, E., *Identity and the Life Cycle*, International University Press, New York, 1959.
6.   Futterman, E. H. and Hoffman, I., Transient school phobia in a fatally ill child, *J. Amer. Acad. Child Psychiat.*, 9 (1970), 477–494.
7.   Binger, C. M., Albin, A. R., Feuerstein, R. C., Kushner, J. H., Zoger, S. and Mikkelsen, C., Childhood leukemia, emotional impact on patient and family, *N. Eng. J. Med.*, 280 (1969), 414–418.

8. Friedman, S. B., Chodoff, P., Mason, J. W., and Hamburg, D. A.,
    Behavioral observations on parents anticipating the death of a child,
    Pediatrics, 32 (1963), 610–625.
9. Natterson, J. M., and Knudson, A. G., Observations concerning fear of
    death in fatally ill children and their mothers, *Psychosom. Med.,* 22
    (1960), 456–465.
10. Hamburg, D. A. and Adams, J. E., A perspective on coping behavior:
    seeking and utilizing information in major transitions, *Arch. Gen.
    Psychiat.* 17 (1967), 277–284.
11. Sabshin, M., Psychiatric perspectives on normality, *Arch. Gen. Psychiat.*
    17 (1967), 258–264.
12. Benedek, T., Parenthood as a developmental phase, *J. Amer. Psychoanal.
    Assn.* 17 (1959), 389–417.
13. Lazarus, R. S., *Psychological Stress and the Coping Process,* McGraw-
    Hill, New York, 1966.
14. Haggard, E. A., Psychological causes and results of stress, in *Human
    Factors in Undersea Warfare,* National Research Council, 1949.
15. Bozeman, M. F., Orbach, C. E., and Sutherland, A. M., Psychological
    impact of cancer and its treatment—adaptation of mothers to threatened
    loss of their children through leukemia I, *Cancer,* 8 (1955), 1–19.
16. Hamovitch, M. B., *The Parent and the Fatally Ill Child,* Delmar, Los
    Angeles, 1964.
17. Richmond, J. B. and Waisman, H. A., Psychological aspects of manage-
    ment of children with malignant diseases, *Amer. J. Dis. Children,* 89,
    (1955), 42–47.
18. Orbach, C. E., Sutherland, A. M., and Bozeman, M. F., Psychological
    impact of cancer and its treatment—adaptation of mothers to threatened
    loss of their children through leukemia II, *Cancer,* 8 (1955), 20–33.
19. Chodoff, P., Friedman, S.B., and Hamburg, D.A., Stress, defenses and
    coping behavior: observations in parents of children with malignant
    disease, *Amer. J. Psychiat.,* 120 (1964), 743–749.
20. Hoffman, I. and Futterman, E. H., Coping with waiting: psychiatric inter-
    vention and study in the waiting room of a pediatric oncology clinic,
    Compreh. Psychiat. 12 (1971), 67–81.
21. Ross, E., *On Death and Dying,* Macmillan, New York, 1969.
22. Glaser, B. G. and Strauss, A. L., *Awareness of Dying,* Aldine, Chicago,
    1965.
23. Futterman, E. H. and Hoffman, I., Shielding from awareness: an aspect
    of family adaptation to fatal illness in children, *Arch. Thanatol,* 2 (1970),
    23–24.
24. Vernick, J. and Karon, M., Who's afraid of death on a leukemia ward?,
    Amer. J. Dis. Child. 109 (1965), 393–397.

The Doctor and the Dying Child*

N. Alby, Ph.D. and
J.M. Alby, M.D. (France)

Introduction

This work, which is an evaluation of the dimension and nature of the psychological needs on an hematologic service, has been undertaken and continued in spite of the inherent difficulties in the management of leukemic children and their families at a specialized center. Eighteen years ago, the initial concern of the department chief, Professor Jean Bernard, was to make the living conditions and treatment more tolerable and to study the psychological repercussions of the illness. At that time the therapeutic activity was minimal both in its efficacy and complexity. One of us (J. M. A.), a resident in the department and already oriented toward psychiatry, felt a similar need to do something about the psychological aspect. Thus, research was then undertaken in collaboration with the co-author of this article (N. A.), a clinical psychologist who is now completely in charge of it. Needs and demands have been modified and so has the disease and its treatment. The increased duration of the remissions, the effectiveness of an aggressive therapeutic approach, and the "psychological presence" have sensitized the medical team.

*Translated by E. James Anthony, M. D.

The "Psy Function"*

We are conscious that "psychological presence" is an imperfect term to describe what we mean, but we will use it as a global indication of the overall psychological impact and activity of someone who is functioning at the level of relationships. This "psy function" can be exercised by a psychiatrist, a psychologist, or an internist, but it is a psychoanalytic orientation that prepares an individual best for a role involving a mutual identification with members of the medical team, and the maintenance of relationships in which the degree of closeness is determined by its usefulness to the individual concerned.

Two points must be emphasized: first, it is not necessary to function according to the psychoanalytical model; and second, the personal involvement and the sharing of the real experience, the raw material reality, is imperative, otherwise the medical team which has its own obligations regarding technical procedures and psychological conduct is likely to react to psychological interventions as either absurd or attacking.

We have inquired into the usefulness of the "psy function" under such conditions and it would seem that a knowledge of the child's defensive and coping mechanisms and those immediately concerned with him can be presented to the medical staff as the only possible intervention model with the implication that no one can substitute for the physician with sole clinical responsibility for the case [2].

The role of the "psy person" can be very frustrating; while participating in the stresses and strains of all that goes on, he does not have the field of action of a doctor and yet at the same time he must tolerate the same aggressive projections. His motives as well as his reactions must be carefully and constantly evaluated to ensure that his work is effective and enduring.

The Center

Four hundred leukemic patients a year are treated there, half of them being children. Depending on their conditions, the sick are treated either as outpatients with day-care, or inpatients in the 120

*"Psy" is used as the common prefix for both "psychiatrist" and "psychologist." (Editor's note.)

beds of the department. The duration of hospitalization is variable, but the aim is to keep it as short as possible; at the present time for a child, the first stay is from four to five weeks. In 95% of the lymphoblastic leukemias (the most frequent type seen at the center), the treatment brings about a lasting remission of good quality. The preventive and maintenance measures are necessary to keep control of the disease and are more or less painful and restrictive. The goal is to avoid, as much as possible, rehospitalization, the child being treated near his home or at a day hospital.

The treatment center is linked to a research unit that is itself in constant touch with similar international units. This association between the scientific research and the treatment gives a feeling of security to the patients, the families, and also to the doctors. The rule is that the physician must undertake some work in the research unit that is independent of the center's activities or those of the medical service; this scientific activity is an effective safeguard against the built-in tensions that are inevitable in the care of the leukemic child. We are tempted to attach as much importance to the activity of the center as to progress in therapeutics for bringing about certain improvements in the relationship between the family and the center. The influence of the latter prevents parents from giving up treatment or turning to faith healers and quacks.

The greater therapeutic effectiveness has resulted, paradoxically, in an aggravation of the situation in the wards where new cases are once again being put together with complicated ones, resistant ones, or treatment failures. This state of affairs is recent and its consequences are already observable in the department where the accumulation of serious patients, some of them in a terminal phase after a prolonged course, have produced conditions that are very difficult to tolerate. The tensions experienced, particularly by the nursing personnel, tend to reach a breaking point when several deaths occur simultaneously. The tradition of the service is to accept patients beyond therapeutic reach when the demand is made by themselves or their parents.

The role of the nurse, particularly, is becoming more difficult; her responsibility is greater because both the cases and the procedures are increasing in complexity. In addition, prolonged contact with chronic cases creates bonds whose emotional intensity is not only burdensome in itself but even more so in proportion to the hopes and disappointments engendered by treatment.

Any specialized center using advanced techniques for the extremely ill will recognize a similar situation. Lately we are witnessing an increased demand for "psy function"; originating from the medical staff, it is seemingly understandable as an increasing concern for the patients and their family; actually it reflects the unbearable anxiety of the physicians. It seems good that a highly technical group of doctors can paradoxically ask for help with this anxiety at a time when this therapeutic armamentarium has become considerable; it is undoubtedly harder for the top-rank specialist today to accept failure. Furthermore, he is being made to realize, with much uneasiness, the gap between his technical proficiency and his ability to communicate meaningfully with his patients.

PSYCHOLOGICAL INTERVENTION AND THE MEDICAL TEAM

In 1956, one of us came to the conclusion with Bernard [3] that our task was to protect the child from anxiety and allow the families to adjust to a psychologically traumatic situation. Their mechanisms of defense were respected since these allowed them to face up to the idea of possible death. Ten years later with Chassigneux [1], the focus was on the needs of the nursing staff.

Today the duration of the illness and the condition on admission have compelled us to take into consideration the importance of the relationship factor and its bearing on intervention. It now appears to us that a better level of communication reflects the increased tolerance of both individuals and groups to pathogenic situations occasioned by some demand.

How does this show itself? It may be formulated under different kinds of rationale, but in the first analysis, it may involve some realistic situation such as a difficulty on the part of a family to accept the diagnosis; symptomatic reactions in the child, like anorexia or mutism; or the effects of modifying some aspect of the therapeutic regime as was the case with regard to sterile rooms and the attitude toward opening them during treatment period. The obvious request, made by a member of the medical team, always includes a latent meaning, the recognition of which enhances our effectiveness even though we would not wish to interpret it.

What then is this real need? The anxiety of the group is the principal motive force; someone or other is going to be the spokesman when a formal request is made for an interview with a child or his parents.

The need is in the doctor or in the nurse; the evidence for this is based on certain almost deviant requests—for example, the evaluation of emotional difficulty in an unconscious patient whose physical condition is of primary urgency. Even with a superficial consideration of this, it becomes very obvious that the sort of thoughtless behavior on the part of a member reflects the tension of the group.

However, things progress. On the first occasion, the request for intervention tends to be applied almost exclusively to cases in which the manifestations are blatant without being, for all that, justified. Following this, a selection is made in favor of those cases where a real need for help is expressed in some indirect fashion. As the situation develops, so does the willingness of the medical team to present the "psy person," without ambivalence, as one of them.

Although well aware of all this, we have had to come to terms with the gratification afforded us, on the one hand, by their expression of strong emotional needs, and on the other hand by the feelings of belonging to a team where the need for evidence is indispensable. A certain degree of adjustment is necessary otherwise; from whatever source the approval comes, the "psy person" runs the risk of either becoming "encapsulated" in the team or of attempting to take over the doctor's role in relation to the patient or of withdrawing into an unrealistic psychotherapeutic attitude.

The demand must always be recognized for what it is, but the response and the relationship that stem from it must be handled with tact. A good test of whether it works is the reestablishment of communication between the caretakers and those who are cared for following the "psy" intervention but without us functioning as intermediaries.

Authors like Raimbault [5] have insisted that the specific psychological needs of patients themselves, because of the organizational structure of the hospital, cannot and perhaps should not become a therapeutic goal. Without challenging this reality, we would keep some reservations about it: The gravely ill have a right to be relieved both of physical pain and of the fear of death. However, even when the "psy" demand is given free expression, whether solicited or not, we are doubtful whether anyone can completely meet it.

Such reservations would lead us to prefer, in most cases, an intermediate type of intervention dealing with real situations of conflict and anxiety in the context of everyday life. The dynamic power to this comes from the realization of the difference between individuals in the variety of their responses. Thus, one assesses, in the manner of Raimbault [6], Solnit and Green [7, 8], and Friedman [4], the difficulties of communication with the child and with those around him and the importance this factor holds for his recovery.

THE DOCTOR AND THE EVOLUTION OF THE ILLNESS

The doctor, along with the patients and their families, is pressured by all the unpredictable changes of leukemia.

The admission into the department imposes the reality of the diagnosis on everyone excepting the child. It still signifies death in the end but mitigated more by the now expectable prolonged first remission than by any hopes engendered by the immediate but precarious therapeutic response. In the department, the parents are informed of the diagnosis except in those rare cases where one of the parents themselves is afflicted with the same illness.

The traumatic emotional reactions to the diagnosis are known and expected by the medical team. One of them, however,—the apparent incapacity to understand, bordering on intellectual inhibition—may nevertheless take the doctor and nurses by surprise. Some of the younger doctors, already worried by the part they are playing, are intolerant of not being understood, or rather of not being heard, and without realizing it they cover their uneasiness by the use of technical jargon that reinforces the lack of understanding.

The doctor who informs the parents of the seriousness of the child's illness nevertheless feels a sense of relief in spite of the inevitable initial tension. In sharing his burden with the parents, he finds that he is no longer alone in the situation. He knows, furthermore, that he has laid the basis for collaboration throughout the remainder of the illness.

As a counterpart, the parents (the mother especially) need to be accepted the way they are; with their regressions, their opposition, and their denial. The doctor tries to evaluate the type of personality with which he has to deal. The "psy" intervention, which often consists of showing the doctor that he can appeal to the patient's ego, may frequently lead to a reintegration and a wish to communicate. If the doctor was previously able to support the parents' emotional reaction until its intensity brought about a loss of control, then the resumption of contact with someone else in the team is sometimes sufficient to reestablish control.

Once the critical period of diagnosis is over, the medical team will be importuned over and above the requirements of care to participate in more emotional ways and not to remain uninvolved. There is an obligation to support the limited identification of the parents with the routine and regulations of the hospital so that they can shape their lives to the rhythms of examinations and treatment, and to recognize the unconscious identification with the therapists to control the situation by magical means. When the mechanism entails an identification with the aggressor, tolerance comes harder, particularly for the nurses.

The parents' hysterical reactions, often noisy and histrionic, may lead either to characteristic neurotic disorders or to angry denials of the disease and its consequences; these outbursts are better tolerated if they do not last too long.

Bringing to light the defensive character of these behaviors helps to reduce the aggressive and guilty responses of the medical team and to avoid the rigid and even rejecting attitudes that tend to deflect the vital force of the members into the areas of conflict at the expense of the therapeutic work that needs to be done.

The team is especially likely to get involved with mothers. The behavior of certain fathers is sometimes severely criticized in proportion to the medical team's unconscious reactions to irresponsible or authoritarian attitudes that activate feelings of powerlessness and profoundly threaten the integrity of each one in the group.

During the period of remission, when it is struggling to resolve the impossible dilemma between projecting into the future with hopefulness and preparing to mourn its loss, the family may behave in an "as if" manner, crediting the physician with special powers apparently justified by his therapeutic capacity but actually based on quite unrealistic magical needs for assurance.

As a result, the relationship is easier, but at the price of an increased vulnerability to any provocations or relapses. Being on guard, the doctor can preserve the rapport without being seduced or taken in. He must also be alert to the overprotection of the child by the parents and to the omnipotence that the child displays as the result of becoming a very precious object set at a distance and idealized.

The most favorable circumstance—and the doctors in the department are very aware of this—is to induce the parents to accept a return to normal family life. However, this is much easier to write about than to achieve, and it is perhaps the peculiarity of the surroundings that militates against such a development.

At the time of relapse, the emotional aspect of the relationship finds itself suddenly under increased tension. The tie of dependency is certainly a support but its inescapable ambivalence cannot be overlooked when put to the test by provocative incidents and treatment difficulties. It is hard for everyone (the doctors included) to admit that the shared illusion disappears under the impact of reality.

If, in these same exigencies, the family group manifests a quasi-megalomanic attitude that is tolerated for a time because of guilt, intervention becomes necessary to prevent the tension from reaching the breaking point. One can interpret this attitude as a defense against depression. In our opinion, this is the only tolerable kind of intervention by the medical team considering the overwhelming repression of aggressiveness by every adult when confronted by his powerlessness in the face of a child's death. It is even more difficult for anyone to accept the fact that a child, already the victim of his disease and of the treatments imposed by it, can himself become an aggressor when brought up against the adult's impotence.

One can observe the eruption of catastrophic reactions in cases, seen more and more frequently, where relapses follow long periods of remission (more than five years). Thus, families have "forgotten" the threat and respond in a manner reminiscent of a traumatic neurosis. The intensity of the anxiety may overflow the regulator mechanism and aggressive outbursts are not infrequent, some of which may be witnessed by the child and some of which may be directed at him. The doctor who is also beguiled by the remission is not far from sharing the same feelings. Even if another remission is obtained, the heart is no longer in it anymore. There are some treasons that cannot be forgiven, even to oneself. The death of a child is one such instance.

How else can one understand how competent doctors try to explain a death by citing a so-called therapeutic error or an imaginary carelessness when the condition of the child left no hope. In most cases, one can guess more or less at the reason for this. Is it not part of a prolegomena to mourning? Distancing and intellectualization, in general, allow ways of avoiding some of the occupational hazards of being a doctor, *but everyone is vulnerable when a child dies.* The guilty attitude of the group can overwhelm the individual defenses especially when identifications are very close as, for example, in the case of a doctor's child. The entire group becomes depressed and looks around for a scapegoat.

THE SECRET AND THE TELLING OF IT

The hospital team, as we have mentioned, has modified its attitude toward concealing any knowledge of his condition from the child. This change, we believe, is in keeping with the introductions of the "psy function," bearing in mind that opinions may differ on this.

In the French medical tradition, the child is allegedly safe-guarded by exclusion, the silence surrounding his illness representing a concrete expression of this. The thinking is circular: "It is not serious"; "It will not be painful"; "There is nothing the matter with you, etc. . ." Who is being reassured? Who is being duped? In the end, those around the child begin to live and act in a completely unreal world.

What should one say to the child? Every team ponders the same question. Vernick and Karon [9] give the diagnosis to the child and "tell the truth." They take their stand on the contention, correct in our opinion, that a child "knows" more about his disease than one believes and, especially, more than one fears. Is it not a matter rather of a "recoiling lie?" To give the diagnosis and subsequently to modify the prognosis by proposing a line of treatment forces one into ambiguity, particularly in a country where faith in the power of science is so strong. Is there not, inevitably, a distortion of the reality of "what has been said" according to the specific conditions of functioning at each center, in terms of its philosophy and microsociology? Who can ever forget Solzhenytzin's "Cancer Ward?"

In order to remain close to our experience, that motivational analysis of someone who "tells the truth" to a child might furnish an adequate answer: the frankness that consists of saying "You have leukemia; perhaps you are going to die, but I am here to help you"; may simply be a means of taking action.

Whether as a rationalization or as an impulsive and unexpected act, "to give" the diagnosis becomes the equivalent of unburdening oneself of anxiety and of shifting the responsibility onto someone else. Here again we find the same projective mechanisms provoked by the threat that a child's death represents for each one of us. We doubt very much that communication with the child can be re-established in this manner. This way of doing things is very reminiscent of the counterphobic attitudes of certain doctors who cannot bear the idea of taking care of dying children.

Silence at any price—the atmosphere of conspiracy that goes with it and the avoidance of every question asked by the child pertaining to his illness—is another form of exclusion. The children understand it so well that very soon they too keep silent for the sake, so some have informed us, of protecting the adults.

Solnit and Green (op. cit.) deal with the child's question according to his age, his physical condition, and his surroundings. We would agree with them. The qualitative and quantitative evaluation of the child's anxiety, indispensable in this matter, tends to reflect his relationship with his parents and cannot be separated from this.

The "conversations" of the psychologist with the child in front of one of the parents are used more and more for this evaluation. Whatever the age of the child, the "psy person" presents himself as someone coming to talk to him about his illness and about his fear, the existence of which is thus implicitly acknowledged. Once the moment of surprise and anxiety occasioned by this unexpected overture has passed, the child seldom refuses to answer on a level appropriate to himself. His response, however, may be manifest or latent and ranging from fantasy to very precise questions. These provide some indication of the quality of his defenses.

Listening at the right moment can, if not impeded by mechanisms of denial or reaction formation, bring about an interchange. At such times, it is possible to talk to a child about his illness and to provide him, without necessarily labeling it, with explanatory pictures of the pathological reality, giving a concrete and real form to the medical terms. Moreover, the approach to any conflicting situation is then made easier. When a child obtains the right to speak and to share the knowledge of others concerning his body, he acquires an intellectual control over his fears and an objectivity regarding his distressing fantasies. This also allows a child, and those around him, to approach more freely the real object of their constant preoccupation, the illness.

At a deeper level, the failure in communication with respect to the illness is tied to the prohibition of knowledge: To know what is frightening, indeed, is but to know what is *forbidden* in the dialectic of the Oedipus complex and castration. The adults unconsciously contribute to it by their counter-Oedipal attitudes and reinforce the prohibition, hence the silence. The misunderstanding by the adult of a sick child's fantasies accounts for it. The content of the child's fears are pictured in relation to their own imagery.

The medical team calls for someone to intervene in the care of the child who "knows what he has" or of the child who says "I have leukemia." Now, this "nosological" anxiety seems quite often of secondary importance. One could even say that a child prefers the adults to have certainty. In return, guilt feelings appear fast: "Why am I sick?" That is to say, "What did I do to get sick?" Certain children do not want to hear about their illness. They make this very clear that it should be the parents who must keep the power and the knowledge and remain their mediators. It goes without saying that this defense must be respected.

When the somatic condition worsens in spite of the usual remission, the anxiety stirs up new aggressive projections tied to the fear of being abandoned. The unconscious attitude of the parents who cannot bear the "treason" of the object reinforces archaic defenses. Members of the medical team are part of it in proportion to the degree of their identification. The doctor, protected by the calls on his services and by the justification of his research, is less vulnerable than the nurses.

Conclusion

The introduction of the psychological dimension as such in a specialized center creates more questions than it can solve. One should individualize the specific situation of the child and of the adolescent: the mechanism of distancing, characteristic of the child, and the adolescent's sensitive self-consciousness to the life threat both put the physician to the test. The adolescent, particularly, would justify a special study.

The demand for help goes to the one who is taking care of the case. What then can the "psy person" do? His specific intervention in the dramatic situation created by the illness could be considered as traumatic and useless, similar to a "wild analysis." We would not regard it thus. The proposed model is not a classical analytic mirror, but the analytic framework is essential to evaluate motives, to facilitate the development of mutual identifications with the doctors in charge, and to tolerate the built-in frustrations. A prolonged and concrete experience of life in a hospital is equally essential, which does not mean that one must conform to the medical treatment model and find a place for oneself within it.

The medical model is geared to high technical standards and increases the level of anxiety, paradoxically, in proportion to the discrepancy between the technical requirements and the patient's needs, between medical efficacy and the ultimate struggle. The functional model that we have proposed is therefore difficult but compatible, in our opinion, with the medical one. It brings in attentive listening, the understanding of implicit demands, and the recognition of an optimal psychological distance between caretaker and patient that allows a tolerable relationship for each.

The medical team knows that it cannot fulfill its task without appealing to someone. The "psy person" must also know this and accept it in order to function efficiently. To emphasize efficiency does not imply competition, but on the contrary, his personal make-up permits the psy person to recognize it and thus to be able to protect himself against the seductive and controlling efforts of the group, both by way of action as well as by communication which is also a mode of action.

All must reckon with *time;* slowly, through all the vicissitudes of the team relationships and the team-patient relationship will come the wish to establish the best conditions for the use of the "psy function," constantly tested by changes of the medical personnel or by the ever-present threat of death.

It would be vain to believe that the existence of the "psy function" can abolish the harsh reality that the doctor must face in such services. Furthermore, the "psy person," by his very presence, stimulates ambiguously worded demands for help that have to be decoded; to meet this need directly, even if it were possible, would go counter to the objective in view which is to help the doctor function better by patiently working through the relationship between the adults involved and between the adults and the sick child which will make conditions more effective and tolerable for everyone concerned.

Bibliography

1. Alby, N., Alby, J.M., and Chassigneux, J., Aspects psychologiques de l'évolution et du traitement des leucémiques, enfants et jeunes adultes dans un centre spécialise, *Nouv. rev. fr. hémat, 7* (1967), 577-588.
2. Alby, N. and Alby, J.M., L'intervention psychologique dans un centre de recherche et de traitement d'hématologie. A paraitre dans, *Psychiat. enf. XIV, 2* (1971).
3. Bernard, J. and Alby, J.M., Incidences psychologiques de la leucémie aigue de l'enfant et de son traitement, *Hyg. ment., 3* (1956), 241-255.
4. Friedman, S., Chodoff, P., Mason, J.W., and Hamburg, D., Behavioral observations of parents anticipating the death of a child, *Pediatrics, 32* (1963), 610-625.
5. Raimbault, E., Recherches psychologiques en cancérologie. Rapport non publié de l'Unité de psychologie médicale. Institut Gustave Roussy, Paris.
6. Raimbault, G. and Royer, P., Thématique de la mort chez l'enfant atteint de maladie chronique, *Arch. fr. ped, 9* (1969), 1041-1053.
7. Solnit, A.J. and Green, M., Pediatric management of dying child II. Child's reaction to fear of dying, in *Modern Perspectives in Child Development*, Solnit, S.A. Provence, New York University Press, New (1963), 217-228.
8. Solnit, A.J., The dying child, *Child Neur., 7* (1965), 693-704.
9. Vernick, J. and Karon, M., Who's afraid of death on a leukemic ward? *Amer. J. Dis. Child, 109* (1965), 393-397.

The Dying Child in Hospital

W. H. G. Wolters, Psychologist (Holland)

Introduction

Confrontation with the dying child generally places a heavy burden on the physician. Is it perhaps that the death of a child emphasizes even more strongly the poignant absurdity of our existence than the death of an adult? The practical and material consequences for the rest of the family when a child dies are almost nil whereas a father's or mother's death may jeopardize its very existence.

On the other hand, the death of a child may cause a grave emotional crisis. For most adults, suffering and destruction are aspects of life not associated with children. This is, perhaps, why the death of a child seems particularly brutal: Children ought not to die. When they do, a crisis can result for all concerned — relatives, nursing personnel, and physicians. The course of this crisis will largely depend on individual attitudes toward death and dying.

These attitudes, in turn, are to a great extent determined by the prevailing concepts of death in a particular society or culture and it is this culture too that provides the means of achieving or helping to achieve integration.

THE GENERAL CULTURE IN RELATION TO DEATH AND DYING

The significance of death and dying is directly connected with the fundamental values that predominate in a given period of history. Borkenau distinguishes three possible attitudes toward death: denial, defiance, and acceptance. Fulton speaks of "death oriented" cultures such as are still found in Spain, Mexico, and Italy. In these cultures "the cemetery stands in close proximity to the church," and attributes of death are handled in a way that would be considered macabre in other cultures. Skulls and bones are common objects in everyday life. In fact, as Fulton says, "for these societies the recognition of death is a prime requisite for life."

In our modern, highly industrialized society the attitude toward death is totally different. Van den Berg speaks of an "absence" of death. Fulton points to the marked avoidance attitude character-istic of American society. The word death is scarcely ever pro-nounced and all sorts of euphemisms are employed to veil the ob-ject of fear. Flowers sent to the funeral parlor are addressed to the deceased "as if he were still alive" and the body lying in state is made to look as lifelike as possible. It takes a great deal of money to eradicate the specter of death from such occasions; consequently, "the American way of death" is costly. These are the collective repressive techniques employed in a "carpe diem" culture, in which the distractions of everyday life stand in the way of any explicit thinking about death and finiteness "(Beerling, 1966). Death be-comes a prohibited area: death is, in a sense, taboo. The object of repression, however, retains its fascination and consequently words and images of death, dying, and destruction emerge in pornographic form. To quote Gorer (1965), "While natural death became more and more smothered in prudery, violent death has played an ever-growing part in the fantasies offered to mass audiences, detective stories, thrillers, westerns, war stories, spy stories, science fiction, and eventually horror comics."

The death taboo is often mentioned in the same breath with the sex taboo and since sexuality is gradually being divested of the most primitive taboo atmosphere surrounding it, we may wonder whether the same might not be done for death?

Undoubtedly there is at present an increased willingness to face problems connected with death and dying. In Holland, as in many other countries, numerous philosophical, psychological, and psy-chiatric studies dealing with these subjects have been published during the last few years. For the time being, however, the discus-sion remains restricted to a very small circle. It seems doubtful whether the death taboo can ever be subjected to more collective treatment and liquidation like the sexual taboo. In the way of direct gratification and visible gain, revision of our concept of sexuality has a high degree of "material" attractiveness. Successful integration of death in one's life, however, requires rather more maturity and the ability to accept the finiteness of one's personal existence.

Traditional attitudes toward church and religion have been caught up in an avalanche of social change and this is especially true in Holland. So strong has been the impact, that many people have seen their faith demolished beyond repair, thus losing both the values and security of religion and the comfort of its outward observances without being given a chance to accommodate themselves to the new situation. Consequently, many, especially of the middle generation, feel completely uprooted. Life's perspective has suddenly been reduced to the present, tangible world while the ritual which used to envelop important social and emotional events has been cast aside as worthless. It may be that new rituals will evolve eventually, but such processes take time.

Ten years ago, before urbanization had penetrated to the rural areas of the Catholic south, a funeral was an occasion in which the whole village participated. A clear traditional pattern prescribed the mode of conduct to be followed. Communal mourning provided a common outlet for emotions. The material side of the funeral too was handled by the community, not by a "neutral" undertaker. Neighbors and friends actually carried the deceased to his grave. The social role of the bereaved was clearly defined and distinguished by outward signs like clothing as well as by set patterns of conduct both for the mourners and for those around them. In this setting the mourner's status might remain visible, and recognized, for a long time.

Such a model of conduct with respect to death and mourning existed in most religious groupings before the process of urbanization and concomitant secularization, having started in the western provinces, spread over the rest of the country. Now, although remnants of these traditions are still to be found here and there, on the whole it may be said that the familiar patterns of conduct surrounding death have disappeared within an unbelievably short space of time.

THE MEDICAL SUBCULTURE IN RELATION TO DEATH AND DYING

A second related factor has undoubtedly also played a part in changing attitudes toward the dying, namely, the altered position of the doctor himself. The forces that have brought about the "dismantling" of religion, of religious practice and religious leadership, are also challenging the position and attitudes, traditionally sacrosanct, of the medical profession. In a recent controversial publication, a psychiatrist, Van de Hoofdakker, has accused the medical "caste" of being only too happy to play the part of "secularised saviour" instead of acting in the first place on the basis of scientific knowledge and technique.

A fair amount of publicity is being given at the moment to this kind of self-critical analysis of the medical profession's role in modern society although neither the doctors nor their patients seem to be happy with the assault on a long inviolate stronghold. There is an unmistakable tendency toward demythologization of the doctor's status and work. As a result the doctor finds himself, like the priest, deprived of the certainties that used to determine his attitude toward the dying patient. More than ever before aware of his own doubts and ignorance and no longer having at his disposal the traditional means of masking them, how can he give the patient the security and reassurance demanded from him?

Parents take their child to the physician with problems of a specifically somatic nature. They come to him with certain expectations, either of restoration of the child's health (even when there is no realistic hope of recovery) or else of comfort in the crisis confronting them. For the parents, and often for the child as well, the doctor is the obvious source of both physical aid and psychological support.

To the physician himself this usually is not quite so obvious. He knows he is no closer to finding an adequate answer to death than anyone else. As far as medical technique is concerned he knows where he stands: In this area the possibilities and limitations are more or less fixed. The psychosocial side of his work, however, is rather more complicated. Little has been done in the course of his training to prepare him for this task. The changes taking place in society, moreover, tend to detract from his role specificity while at the same time he finds himself deprived of the aid and the certitudes formerly provided by ethico-religious systems. With respect to death and dying, the physician suffers as much bewilderment and uncertainty as anyone else. In the medical organizations of a children's ward or children's hospital the consequences of such emotional confusion may be far-reaching, both for the sick child and his parents and for the nursing personnel who equally look to the physician for guidance and support. His behavior and actions in marginal situations may be of decisive importance for his image with the nursing staff and for future relations within the ward.

THREE REACTION PATTERNS

Three reaction patterns seem prevalent in hospital practice:

1. *Death as a Nontopic.* Repression may be so complete that the doctor or nurse in question is not aware of any problem. Ostensibly, death is a part of everyday routine. No mention, or as little as possible, is made of it in oral communication. Certain "critical" words are avoided. Little or no communication about this child occurs with others outside the ward with whom, normally, questions and anecdotes about the children would be shared. This attitude has an isolating effect both within the ward and in relation to the outside world. It reduces the possibilities of lending support and increases the risk of tensions. The desired integration and coordination of activities are impeded.

2. *Death as a Challenge to Medical Technique.* In these cases there is a conscious effort to face the death of the child, but there appears to be no adequate answer. The physician will attempt all sorts of partial solutions to the problem. He may approach it as purely a matter of medical technique, a battle that has to be won. Death, when it occurs, is regarded as a manifestation of the failure of this technique, dying as an incidental happening requiring a particular kind of engineering. Personal involvement and subjective emotion are eliminated. In this situation procedures may be carried out to the very end even when there is no longer any medical need. Technical perfectionism clearly becomes an escape.

   With so much stress on defenses, it is difficult to give children and parents the necessary support and guidance. The child's signals are not perceived or recognized, and he remains

alone with his ever-growing fear and insecurity. All sorts of
rationalizations are employed to justify the situation: that
the child does not realize, does not understand. Where communication is thus absent, it is hardly possible to maintain adequate relations with the parents. The fact that such contact is
avoided will increase their anxiety and fear, often causing
them to adopt an aggressive posture, especially if information
does reach them through side-channels. In other cases the defensive attitude of the parents is reinforced by the avoidance
reactions of the physician. Inevitably the child's own attitude
will be affected.

3. *Overidentification with the Dying Child.* Confronted with a
dying child, the doctor, nurse, or occupational therapist may
become emotionally involved to such an extent that a kind of
symbiotic relationship develops. Pain and distress suffered by
the child are experienced very keenly by the other person. The
child comes to depend too much on this one relationship to
the exclusion of other possibilities. Consequently, he will react very strongly to temporary absence of the person in question during weekends or off-duty periods. Outbursts of anger,
depression, or panic may occur. Especially in a terminal phase
the child may demand his familiar presence. Such close involvement may lead to strong reactions after the child's death
manifested in depression and feelings of guilt, rebellion, and
helplessness. The mourning reactions of the "professional"
survivor are almost indistinguishable from those of the relatives.

Like the two patterns previously described, therefore, this
reaction pattern also prevents an adequate relationship with
the dying child and his parents and may impede communication with fellow workers.

The Management of the Terminal Phase

THE GENERAL PLAN

Where there are several physicians working on the ward, it is important that one person should be in charge of coordinating all aspects of treatment and psychological assistance. There should be
explicit agreement about whether the physician is to function

exclusively as the source of medical information or is also to extend psychological support. Preferably one person should fulfill both functions.

Certain subsidiary tasks may be taken over by psychologists, psychiatrists, or social workers. This will depend on a number of factors, such as on the amount of time that the physician can spend on the case himself, on the degree of his emotional maturity, and on the specific psychological requirements of the situation. If these are crucial, it may be preferable for a psychotherapist or psychiatrist to occupy himself directly with the child. Relations with the parents concerning nonmedical aspects of the case may best be left to a psychologist or social worker.

Particularly in cases of protracted illness with fatal prognosis, a coordinated approach, based on a detailed plan, is essential to the interests of the child and his parents as well as of the hospital staff. Only in this way is it possible to support one another, resolve tensions, and together devise solutions that the individual is no longer able to find.

In the case of a three-year-old leukemia patient in our hospital, regular group discussions with all concerned provided relief in extremely difficult situations. The methods developed, often pragmatic rather than theoretical, proved very satisfactory in practice. During the last weeks preceding his death the child was not capable of much activity. He grew depressed and totally passive though mentally remaining quite lucid. A bowl of goldfish placed in his cubicle brought about a remarkable change in the child's mental condition. He became more cheerful, less depressed, and, above all, less preoccupied with his badly wasted body. Communication, which had been blocked, again became possible.

A few special aspects in the child's situation deserve attention. The environment is of great importance to the child, the other children, and the parents. If deaths occur regularly in the ward, care should be taken to ensure privacy, permit communication, and prevent stigma being attached to any one locality. Children have an acute sense for these things and react immediately.

HELPING THE CHILD

Depending on his degree of maturity, personal background, and intelligence, it may be advisable to actively involve the child in his treatment and give him information about it. Care should be taken, however, not to offer more than the child can comprehend. A difficult point is whether or not to let the child know how serious his condition is and what it means. I have the impression that the decision to say nothing and to avoid discussion is often too hastily taken. Surrounded by vague silence or false optimism, the child can become extremely apprehensive.

There is little point in trying to conceal the death of a child from the other children in the ward. Usually they are perfectly aware what has happened and know quite well what it means when a child is said to have gone to another ward or another hospital. Even when the death occurs at night, the information may spread imperceptibly from cubicle to cubicle.

Fantasies and discussions about the hereafter, about dividing possessions among brothers and sisters, or planning the funeral are not unusual. Evidently children can talk about death easily, directly and openly when the question is broached. "It is a grave error to think that a child over four or five years of age who is dying of a terminal illness does not realize its seriousness and probable fatality" (Binger, 1969).

A group of children were talking about what they were going to do after primary school, a seven year old who was seriously ill said: "After primary school I'll be going to the cemetery."

A high degree of sensitivity is required in the person directly in charge of the child, to recognize and adequately interpret any signals he may give. Too soon or too direct a confrontation with the problem may be as harmful as denying the reality.

HELPING THE PARENTS

The effectiveness of his help depends to a large extent on the doctor's ability to treat the parents as mature and responsible partners in a common task. This means keeping them fully informed about the child's treatment, about the progress of the disease and any procedure applied. Parents may find some relief in being allowed to aid in the care of their child. Again their individual capacity for such participation should be taken into account. Many problems arise if the information process is not sufficiently supervised. Information must be given with the greatest frankness. Emotional distortion of information by drawing conclusions from examinations too hastily, by postponing reports, or by assuming an overemphatically matter-of-fact attitude during interviews can have adverse effects.

The parents of a leukemic patient had been told in a previous hospital that the child had no more than four or five months to live. Eight months later he was still alive. The mother found this hard to accept. She wished he had died within the set term because in continuing to live he prolonged and intensified the parents' personal crisis. This thought or wish increased her already existing guilt feelings towards the child. The patient, whose body was badly wasted away, did not want his mother to see him like this and would only permit her to come as far as the adjacent cubicle.

In addition to the regulation of the information process it is essential for the physician in charge to know to what extent the parents are able to assimilate the information that is given. This is where the family physician should enter the picture. He should be invited to the group discussions held in the ward, both because he has important information to give and also because he has an important task in sustaining the other members of the family.

The emotional tensions and reactions of the parents are closely linked up with the attitude of the child and with the reactions of the hospital staff. The child's reactions may drive the parents to despair. In a fiercely aggressive way, he may accuse his parents of being responsible for his illness and approaching death. Sometimes he can become extremely demanding and dependent on them, and at other times refuse to see them altogether, or see perhaps only one of them.

GROUP DISCUSSIONS

To be able to take proper care of the dying child and its parents in the organization of a hospital or children's ward, it is necessary for everybody concerned to be well prepared in advance. It proves very rewarding in practice to treat various aspects of death and dying in group discussions. This is very valuable also for nursing staff and occupational therapists.

These group discussions should not be incidental occurrences but need to be integrated in training programs. Another useful measure may be some sort of selection of the person who is to be directly in charge of the child's psychological guidance. Not every nurse or occupational therapist will be able to endure being the central figure to a dying child for long. At all times, it should be possible for them, as well as for the physician, to fall back on the psychologist or social worker. In this way the hospital staff may come to understand more fully the problems surrounding death and dying so that eventually they may avoid the situation Natterson and Knudson (1966) note as one of the conclusions of their investigation, namely, that "in contrast to the mothers, the reactions of the staff were at least well integrated during the terminal phase."

Bibliography

1. Beerling, R. F., Denken over de dood., *De Gids.*, 129 (1966), 4/5.
2. Berg, J. H., v. d. *Metabletica*, Nijkerk, 1957.
3. Borkenau, F., The concept of death, in *Death and Identity*, 2nd printing, New York, (1966), 42–56.
4. Fulton, R. L., The sacred and the secular: Attitudes of the American public toward death, funerals, and funeral directors, in *Death and Identity;* 2nd printing, New York, (1966), 89–105.
5. Gorer, G., *Death, Grief and Mourning in Contemporary Britain*, Cresset Press: London, 1965.
6. Natterson, J. M. and Knudson Jr., Observations concerning fear of death in fatally ill children and their mothers, in *Death and Identity*, 2nd printing, New York, (1966), 226–240.

Symposium: The Dying Child in an American Hospital

Jimmy – A Clinical Case Presentation of a Child with a Fatal Illness*

C. M. Binger, M.D. (U.S.A.)

Jimmy was nine years of age when first admitted to the University Hospital. For some ten months he had had symptoms of recurrent leg and abdominal pains, the etiology of which had not been determined.

He came from a lumbering community some three to four hours drive from the hospital where he lived with his 15-year-old sister, mother, and stepfather of two-years duration. Both mother and stepfather worked as laborers in a lumbermill. Their income was marginal.

Jimmy's natural father was reported as alcoholic, unemployed, recurrently in jail for drunkenness, and having infrequent contact with Jimmy or his sister.

Max, the stepfather, was a tall, lean, high-strung, red-haired, tense man in his early thirties, divorced from his first wife who had custody of his children. He infrequently visited his own children because it was so "painful" to leave them at the end of a visit. He and Jimmy had a warm relationship. Among other things Max had taught Jimmy how to hunt and fish—things his own father had never done.

*The author wishes to express his appreciation to the following—A. R. Ablin, M. D., R. C. Stein, M. D., J. H. Kushner, M. D., S. Zoger, M. D., and Cynthia Mikkelsen, M. S. W. (University of California, San Francisco, Medical Center, Dept. of Pediatrics) who made this study possible.

Mother, also in her early thirties, appeared worn, tired and frail. She and Jimmy seemed to have a close relationship. The 15-year-old sister was reported as "inner directed" but did well in school and got along well with mother and Max. She and Jimmy were somewhat distant from each other.

When Jimmy's mother and natural father were divorced, she told Jimmy that he was now the man of the house, a responsibility he assumed with all seriousness. When Max moved into the home, Jimmy soon realized this was not so, but he did not relinquish his inner responsibility of protecting and supporting his mother. Up to the present illness Jimmy had been in good health and had done well in school. None of the family members appeared to have close friends, nearby relatives, or meaningful group or church affiliation.

Initial Conference

Diagnostic tests revealed that Jimmy had a fatal disease—acute leukemia. These findings were shared with Max and Mother by the ward pediatrician. They reacted with shock, disbelief, self-blame, and anger. They insisted that Jimmy be kept in ignorance of the diagnosis. He was told that he was in the hospital for diagnosis and treatment of "anemia." They also expressed their desire that he have both inpatient and outpatient care at the University Hospital and clinics and utilize their local physician for supportive or emergency care in collaboration with the medical center specialists.

The following day, an initial conference was arranged with Max, Mother, the ward pediatrician, pediatric hematologist, social worker, and myself, a child psychiatrist, all members of a team working together on this problem for several years. It was suggested and they agreed that Jimmy's father be present.

It was at this conference that I met Max, Mother, and Father. I was introduced by the hematologist as a child psychiatrist who, like the social worker, was a member of the clinical team and that we worked closely together. It was explained that we would be available to them and Jimmy to assist in whatever way we could during their visits to the hospital. During the course of the conference they agreed to my meeting with Jimmy in a confidential relationship but again stressed that he did not know the diagnosis and understood that he would be coming to the clinic for treatment of anemia. They saw no reason that he be told differently.

This "initial conference" was particularly stormy. As the hematologist proceeded to answer their questions concerning the diagnosis, anticipated course of the illness, treatment, and its fatal prognosis, Mother raised many questions having to do with self-blame. Max was tense and rather quiet but suddenly verbally exploded at Father for not really caring about Jimmy or his daughter. Father was teary-eyed as he verbally defended himself. It was finally agreed that he could come to visit Jimmy and he in turn offered to resume support payments. (In actuality, this didn't come to pass since he apparently became increasingly depressed, drank more heavily, spent more time in jail, rarely came to see Jimmy, and was unable to provide the support payments—in retrospect, we felt that we should have met with the natural father alone.)

FIRST INTERVIEW WITH JIMMY FOLLOWING THE INITIAL CONFERENCE

Following the conference it was agreed that I would work with Jimmy and the social worker would mainly work with the parents. The social worker, I, and the hematologist would collaborate regularly. Subsequently, I introduced myself to Jimmy stating that I was a child psychiatrist working with the hematologist and social worker and would be available to him both in the hospital and at his clinic visits. It was further pointed out that I saw a number of young people who came to the medical center with all sorts of illnesses and most had many worries and concerns about themselves and their illnesses. I further pointed out that what he and I should talk about would not be shared with his parents since I well realized that young people have many thoughts or feelings which are difficult to discuss with people close to them but that talking them over with someone outside the family could be helpful. I also pointed out that I, the social worker, hematologist, and pediatrician had met with his parents so I already knew something of his family and of him secondhand. He said he already knew that. I then stated that I wasn't really clear as to what his illness had been like for him and what he understood about it and the treatment. His first comment was "Don't you dare tell my mother what I have to say." I again stated that what he shared with me would not be conveyed to his parents. He then proceeded to state "I have a blood disease—anemia." He pointed out that he was worried but could not tell his mother since she would be upset if she knew he was worried, and he couldn't tell his sister since she would tell his mother. In a most serious manner he proceeded to state that several years ago he knew a boy who had "anemia." He recalled that this boy has passed out during a baseball game and had subsequently died, "I'm afraid it could happen to me also." He went on to talk of his family, his life at home, and his loneliness. I had to remind myself that this young man, who was so concerned about protecting his mother from worry, was only nine.

Jimmy had a good response to medication and within a week was discharged. During the hospitalization, the social worker had several interviews with Max and Mother around financial arrangements, transportation funds, and in general helping them to begin coping at least with material matters in a positive manner. They pointed out that Jimmy's 15-year-old sister knew the diagnosis. They were concerned that she kept her thoughts to herself. It was suggested and they agreed that she come with them when they brought Jimmy back to the clinic in a week or two so that she might get to know the staff caring for Jimmy and have a chance to talk with the psychiatrist if she wished.

First Clinic Visit by the Family (A Week Later)

When I met alone with the sister a week later, she appeared as a stout, timid, 15-year-old girl. She talked of high school, her friends, and generally doing well. Tearfully, she described her inner pain and grief upon learning of the seriousness of Jimmy's illness. "It bothers me to think about it—so I don't." She was concerned about compulsive eating and gaining weight. We did not see her in clinic for the next couple of years when Jimmy was doing relatively well though she knew she was welcome, but we did see her on occasion during the last year-and-a-half of Jimmy's illness. According to Mother, in the interim when she stayed away, she became increasingly obese and kept more and more to herself.

During that same first clinic visit following hospital discharge, Jimmy readily came to the office with me and began, "I have no problems." He described his day at home. Several times he warned me not to tell his mother what he said. He told of having made up his mind not to worry. "What can I do about it?" "I come to the clinic, the doctors check me, tell me to restrict my diet, and take some pills—why worry?" He angrily described being teased at school by a boy who called him "sickly." "I'll pound him if he does it again." "Sure it hurts." He was tearful.

Regarding his father he commented, "Sure I like him"—"But don't tell my mom." "He had a rough life,—was beat up as a kid, never knew how to be good." He lowered his eyes and looked at the floor as he said he hadn't seen his father since he was discharged from the hospital.

He guardedly stated that Max seemed different. "He doesn't seem the same." "Always angry." "Not want to do much with me." He stopped short—"I can't say more." "All I have is your word." I commented that I guessed he really didn't trust me yet.

That same day Max and Mother were seen by the social worker. After some initial defensiveness they began talking of an area of conflict between themselves. Max complained that "she babies Jimmy." "He needs discipline—sick or not." "Gotta face fact— death is death—gonna lose him—no sense hovering over him." As he said this his eyes appeared moist and his hands moved agitatedly. Mother remained calm—too calm—with logical reasoning. The social worker was concerned about Max's handling his inner pain by distancing himself from Jimmy and Mother, and by Mother's cool acceptance.

Second Clinic Visit (A Month Later)

Another month went by before the family returned to the clinic. Max and mother told the social worker that Jimmy had been ill with the chicken pox. Both had been very worried. Again Max was critical of Mother for worrying, crying, and looking sad. He felt that Jimmy "fakes his leg pains." He just wasn't going to pay that much attention to Jimmy. "You gotta treat him normally." Both commented that Jimmy didn't seem worried about his illness. "He never asks any questions about it."—"But he is getting mean." Mother then went on to ask "How do these kids die?" She related that a neighbor boy died recently of a tumor. "Do they die suddenly or linger on?"

That same day Jimmy seemed somewhat reluctant to talk with me. In response to questions about school and how he was feeling he would simply answer "fine." He stated "I'm bored with school." "Can I say something"—"Don't get mad." "I don't feel like talking to anyone." "Just feel like sitting." I commented that he appeared tired and sad. He went on to relate he had had chicken pox—was seen by the family doctor—no shots. "I may have to come back here more often because of having had the chicken pox." "I don't worry about my blood count." "Why worry." "Nothing I can do about it." I asked if any of his schoolmates still teased him. "One guy teased me and I hit him on the jaw." "If he were an older person I would beat him with a club." He related that he still hadn't seen or heard from his father. He hesitated in leaving my office and began asking about my favorite hobbies and sports. He then related that he liked hunting, fishing, and building models and proceeded to elaborate on each of these areas.

Three Months After Hospital Discharge

A month later Jimmy again began by saying everything was fine. I noted that he was cracking his knuckles. He responded "to make them larger." He said he had had two fights with guys who pushed him around. "No one is going to get smart with me." Later, when I asked if he had seen or heard from his father he said "I don't know where he is." He paused "I really do"—"He is in jail for drunk driving." "I'm not proud of this." He again asked for confirmation that what we talked about wasn't shared with his parents. When I reassured him of this he again stated "all I have is your word." He went on to talk of having more enemies than friends.

Later in the interview I asked how he felt about his blood disease, all the lab tests, and having to come back to the clinic. "I used to worry that I had cancer." He related having overheard Max and a friend use the word cancer but hadn't heard the rest of the conversation. He told me of an aunt back in Georgia who had died of cancer. He then reflected on his early life on a farm in Georgia and a desire to return to the farm in "later life." I again asked what happened regarding his concern about cancer. He said he had asked the resident in the hospital if he had cancer and had been told he did not. "All you have is one's word." (I sensed a certain amount of mistrust in this answer from the resident.)

That same day, Max talked of his pain and sense of loss of his own children around his divorce. He was able to relate this to the pain of facing the eventual loss of Jimmy. Again it was clear that he was pulling away from his own disturbing emotions and therefore from Jimmy and Mother. Mother talked of feeling deserted by Max. She then went on to describe recurrent thoughts as to what it would be like when Jimmy was gone.

First Two Years

For the first two years after the diagnosis Jimmy did well. His blood count remained normal and he attended school regularly. He remained on chemotherapy and came to the clinic monthly for evaluation. Jimmy mainly talked of school, hunting, and fishing. He described feeling lonely. It was clear to me that though he wouldn't say so he was eager to visit with me on his trips to the medical center. Several times, if our visits had been inadvertently cut short, or if I spent time with other clinic patients, he would refuse to talk with me.

Max began to doubt the diagnosis. "Maybe he doesn't have leukemia after all." "Maybe he is cured." Mother would react with anger to such statements.

On one visit we learned that Mother had had an ear infection which resulted in temporary facial paralysis. Jimmy had responded by becoming quite dejected and worried about her.

Although I made it clear to Jimmy that he could talk about whatever he wished he avoided the subject of his illness, or concern about it both to me and to the hematologist. However, we were quite aware that Jimmy had gotten to know a number of children with the same disease who were receiving similar medications and diagnostic tests. Frequently, Jimmy would be sitting next to his mother who would ask the social worker what had happened to a particular child. The answers were always truthful such as he or she was admitted to the hospital or he or she had died. It seemed apparent that Mother knew what the answers would be and used this interchange to indirectly convey the seriousness of his illness to Jimmy. At the same time, however, Jimmy would neither ask me such questions nor follow through on what he had heard from the social worker. Whenever I would comment that perhaps he was worried that he too might die he would reply, "Why worry." "Nothing I can do about it."

On one occasion when Max and Mother were talking alone with the hematologist, the social worker asked Jimmy if he wondered what they talked about. He replied, "I know—me." She stated to him that if he had questions about himself he should ask the hematologist. Jimmy replied, "Yes—but I wouldn't get the truth." She commented that she was sure he would get truthful answers. What sort of questions did he have? He hung his head and didn't reply.

Third Year—Exacerbation of the Illness

During the third year of illness Jimmy suffered from recurrent joint pains and swelling due to the exacerbation of the leukemia. Medications were changed. There were two brief stays in the hospital for further diagnostic procedures—bone marrow, knee taps, x rays, and radiation treatment. Max and Mother were again faced with the reality of Jimmy's illness and its terrible prognosis. The family moved to a trailer home adjacent to the mill where the parents worked. Max made fewer trips to the hospital with Jimmy and Mother saying he couldn't take more time off from work. Although Mother recognized the reality of Max's work and that he couldn't face the probable loss of Jimmy, she was angry at him for increasing distance from the family, his tenseness, and angry outbursts. There were more arguments and conflicts between them. Jimmy's sister was fearful that the family arguments would hasten Jimmy's death. Mother regularly discussed these problems with the social worker in addition to the practical realities of obtaining funds for transportation to the hospital and covering hospital bills and medications. Mother expressed her need to encourage and protect Jimmy, "I put on a strong front." At the same time she was increasingly worried and depressed about his illness, exhausted from her own work at the mill, household chores, increasingly frequent trips to the hospital, and marital tensions. On a number of occasions she openly cried within the confines of the social worker's office.

During the early part of the above third year I met with Jimmy fairly regularly. Although I found myself commenting—"it must be upsetting to have such a disease"—"I wonder what sort of things you worry about." "Most young people worry about what will happen." He talked very little of his illness and its exacerbation. He continued to relate concerns about his mother and his need to protect her from worry. He, like his mother, was putting on a "strong front." On several occasions he described his many live pets at home—canary, bees, fish, snake, and dog. He would then talk of pets he had lost, "I don't like to see anything killed or die." This sort of statement, said despondently, came up recurrently in our interviews. The words death, die, kill, were used with increasing frequency and in many contexts.

One day toward the end of this third year Mother related that Jimmy now knew his diagnosis. She related that she had gotten into a struggle with him over his refusing to take his medications. In desperation she had told him he had leukemia and would be very sick and could die if he didn't take medication. She went on to say she felt relieved at having told him—She no longer had to avoid the word or subject—could be more direct and more supportive.

That same afternoon I met Jimmy, Mother, and the social worker in the hallway where they had been talking about another clinic patient with leukemia "like Jimmy's" who was now in the hospital doing poorly. The social worker commented that Jimmy had just stated that he didn't like people talking of his leukemia.

As I met alone with him he commented on his worry about a sore throat and painful knee—"the leukemia is getting worse." I asked what the word leukemia meant to him. In a serious matter-of-fact manner he described his illness as a cancer of the bone marrow for which there was currently no known cure. He went on to relate that he had known this since his first hospital admission when he had overheard the doctors talking about him. "My ears are very big." "I listened when I shouldn't have." He again told me that when his father left he became the man of the house. "But I resent Max's treating me like a little kid." "If my mother had known that I knew all about my illness she would have worried." "I couldn't let anyone know what I had overheard, not even you." He again went on to say that he recurrently tried to cheer his mother by reassuring her that he would be OK. He commented "they gave me three to four years." "Everyone has to go sometime." "I think it is just a matter of months." "I feel better now that it isn't a secret and I can talk about it." He then went on to talk of his resentment towards his teacher who had told the class he had leukemia. "They all treat me differently." He commented on his loneliness, and went on to talk of his pets, model cars, himself, and in one context or another recurrently used the word death or die. He then let me in on another secret—"You know what I like to do best of all—give gifts to people."

Fourth Year—Terminal Phase

Jimmy was then twelve years of age. Over the next year prior to his death his disease progressed. He suffered from recurrent pains—bone and joint—and toxic reactions to the drugs—loss of hair, cushingoid appearance, and month ulcerations. His bone marrow picture worsened and did not respond to chemotherapy. He had to be hospitalized several times for blood transfusions, diagnostic tests, and intravenous chemotherapy. Jimmy's own personal courage amazed me. He continued to have utmost confidence in the hematologist and medical staff responsible for his care.

At times of hospital admission the social worker, hematologist, and myself found ourselves lending support to the ward staff—nurses, technicians, and young physicians who invariably found it upsetting to care for a teenager in the last months of a terminal illness. Such support consisted of listening to their experiences and conflicts in working with Jimmy and similar patients and sharing our own experiences with Jimmy. Our hope was that through such collaboration our individual efforts to help Jimmy and his family would be mutually reinforcing of each other. We were also quite aware of the value and necessity of talking over with other professionals one's own grief, pain and conflicts which were aroused in all of us in working with terminal patients. The fact that Jimmy knew his diagnosis and prognosis made our task somewhat easier in that the staff wasn't caught up having to avoid certain words or subjects.

Much of my own effort with Jimmy consisted of continuing to be available to him, to listen to his concerns, to encourage when possible, and not to desert him. I vividly recall visiting him on the hospital ward during one of the final months. He had just been readmitted to the hospital and had been placed in reverse isolation because of a low blood count and the danger of his picking up infection. There was no TV or radio. He was tearful, lonely, and obviously in pain. "I want to die"—"now"—"I can't stand this"—"It's all over"—"the drugs just prolong it." As I listened I wondered what I could say. I commented that I had seen him pull through worse periods than this. I knew how miserable and discouraged he felt but he would feel differently in a day or two. We weren't giving up—neither should he.

I shared with the ward care staff my concern about Jimmy and the effects of reverse isolation upon his emotional wellbeing. Plans were made to obtain a TV set and radio, for the play lady to take a program to him when he was ready for it, and for ward staff to make a concerted effort to spend more time with him. All limitations on visiting hours were withdrawn. The social worker continued to be available to Mother who also appeared lonely and ready to give up. At one point the social worker called Max and insisted that he come to the hospital more frequently. In an interview that followed she was most supportive with Max acknowledging what he was going through but pointing out that his method of coping—by avoidance—was anything but helpful to Jimmy and his wife. He agreed to try to alter his ways which he did with some success. Together they were able to offer increased support to Jimmy (just being there and emotionally available).

Jimmy rallied through several such low points and returned home. When I saw him in outpatient clinic he appeared cheerful. He had not been able to attend school and had to spend each day at home while Mother and Max worked in the adjacent lumbermill. In describing how he spent his time he reminded me that he wasn't really alone. He went on to talk of all his pets and his interaction with them. He then let me in on another secret. "Don't tell anyone for they would make fun of me." With considerable elaboration and excitement he described how he would pretend he was a big game hunter. Each day he would set up tents with blankets, make caves from piled up chairs, and take his play rifle on his daily dangerous hunting missions. He would come face to face with lions, tigers, elephants, and snakes and wipe them out one by one.

Jimmy's leukemia became unresponsive to chemotherapy. He knew, his parents knew, and the staff knew the end was near. After long, careful, concerned deliberation, the hematology staff decided to stop all further chemotherapy but to continue with supportive therapy—blood transfusions and pain medication. This was based on the fact that he was no longer responding to these drugs and the quality of his limited remaining life was worsened by their toxic effects. Jimmy seemed ready but not desperate to die.

In the next several weeks Jimmy and his mother made weekly trips (6–7 hours round trip) to the medical center. With help from the social worker, Mother verbalized her ambivalence about these weekly trips—she was sure the local doctor could give what supportive medical care was needed. It was obvious that the next hospitalization would be his last.

Our own clinical team—hematologist, social worker, and psychiatrist—discussed the advisability of having the family make these long, tiring trips on a weekly basis. After all we didn't have new drugs to use and were entirely focused on supportive medical care. No heroic services were contemplated. On the other hand, what we could offer was whatever hope and support the family could gain by coming back weekly and our being available to them. It was also clear that Jimmy was increasingly turning to his mother for the emotional support he so needed. She in turn needed what support we could offer her. We openly discussed with Max and Mother our desire to see them regularly in the clinic. They agreed and seemed relieved. Jimmy had told his mother he wanted to stay home as long as possible with his family and avoid his final days in the hospital. We listened and agreed to this. That day was the last time I saw Jimmy and his parents. He was pale, weak, and feeling low. We talked briefly and said goodbye—"see you next week."

Several days later we learned that Jimmy had been admitted to the local hospital where he died that same day.

Discussion

Albert J. Solnit, M.D. (U.S.A.)

This is a poignant presentation of the assistance provided by a child psychiatrist as a member of a clinical team caring for a child and his family over a three-year period as they all cope with the course of their lives while the son is dying of acute leukemia. The evaluation and treatment of Jimmy and the assistance provided to his family reflects the superb sensitivity and cooperation of the clinical group as well as the limitations of our knowledge and resources in proffering assistance to the patient and his family. Jimmy was eager to stay in contact, but the pace at which he could acknowledge his illness and accept guidance and psychological support was subtly determined by many influences. These included his capacity to cope with knowing the consequences of his illness, his tolerance for the anxiety that was generated by the family's recognition of the illness and its outcome, and by the psychological and somatic depletion caused by the illness and its treatment.

Dr. Binger's report requires us to accept the need for group care for Jimmy and his family, the group consisting of physicians, nurses, and a social worker. Can such group assistance retain the strengthening influence of person-to-person care while offering the knowledge and energy that no one professional can be expected to provide in the 1970's? This report describes one such effort, largely successful, without minimizing or glossing over the difficulties or the failures to be effective.

When a nine-year-old boy confronts death and dying as Jimmy did over a three-year period, his anxieties will center not only on the fear of pain and the unknown, but also on the impotent rage that is associated with feeling cheated because his present life is crippled and his future expectations are dismal. Family difficulties heightened Jimmy's sense of impotence and apprehension and magnified his feelings of helplessness. He felt blocked from protesting or taking effective action to gain hope or find relief. The relief of taking action on his own behalf seemed unavailable to him because of the physiological depletion and because of the conspiracy of silence imposed by the adults. The adults were manifestly motivated by their wishes to protect the child.

However, it often happens, especially in leukemia, that the child knows about his fatal illness but also knows that he is not supposed to know. This prohibition heightens the child's sense of helplessness and bewilders him, often to the extent that he feels cut off from his parents and siblings. In this connection the fatally ill child tends to lose confidence in his ability to understand and cope with his fears and anticipations. Dr. Binger's presentation emphasizes the importance of individualizing the plan to inform or not to inform a child about the immediate and long-term expectations he can have about his illness and its treatment.

The medical group often finds themselves particularly thwarted in helping a Jimmy to cope because they are aware that the family problems may be heightened rather than miraculously resolved or deferred as they unite to cope with their son's fatal illness. Though some families are able to mobilize their resources, functioning beyond their usual capacity in order to help their child and themselves cope with the diagnosis, treatment, and outcome of a fatal illness, just as often the challenge presented by their dying child complicates the preexisting problems of the family and further weakens their capacities to function effectively.

The wisdom that is modestly expressed in Dr. Binger's study and report is that health personnel can be helpful to a child who is dying and to his family, if they are patient, tolerant of their limitations, able to work together rather than compete in their care of the patient and his family, and eager to convey relief and assistance through understanding. As Freud so clearly demonstrated, therapeutic zeal is no substitute for the healing qualities of insight and comprehension. Truth is liberating and ameliorative when it is administered with due respect for tolerances and in the context of care and support.

Reginald S. Lourie, M.D. (U.S.A.)

This sensitive and poignant case report highlights the importance of active participation by mental health professionals on the medical team which carries responsibility for the management of the child with a terminal illness. The support provided is needed not only for the child himself but also for the family and the medical and nursing staff.

With this family, the help necessary was to assist them with the process of grieving long before the child died, as well as assisting with less productive defenses such as denial. With the child-care staff, it was to support them when there was the understandable tendency to avoid and withdraw when valiant efforts to save life began to fail.

With the child himself, there was the need to help him maintain his defenses, never taking away hope, and preserving the fantasies of strength and ability to continue to protect his mother.

In some experts' opinion, the child who can understand should know his diagnosis of leukemia. Others sharply disagree. This case would seem to reinforce the position of those who would tell the child. Jimmy knew his diagnosis from the beginning and gave the psychiatrists hints of this. However, he respected the adult's conspiracy of silence until his mother's anger and frustration ("but you don't die") brought it out into the open. However, one should not generalize about this type of communication. It should be individualized in terms of a given child, in a given family.

One important missing piece in the handling of this case is the lack of a resource that could reach out into the patient's own community and the outlying hospital. Continuity of support even with patients from rural areas can be structured by making the visiting public health nurses, a physician, a social worker, or a clergyman, an extended member of a network working in collaboration with the medical center team.

Howard Hansen, M.D. (U.S.A.)

The brevity imposed on this discussion limits my remarks to the following salient issues:

I find most unsettling the still existent delusion among adults that one "can be kept in ignorance of—diagnosis"-the purported *secret*. Some level of cognitive awareness most assuredly is present in any one of any age afflicted with fatal illness. Knowledge of unconscious processes and covert communication renders the possibility of "ignorance" indefensible. When the deceit had finally ended well into the third year, Jimmy shared an inner world of fantasy he had found necessary to construct. As a big game hunter he was able, one by one, to wipe out his adversaries. He identified with those aggressors toward him—better to wipe out than be wiped out. Can there be doubt who in displacement was represented in the threatening dangerous monstrous predators! In even the initial interview with Dr. Binger, Jimmy probed for an invitation to learn more of the concerns he had of his illness when he related "in a most serious manner (that) he knew a boy who had leukemia—and subsequently died."

As Dr. Binger did, I too have entered into a *contract* with parents and colleagues of "keeping the child in ignorance." No longer is such a contract tenable to me. The very nature of the psychodynamic inherent in a "truly confidential relationship" precludes such a restrictive bind. It is nondynamic and nontherapeutic.

Brief mention of *age* is relevant. Approaches and responses must be couched by age groupings along established psychoanalytic and developmental phase constructs. Jimmy at nine had acquired logical thinking and his potential for understanding reality was greater than that for which he was given credit.

The psychological responses and needs of *staff* working with the fatally and terminally ill calls for improved avenues of collaboration and communication to be found and maintained if we are to retrieve from attrition those who develop that very expertness required for maximal therapeutic effectiveness.

Noteworthy was Dr. Binger's and his colleagues' ability to reach a decision in *terminal phase* when further "heroic services" were to be abandoned. This is an ethical and humane position that should be mandated as the *dénouement* of a death challenging engagement. Enlightened medical realism declares when this point is reached. Then, support, relief of pain and panic producing symptoms and situations, presence, and love supersede all other considerations.

The mourning process, though in modified form from the event of death itself, is initiated with the pronouncement of fatal disease. Our present understanding of this process permits temporal prediction. If we accept approximately one year as usual for the work of mourning, what then occurs when the mourning work has been partially satisfied and the mourned one yet survives? Ambivalence results and that ambivalence seems reasonably well substantiated in the reactions of the family members in the case presented. Decathexis of the loved object occurs gradually whether the loss is relative or in fact. This factor complicates the clinical course and management of fatal illnesses of unpredictable duration.

One element of the case haunts me as it has before. Jimmy's illness began some ten months prior to the assignment of a diagnosis. The several years preceding those initial symptoms were troubled and disturbed ones. Our experience, as that of others, suggests that significant life events most often related to loss appear more frequently in these histories than one can comfortably accept as coincidence. What then are we yet to learn of the contribution—minor or significant in the possible *psychoetiology* of oncological processes? Immunologic and hematologic advances have now established the possibility of cellular ravage in all of us. What precisely is the composite that triggers the morbid process that results in malignant manifestation?

I sorrow for Jimmy and the Jimmys and Jeanies I have known. Their journeys have too often been lonely ones. I cannot but linger with the thought that until cancer is conquered, as I believe it will be, we can better apply what we now know in making that journey more tolerable for all.

Cyrille Koupernik, M.D. (France)

I want to make several comments on different levels. The first has to do with the overall feeling generated in the reader that life is (in Camus' sense) fundamentally absurd. Here we have an intelligent and generous child who, when his natural father leaves the family, is ready to take over and who, when he discovers that he has a fatal illness, keeps this knowledge to himself, with the stoicism of a Roman patrician, in order to protect his mother's feelings. Why should such a superior individual be sentenced to death? In my opinion, this problem of justice, illness, and death is a major issue. It appears very clearly in the reactions of the family to the news. The shock is, of course, understandable and so is disbelief though this implies that for some reason they would have expected to be protected against this kind of major catastrophe. But then we come to the irrational feelings of self-blame and anger. This particular response has been nurtured by generations of physicians constantly on the hunt for causal factors within the family so that parents have learned to blame themselves for their bad genes, their bad feelings or their bad child-rearing techniques. They have been sensitized to feel guilty.

The second comment has to do with the reaction of the peer group to Jimmy's illness. Characteristically, they show themselves unfeelingly cruel in the first stage, teasing him for being "sickly"; then, when they know that the illness will be fatal, they become respectful and somewhat fearful, attitudes that hurt him just as much.

The third remark would concern the dynamics of the family group. The mother seems rather self-concerned, if not hostile, as if she would rather have Jimmy die at once because she is not sure that she will be able to tolerate his prolonged agony. Her second husband, Max, is ambivalent and insecure in his feelings toward the dying child who is not his son and of whom he is undoubtedly jealous because of the attention he receives from the mother. The same probably holds true for the sister.

The fourth remark deals with the traditional and long-standing argument between American and French doctors. We, on this side of the Atlantic Ocean, rather tend not to tell the truth even to adults when we know that they are going to die which fits in with the unconscious wish of the patient himself. We find an example of this in Solzhenytzyn's *Cancer Ward* where a specialist in cancer denies frantically any evidence of this disease once she herself gets it. Yet, in the present case, it is obvious from the beginning that Jimmy knows he is going to die and, therefore, the "conspiracy of silence" is manifestly a mistake. This need not be true for other cases.

Finally, I would like to comment on the very difficult role of the child psychiatrist in such a situation. I can only admire Dr. Binger's tact, devotion, and refusal to interpret along theoretical lines, preferring to offer Jimmy his friendship and help him to die not in complete aloneness.

May I add that this type of case should be presented very often to students and perhaps even to doctors since it emphasizes one of the main and most useful tasks of psychiatry and, in particular, of child psychiatry.

DEATH AND MOURNING

Editorial Comment (Section IV)

Loss is the common denominator of this chapter and of course the most radical example of loss is death. Loss through death may be experienced currently with grief and mourning or it may be experienced indirectly in terms of an increased susceptibility to mental disorder or suicide many years after the original loss. For death to be an impact through successive generations, the loss would need to be of a catastrophic order, disrupting not only the lives of those contemporary with the experience but also the offsprings of such individuals who have had no immediate contact with the circumstances of the loss. A heinous example of a cross-generational effect would be the large-scale exterminations that took place in the Nazi concentration camps. The impact of this type of experience upon children born many years after to survivors is well illustrated in Furman's paper where the psychological continuum between the generations is exemplified by the way in which the mother's guilty feelings and horrifying memories generate a prepsychotic attitude in the child.

This is only one of many examples demonstrating how fragile is the state of equilibrium that we label normalcy. It should not surprise us, therefore, when a disturbing event like death creates a disequilibrium in the individual or in the group but as members of the therapeutic profession, we have to learn that we ourselves may become part of the disequilibrium and that we need to manage, first and foremost, our own reactions which may be strikingly similar to those manifested by the persons directly involved in the loss. We can become as deeply concerned and dream about it like Schowalter's nurses, as guilt-ridden by our failures and as prone to denial as the relatives themselves. If we feel guilty, can we be surprised that the siblings of leukemic children studied by Binger should often be inundated with guilt? Another factor affecting the equilibrium of feeling is the alteration in the death process brought about by technical advances. This means that the terminal phase of the illness takes place more frequently in the hospital so that the loss is sustained within an unfamiliar and sterile environment. For this reason, as Solnit emphasizes, we must do our best to ensure that the mourning process of the family as a group is not interfered with, interrupted, or prevented. All of this goes to show that if we are to help in the tragedy of death, we must comply with the requirement laid down by the poet Horace (and quoted by Paul) that we feel pain ourselves.

Mourning is the ritualized way to deal with loss. To use Laing's terminology, it is "a trip" in the way he sees every mental disorder as representing a trip into one's own unexplored depths to find solutions. Without sharing all of Laing's views, it seems important to regard mourning not as an empty ritual but as a most effective way to normalize death and include it into life. To this extent, Homer's characters seem wiser and more humane than the Platonic Socrates who, as Paul reminds us, can only counsel us to adopt a stoical and contemptuous attitude toward death.

There is no doubt that therapeutic progress in recent years may have a disrupting influence on traditional mourning modifying both its content and its sequence. As a result of remissions, anticipatory grief tends to be postponed or replaced by hopes which actually constitute a denial of reality. At the same time and for the same reasons, the process of death is removed from the home, its natural place, into the hospital.

The loss of the loved object, even though partial, can be equally damaging in the case of the mentally ill. As shown by Anthony, a chronic psychosis profoundly endangers the idealized image within the child. This again is a price paid for technical progress. In previous decades, psychotics were committed to mental hospitals and the commitment was the equivalent of civil death. Today a great many of these patients are treated on an outpatient basis. They may, therefore, exhibit disturbing behavior resulting from drugs or from the disease itself and this may give rise in the child to two types of reaction, namely, alienation (with the bizarre parent) and abandonment (with the withdrawn, inaccessible, and remote parent). When studying the effects of schizophrenic illness in the parent upon the children, we have, therefore, to weigh three possible channels of influence—heredity, the distortion, and alienation of the parental image and subsequently identification with it.

All these situations of loss tend to mobilize coping mechanisms. With bereavement through death, one can compare the ritualized traditional mourning organized by culture with the unassisted and idiosyncratic effects of personal mourning and attempt to evaluate the efficacy of either approach in preventing later disturbances. As a profession we must be fully aware of our duty and obligation in this important sphere and we can be extremely helpful only if our clinical knowledge is adequate and our measure of empathy is sufficient.

Cyrille Koupernik, M. D.

Childhood Leukemia – Emotional Impact on Siblings

C. M. Binger, M.D. (U.S.A.)

Introduction

Few other human experiences involve as much anguish and suffering for families as the death of a child—the permanent premature termination to an unfulfilled life.

In a previous publication the results were reported of a retrospective study within a pediatric hematology clinic of some twenty families who had lost a child from acute leukemia. In half the families studied, one or more members ultimately required psychiatric care, and in more than half, one or more previously (and seemingly) well-adjusted siblings showed altered behavior patterns that indicated considerable difficulty in coping. Although these symptoms generally became manifest during the course of the sibling's terminal illness, the more severe reactions followed the actual death of the sibling and persisted. Disorders reported by parents included enuresis, headaches, poor school performance, school phobia, depression, severe anxieties, and persistent abdominal pains. The following vignettes demonstrate some of these reactions.

CASE 1–JIM

Jim was seven at the time his eight-year-old brother, Mike, was diagnosed as having leukemia. Approximately one year later Mike died. Jim, who had always been close to his brother, had been informed of the seriousness of Mike's condition. He had seemed to function adequately during the course of the illness, but after his brother's death he began withdrawing into a world of his own. He went to stay with his grandparents and protracted his visit to about a month. He allowed no one to mention Mike's name. He blamed his mother for his brother's death and declined to do anything she requested of him. He became prone to angry outbursts and was physically aggressive toward his younger sister. These symptoms were still in evidence one-and-one-half years later at the time of the retrospective interview.

CASE 2–JERRY

Jerry was five when his six-year-old sister developed leukemia. During the succeeding 15 months before her death he had seemed somewhat sullen but otherwise functioned adequately. His relationship to his sister was quite close. The parents had chosen not to tell either of the children how serious the illness was, but following the girl's death they did share with him the fact that she was dead and "had gone to heaven." That same evening he developed so severe a headache that the family doctor was called. Jerry did not grieve openly but increasingly withdrew into himself. The headaches continued and did not respond to medication. He was referred to a neurologist and had a comprehensive neurological evaluation including a pneumoencephalogram, but no psychiatric appraisal was made. At the time of the retrospective interview, some three years later, the headaches still persisted.

CASE 3–JILL

Jill was eight months of age when her two-year-old brother developed leukemia. Ten weeks later he died. During the course of his illness he remained in the hospital continuously except for one week. For this period Jill was cared for by her grandmother and a baby-sitter since her parents, who were quite upset at the time (and for several years after), spent most of their time at the hospital. From time to time, Mother made visits home but Jill seemed not to recognize her although she became distressed when her mother left for the hospital again. Following the sibling's death, Jill experienced sleeping difficulties—recurrent awakening and crying. She markedly regressed in all areas of development and clung excessively to her mother. These symptoms persisted for well over a year.

COMMENTS ON SEVERITY OF SYMPTOMS

Reactions of a child to the fatal illness and subsequent death of a sibling include not only immediate physical and psychological symptoms associated with grief but, in a number of children, continue toward enduring symptoms and distortions in character structure.

Cain et al. [1] reported the complex pathological distortions involved in children's disturbed reactions to the death of a sibling to include such areas as affect, cognition, belief system, superego functioning, and object relationships (1964).

This presentation would fully support these conclusions and the implications they have for preventive mental health.

A child's transient and persistent responses to the threatened and subsequent loss of a sibling is multidetermined in differing parts dependent on the individual stage of development, the total response of the family, the "natural history" of the illness, and the extent to which the illness becomes intertwined with the family conflicts. What is of special importance is the sequence of events which the family experiences from the onset of the leukemia through to the death of the patient. When the initial diagnosis is made, the family members invariably experience some "anticipatory grief reactions." The illness may last weeks to years. Frequently, during most of the illness, the child is, in remission, completely free of symptoms and lives a normal life apart from making periodic clinic visits and taking medications regularly. At these times, it is quite easy for families to deny the seriousness of the disease and to continue with little or no change in their life style. However, when relapse occurs, or side effects from the medication develop, defenses such as denial no longer prove adequate and the anticipatory grief reaction becomes more manifest within and between family members. A fatal outcome appears inevitable at some undetermined time and this reality constantly and profoundly affects the adaptation of the group both individually and as a whole.

Each member tends to react in a manner consistent with his own personality structure, past experiences, current adjustment, and the special meaning that the future loss has for him in particular. During this preterminal period of illness, the dying child continues to remain very much a part of the family. His reaction to his illness, the nature of the condition, and the form of communication established between him and his relatives markedly influence the family dynamics. Most families, however, manage somehow to cope with the demands of this phase, whether brief or prolonged. It is the terminal sequence that puts the family to its severest test when they are often found wanting—the death of the child, the funeral, grief and mourning, and the subsequent reintegration of the group, less one member. The absent one remains very much in evidence through photographs, associated possessions, memories, family discussions, anniversaries, trips to the cemetery, etc., and each experience exacts its toll. The reactions to the death crisis vary considerably from group to group in terms of the intensity and persistence of grief, but there is no doubt that the children, to some extent, take their cue from the parents. The following is an example of a family with a limited capacity to cope with the trauma of death but this inability is foreshadowed in the reaction to childhood losses.

The Case of Eric

Mr. and Mrs. Jones applied to the Child Psychiatry Service because of their concern over their 13-year-old son, Eric. They described him as becoming increasingly isolated from the family, moody, sensitive, difficult to talk with, prone to crying spells, underachieving at school, accident prone, and "possibly suicidal." They linked the onset of these symptoms with his younger sister's death from leukemia four years previously.

Eric was Caucasian, Catholic, and attended the seventh grade of a parochial school in a small town about an hour's drive from the clinic. The family constellation included his father, aged 38, a sales representative for a small industry; his mother, aged 36, a secretary; a 62-year-old maternal grandmother who had lived in the home since the birth of his sister Susan some nine years previously; and his eleven-year old brother, Bob.

My initial acquaintance with his family had been four years previously during the course of a retrospective study within the pediatric hematology clinic of families who had lost a child from acute leukemia. At that time I had a two-hour interview with Mr. and Mrs. Jones during which they expressed concern about Eric's behavior and had been referred to a local counseling agency but this had discontinued when their counselor left the district.

In order to obtain some understanding of the genesis of Eric's disorder and its relation to his sister's death, it is pertinent to discuss the family situation prior to the illness as well as the subsequent eight months ending with the death and the family's struggle with its sense of loss. Before we look at the family as a whole, we will examine the life experiences of each member separately.

A. THE FAMILY CONSTELLATION

Mr. Jones had had a hectic and unhappy childhood. His father drank heavily and frequently beat his mother. Following high school he left home and moved to California to the town where he now lived. Soon afterwards his parents separated and his mother and sister joined him. At 23, he met and married his wife. The marriage was described as uneventful. His mother was in her 80's, suffered several minor strokes and talked openly of being "ready to die." Yet she remained independent and active and made no attempt to interfere with his family life. His sister died of an acute heart attack four years after Susan's death. He seemed to accept this in a matter-of-fact manner and likewise his father's death some years previously. He frequently referred to himself as a "complete failure," a "nervous wreck," and one who kept his thoughts and feelings to himself.

Mrs. Jones also described her childhood as chaotic and unhappy. Her parents fought constantly and she recalled her father physically attacking her mother on numerous occasions. Once after accusing her of infidelity, he attempted to kill her with a razor and then cried on his daughter's shoulder in shame. Her parents separated when she was eleven and she continued living with her mother. She soon found herself emotionally replacing her father with her uncle who subsequently died of throat cancer five years after Susan's death. During her adolescent years she was locked into an emotional struggle with her mother, and at eighteen left home to go to work because she felt that either she or her mother would have "an emotional breakdown" unless she got away. Two years later she met her husband and married him. They settled in the small town in California where Mr. Jones had been living along with his mother and sister. She saw herself as nervous and worrying, but efficient in her work.

After three years of marriage, Eric was born without complication. Two years later Bob was born, and after another two years, Susan. It was at this time that the maternal grandmother, divorced from her husband, came to live with the family to help in raising Susan. Mrs. Jones had not liked this but was unable to say "no," and so the ambivalent relationship was resumed. The grandmother was critical and nagging of everyone except Susan whom she treated "as her own daughter" much to the resentment of Mrs. Jones who could not bring herself to the point of asking her to leave. "I wouldn't know if she were all right." Mr. Jones in turn accepted this situation without comment. At this point in time Mrs. Jones again escaped from her mother by taking a full-time secretarial job, leaving the housework and cooking to her mother and husband. When home, she withdrew from the situation by obsessively reading "novels which always had a happy ending." Both the children and her husband complained irritably of her complete preoccupation with her reading. She isolated herself even further from the family by harping on her inner religious life and faith in God as a source of support and comfort. This awkward, tense family relationship continued without interruption and was no doubt responsible for Eric's growing difficulties.

Mrs. Jones recalled that Eric was a "cute baby." She held back full expression of love for him so as not to spoil him. She recalled the struggles over his toilet training and the angry beatings she administered when he soiled. Apart from this, his early development seemed otherwise normal. The kindergarten teacher regarded him as immature and was hesitant to pass him on to the first grade. However, he did perform adequately in the first grade and was in the second grade when Susan became ill. In contrast to Eric's quietness and moodiness, his brother Bob was described as being "open and outgoing." Susan's early development was also said to have been uneventful.

Thus, at the point in time when the terminal illness began, we find Susan, aged three, closely attached to an elderly, depressed, and nagging maternal grandmother who was essentially running the household; Eric, aged seven, inhibited and introverted; Bob, aged five, spontaneous and extroverted; Mrs. Jones, caught in a stressful, ambivalent relationship with her own mother and escaping through obsessional reading, religious preoccupations, and outside employment; and Mr. Jones who tended to let things take their course but was disgruntled and nervous and regarded himself as a complete failure.

B. THE ILLNESS

Susan's illness began in late May with a low-grade fever and vomiting. She became increasingly listless and two weeks later complained of her legs and feet hurting. Mrs. Jones, who was at that time working for an orthopedist, thought of the possibility of a bone infection and took her to an orthopedist who, upon noting an enlarged spleen, referred her to a pediatrician. The white blood count was found to be elevated. Both parents recalled the pediatrician commenting that this could be a toxic reaction, infection, or possibly leukemia. "When we heard the word "leukemia" we were scared." Mother thought, "Oh no! It can't happen to us." They went to a nearby lab for a bone marrow study. That same afternoon the pediatrician called them and said that Susan had leukemia. He recommended referral to the University. "We cried; it was a shock. We knew there was no cure from the beginning. It was the most painful aspect of the entire experience." Father recalled, "I accepted the diagnosis immediately. There were just too many facts that fitted the picture." Both parents said they had been familiar with the word "leukemia" through magazine articles they had read. Father commented, "It is just one of these things that you let pass by at the time and think it could never happen in your own family."

They recalled their first visit to the University Hospital. "We kept hoping that the specialists at the University would find that Susan did not have leukemia." However, the diagnosis was confirmed. They recalled a lengthy conference with the hematologist where the diagnosis was confirmed and they discussed their various concerns regarding prognosis and treatment. This had been most helpful to them in that they had some idea what to expect and quickly gained confidence in the specialist. Susan had a good initial remission to drugs and was discharged by the hospital after ten days "feeling like her old self again." She was followed by her local pediatrician along with periodic visits to the University and continued to do well until four months later when she developed headaches, nausea, and a marked change in personality, becoming fretful and irritable. Lumbar puncture revealed that she had central nervous system leukemia and once again she was admitted to the University Hospital in November where she responded well to medication.

Eight days later, she was home, "feeling like her old self," but the bone marrow and peripheral blood picture revealed that the leukemia was in exacerbation. Various changes of medication were instituted. In March the following year she developed chicken pox and was readmitted to the hospital. Both parents recalled how terribly sick she was with high temperature, deep black pox marks, etc. They began to question the necessity for further treatment with the probable prolongation of her suffering. Although she recovered from this acute episode and was sent home after she had no further remissions. She became increasingly weak and lethargic, and made no response to medication. For most of the month of March and early April she was confined to bed at home. Finally, she was taken back to the hospital for the last two weeks of her life, the last five hours of which were in a state of shock.

Both parents regretted that they had not been with her when she died. They had stayed with her for five days and, since her condition seemed stable, decided to return home for a night. While there, they were recalled to the hospital. "We knew the end had come."

Susan had known that she had a blood disease called leukemia but it was doubtful whether she understood the implications of this. However, her mother felt that she knew she wasn't going to live long. She recalled her asking, "When am I going to die," and "When I die I'm going to heaven and kiss President Kennedy." Susan had been in the hospital during the Kennedy assassination and had reacted strongly to this with crying. She frequently and freely talked of death. Her parents recalled that "she seemed to grow up overnight," in fact, she insisted that she was "grown up and through with high school." They finally went along with this delusion. "It was almost as if she felt she had to live her whole life in a short time. It was a supernatural type of reaction."

Both parents reflected on their own reaction to the diagnosis and the following eight months leading to Susan's death. After the initial shock and grief they found themselves "taking one day at a time." There were the trips to the pediatrician, to the hospital, and to the hematology clinic. With each visit, until the last, they had a magical expectation that everything would come out well and that Susan would respond. It was during what turned out to be the final trip to the University that both realistically conceded that the end was near. During the early stages of the illness, Mother found herself turning to "inner" religion for strength and support. "I became aware of God in everything I did; material things became meaningless." She recalled how, at the time of Susan's death, she had viewed the body, cried briefly, and was suddenly aware of a feeling of comfort and relaxation in accepting God's will. "It was a tremendous calm." Father commented that from the beginning "I couldn't accept it. It was like murder. I found myself mad at God. It was unnecessary suffering for Susan. I no longer accept religion." He felt he had not gone through this period as well as his wife. His work had suffered. He described how every day he would go to work worrying that at night he would come home and find Susan in critical condition. "Sometimes I wouldn't want to come home at all, but I did." What support he gained was through talking things over with his wife. Grandmother would not accept the diagnosis at first, but later she became more obviously upset, had spells of crying, and nagged the family more. She insisted that "the only one who really cares for me is Susan."

The boys were left with the grandmother when Susan and her parents were at the hospital. "It was a worse year for them than it was for Susan. They suffered more. We were gone so much. Friends brought presents for Susan but not for the boys." They had been very open with the two boys about Susan's illness from the beginning. We told them she was very ill and would not be with us for long—that she would die. Mother commented, "I wanted them to be prepared emotionally." Both boys reacted with disbelief and denial and throughout the illness repeatedly asked when Susan would recover. The parents were particularly concerned about Eric who became increasingly sullen and withdrawn. Although he had reacted with little overt affect on being told the diagnosis, he was hysterically upset over the loss of a pet kitten some days later. Unlike Susan, neither of the boys asked questions about death or dying.

C. FOLLOWING THE DEATH

The parents described their return home after Susan's death. The boys had not seen her for the previous two weeks since she had been in the hospital. Eric reacted to being told that Susan had died and gone to heaven by stating, "But I prayed." He turned and walked away. He, like his father, expressed anger at God. Bob seemed to accept what was said without further questions.

They chose to have an open casket at the funeral. "We felt it was real important that the boys realize where she had gone. They hadn't seen her for two weeks." They recalled that upon visiting the funeral parlor Eric held his mother's hand, briefly peeked in the coffin, shed a few tears, and pulled back. "He never has really grieved her loss. He keeps everything to himself."

Bob reacted differently. He went to the casket, touched the body, and seemed fascinated. He asked why she was so cold and hard. Mother told him that the soul leaves the body, goes to heaven and that the remains of the body are cold and hard. He seemed content with this explanation and was appropriately tearful.

Grandmother reacted most strongly. She grieved hysterically. Her own real reason for existence was gone.

At the funeral, Eric did not cry openly but was teary-eyed. He turned to his mother and asked her not to cry. Bob allowed himself to cry.

Although Susan was dead and buried, she remained very much a part of the family. Over the years leading to this psychiatric evaluation of Eric, there were frequent trips to the cemetery to place flowers on the grave. Grandmother's depression remained. She had recurrent crying spells, talked of her loss of Susan, and openly talked of leaving or just dying since no one really cared for her. Recollections of Susan were recurrent themes of family discussions. All cherished every moment they had had with her. Mother returned to work, her obsessional readings of happy novels, and continued to find solace in her religious thoughts. Like her mother, she experienced another grief reaction when her uncle (the man who had, in effect, replaced her father in her life) died of throat cancer. Father felt he had never been the same since Susan's death. He reacted to the death of his own sister with little affect. "I felt emotionally exhausted." Eric increasingly withdrew into himself and his grades in school dropped markedly. Both parents felt that he blamed God and himself for Susan's death. In spite of the recurrent conflict with his grandmother he seemed extremely concerned for her and worried that she might go away and die. He would occasionally get into bed with her and express a desire to lie close to her. He asked his mother "do you love me?" so many times that she would get irritated.

D. PSYCHIATRIC EVALUATION

Eric's first visit to the Child Psychiatric Clinic was approximately five years after Susan's death. It began with a conjoint family interview consisting of the Child Psychiatrist, a resident in child psychiatry, Mr. and Mrs. Jones, Eric, and Bob. The boys were told that their parents had been seen four years previously and had talked about their concerns at that time. Since then the family had passed through a difficult period, and the reason for the present meeting was to talk about any unhappy feelings or misunderstandings that might have arisen as a result. It could be helpful to discuss these. In between the two meetings with the family as a whole each of them would have an individual meeting focusing on problems that they were unable to express in the group. In addition, it was arranged for Eric to be seen diagnostically by a clinical and educational psychologist and to have a physical and neurological examination to find out what might be contributing to his learning difficulties. An individual interview with the grandmother was also added since she was very much a problem member of the family.

During this first conjoint interview Eric appeared tense and anxious and his mother, on several occasions, and with some frustration, pleaded with him to open up. "The problem is that you don't talk to us—how can we help you?" Mr. Jones also expressed irritation with Eric's sullenness. Bob, as usual seemed more relaxed and spontaneous. To all his parents' overtures, Eric responded with disgust and silence. The parents then complained that Bob too was becoming a behavior problem in school and not attending to his school work. At this, Eric and Bob both verbalized their irritation at Mother's obsessive reading, Father's moodiness, and Grandmother's nagging. This led, it seemed, inevitably to a review of the cirumstances around Susan's illness and death, and Eric became tearful. He seemed to have "forgotten" a considerable part of the past history which Bob was quick to fill in.

In his individual sessions, Eric initially showed considerable denial of problems at home or at school. However, by the third individual session he was more open and relaxed and talked with sullen affect and tears of his concerns for Susan surrounding her illness and death. He appeared depressed and quite constricted.

Grandmother, when seen, was also tense and anxious and quickly revealed feelings of depression and fears of death. She cried openly as she talked of losing Susan and more recently her younger brother. She was clinically depressed.

The clinical psychologist pointed out that Eric appeared to have a potential for intellectual functioning within the bright, normal range and perhaps higher. Within the WISC there was marked contrast between Eric's high level of ability in abstraction and his lower social judgment. He concluded that Eric's conflict had resulted in some distortion of cognitive development. The most prominent aspect of Eric's functioning on the Rorschach test was constriction.

He appeared to be deeply afraid of losing emotional control and was reactively overcontrolled through the use of repression, isolation, and intellectualization. He perceived the mother figure as potentially destructive, and one sequence of associations suggested that in fantasy, he held his mother responsible for the death of his sister. He seemed caught between a fear of his own aggression and a fear of his mother's destructive potential. His father, on the other hand, he saw as depressed and withdrawn.

The educational psychologist found that his overall achievement was within the average range for a seventh grader (he had repeated sixth grade and was currently in the seventh grade). He was two years behind in oral reading and spelling. In viewing his intellectual potential it was clear that he was underachieving.

Physical, neurological, EEG, and laboratory tests were normal, and his past medical history was essentially negative.

During the course of the brief therapeutic contact with the family, resolution of conflict within and between the family members was beginning to take place. This was particularly apparent in the final conjoint meeting when Eric's depression and constriction were shown to be closely related to the conflictual situation within the family, conflicts that had been reactivated and intensified by crisis of dying and death. A therapeutic program was planned for the family, children and adults, who agreed to undertake this at their local psychiatric clinic.

Discussion

A death in a family all too frequently leads to profound and enduring psychopathology within and between family members. Several authors, Furman [2, 3], Weiner [4], and Rosenblatt [5], have described children's reactions to a death in the family. Nagera [6], recently discussed the various factors that determine children's reactions to object loss and concluded that the loss of an important object represents a developmental interference. He commented on some of the characteristic responses of grief in childhood: "The short sadness span; the incapacity to sustain mourning; the massive use of denial and reversal of affect; the inability to grasp the reality of death; the search for substitutes (before the event, if the child was aware of oncoming death, and after, if he was not); the simultaneous (overt and insidious) symptom formation and the creeping character distortions; the fear of "contamination" causing their own death, often side by side with fantasies of reunion."

In our own supportive efforts with the siblings of children with leukemia, we have noted their inner feelings of being responsible for the sibling's death, fears that they will be next, resentment that the parents spend so much time with the ill child, anger at the parents who "allowed" the sibling to become ill, and preoccupation with inner fantasies around death.

The child's reaction to terminal illness and subsequent loss is not only intrapsychic but inevitably also interrelated with the altered family *dynamics*. The sources of disturbance are numerous and difficult to disentangle and each child's reaction is in some ways unique. This is likewise true for the adult family members who together with the child are experiencing a *profound crisis* which will have persisting effects on all concerned. The author's experience from retrospective and prospective studies of families with a leukemic child tallies with that of Cain and his co-workers.

"Reviewing the clinical data, the determinants of children's response to the death of a sibling we found to include: the nature of the death; the age and characteristics of the child who died; the child's degree of actual involvement in his sibling's death; the child's preexisting relationship to the dead sibling; the immediate impact of the death upon the parents; the parents' handling of the initial reactions of the surviving child; the reactions of the community; the death's impact upon the family structure; the availability to the child and parents of various "substitutes"; the parents' enduring reactions to the child's death; major concurrent stresses upon the child and his family; and the developmental level of the surviving child at the time of the death, including not only psychosexual development, but ego development with particular emphasis upon cognitive capacity to understand death. The effects upon the child obviously are not static, undergoing constant developmental transformation and evolution" [1].

The case presented illustrates a great many of these determinants of the response to a sibling's death.

It is not difficult to understand that a fatal illness and subsequent death of a child all too frequently lead to emotional disorder in the remaining siblings. If we keep in mind relevant etiological factors of childhood emotional disorders as emphasized by Szurek [7], it is not difficult to connect the impact of illness and death on the emotional lives of the survivors. These responsible factors are the *intensity* of the external interpersonal influences and their *duration*, and the *maturational* and *developmental* phases of the children on which these influences are brought to bear.

With a disease such as childhood leukemia, family members enter into a period of "anticipatory grief" at the time of the initial diagnosis. Each individual's response may be so overwhelming that their methods of coping may offer little support to other family members. In our experience, parents rarely are able to provide their children with the additional bolstering they require. Even when the patient and siblings have been given no indication of the fatal nature of the illness, they sense that something is drastically wrong and react accordingly. All their individual conflicts are intensified by the Sword of Damocles hanging over their heads, whether they are aware of this or not. Support from the parents includes an open appraisal of the situation and an honest expression of the feelings associated with it.

There are two phases in the total process. The first dealing with the anticipation of death and the second with the stark reality of death. The first should prepare the family gradually for the second but even under the best of circumstances, the reality of inevitable loss can never be completely prepared for or worked through. Furthermore, families that have been sensitized to loss through the experience of emotional losses tend to overreact to death and mourn depressively for abnormal periods of time. Such was the case with the Jones family. Death is the end of life, but it is not the end of relationships, especially ambivalent ones, and mourning may be postponed for several developmental epochs and sometimes for eons. Such children may become vulnerable adults with a disposition to depression.

Bibliography

1. Cain, A. C., Fast, I., and Erickson, M. E., Children's disturbed reactions to death of sibling, *Amer. J. Orthopsychiatry*, 34 (1964), 741–752.
2. Furman, R., Death and the young child: some preliminary considerations, *Psychoanalytic Study of a Child*, 19 (1964), 321–333.

3. Furman, Robert A., The child's reaction to death in the family, *Loss and Grief: Psychological Management in Medical Practice*, Schoenberg, B.. Carr, A., Peretz, D., and Kutscher, A., Eds., Columbia University Press, New York, (1970), 70-86.

4. Wiener, Jerry, M., Reaction of the family to the fatal illness of a child, *Loss and Grief: Psychological Management in Medical Practice*, Schoenberg, B., Carr, A., Peretz, D., and Kutscher, A., Eds., Colombia University Press, New York, (1970), 87-101.

5. Rosenblatt, Bernard, Ph. D., A young boy's reaction to the death of his sister, *J. of the Amer. Acad. Child Psychiatry*, 8 (1969), 321-335.

6. Nagera, Humberto, M. D., Children's reactions to the death of important objects: a developmental approach, *The Psychoanalytic Study of the Child*, 25 (1970), 360-400.

7. Szurek, S. A., M. D., Psychiatric problems in children, *The Langley Porter Child Psychiatry Series*, Vol. 3 (Psychosomatic Disorders and Mental Retardation in Children), Szurek, S. A., Berlin, I. N., Eds., Science and Behavior Books, New York, 1968.

The Experience of Death on an Adolescent Pediatric Ward* (As Experienced by the Nurse in Dreams and Reality)

John E. Schowalter, M.D. (U.S.A.)

Since the creation in 1966 of a separate adolescent unit as part of the pediatric services of the Yale-New Haven Hospital, I have been especially interested in the reaction of staff and patients to seriously ill and dying adolescents [1, 2].

Over the past year I have collected from nurses a dozen dreams which they identified as reactions to a dying patient. This collection began in an interesting way. During a weekly nurses' meeting on the Pediatric Adolescent Ward, there was a discussion of a patient who had just died. One nurse mentioned that the night before she had a dream about the patient, and a somewhat startled second nurse announced that she too had dreamed of the dead patient on the preceding night. I expressed my interest in the dreams, and the nurses were willing to tell them to the group. I asked if nurses had dreams about death or about dying patients that they write them down for me. Following some of the subsequent dreams, I have had

*Supported by U. S. P. H. S.5T1 MH 5442-20, The Children's Bureau, U. S. Department of Health, Education and Welfare, and the Connecticut Department of Health.

an interview with the nurse and obtained her associations, but, more often, the associations I have indicated in this report are group associations expressed by the dreamer and her colleagues during a nurses' meeting. Other than that which was given spontaneously, no attempt was made to get additional personal information about the dreamer.

The Usefulness of Manifest Dreams

Prior to *The Interpretation of Dreams* [3], the manifest dream content was all that was known about dreams. However, with Freud's understanding of the unconscious and with his emphasis on the importance of the latent dream content, the study of manifest dream content has fallen into disrepute in psychoanalytic circles, this despite Freud's 1925 footnote (p. 506) warning analysts against clinging too exclusively to latent content or Erikson's comment [4] on the need, in order to fully understand a dream, for the analyst to "be at home on the geological surface as well as the descending shafts" (p. 16).

For this paper we have included only manifest dream content, but I believe this can prove useful in understanding the emotional stress placed on the staff caring for dying patients. The day residues for the dreams were thoughts about dead or dying patients, and the individual and group associations with the dreams, made by those who also worked closely with the specific adolescent, provide a unique view of a hospital staff's reaction to death.

The Content of the Dreams

There was a remarkable consistency in manifest content of the dreams reported. Undoubtedly, it was this obvious content which caused the dreams to be reported. All but one of the twelve dreams portrayed either a dying patient as well or a dead patient as alive. In the one other dream an old woman, rather than a child, came alive. In most cases the dreams are clear and direct wish fulfillments. They are reminiscent of the dream reported by Freud (1900, Vol. 5, p. 509), which described a father who dreamed that his dead son reproached him for having allowed the boy to catch on fire. The father awoke to find the child's dead body in flames, but the father's dream had, at least momentarily, brought the son back to life.

Undistorted dreams are rare in adults. When they do occur, they are usually in response to an internal physiologic stimulus, an external stimulus, or a very distressing and recent life experience. The nurses' dreams fit into this latter category. All the nurses had been exceptionally distraught about the fate of the child who appeared in the dream.

In most of the dreams the child spoke. As Freud first pointed out (1900, Vol. 4, p. 183), the words spoken in the dream are often those used by the person (in this case the child) in life. The words in the nurses' dreams often formed questions which were characteristic for that patient, i.e., asking for his favorite food or about his treatments or about his illness. The fact that the spoken words so often were questions was interesting. The nurses usually experienced these questions as a rebuke for their inability to save the patient. This reaction seems to substantiate Isakower's statement that "speech elements in dreams are a direct contribution from the superego to the manifest content of the dream" [5].

Typical Dreams

I will first present five typical dreams which nurses had following patients' deaths and then present two other dreams combined with the group associations to them.

1. On the night of the death of a thirteen year old, a nurse reported the following: "David's body is lying in bed. His body is thin and black and blue. The IV's are running out and then he's dead. On the next day I meet David out walking. He looks healthy. He runs up to me, we hug, and we both cry"

2. After a girl died of leukemia, this dream was reported: "Debbie was in the dayroom and called me to bring her a glass of milk. (She enjoyed milk very much and frequently asked for it.) I gave her the milk, and she drank it. Then she sat down in a chair and said, 'Thank you. Now I can die.' Then she went on to die."

3. The night of the day a girl died of cancer, the nurse who cared for her had this dream: "Bobbi's mother phoned to say the girl wanted me to come to her house and see her doll collection. I did. Bobbi's room was in the attic and all along the walls were shelves of dolls from all over the world. After a few seconds Bobbi got out of breath and said, 'Oh, I have to lie down for a moment.' After she caught her breath she asked me to stay a couple of days at her house. I looked at her and said, 'But Bobbi, you're dead!' At that Bobbi began to cry."

4. During the evening shift, a fourteen-year-old girl died of leukemia. One of the nurses went home the following morning and had this dream: "Another nurse and I noticed Cathy and her mother wandering about the hospital. We became petrified because Cathy was supposedly dead. We started running away from her, but she grabbed my arm and said, 'Don't be afraid. I just wanted to thank you all for the care you gave me and say I really had a good time with all of you.' At that point I woke up and heard myself screaming, 'No, No!' "

5. Following the death of an eleven-year-old girl, a nurse reported this dream: "I walked into Madge's room, found her dead, and went out to console her parents. Her parents claimed that she wasn't dead and urged me to return to her room. I did, and she was sitting up, smiling and talking. I returned to the parents and then they entered Madge's room. They came out crying. She was dead. At this point I woke up."

Although in each of these examples the dead child was returned to life, it is notable that the second, third, and fifth dreams end with the death being reaffirmed. Thus, even in these nurses' dreams, reality is returned to.

Group Associations

While a wish to prevent the child's death is the theme most obvious in the manifest content of the dreams, a feeling of guilt for not accomplishing this prevention pervades the associations.

On the day of one dream an experienced young nurse was caring for a thirteen-year-old boy who had been on the ward many months and was now very close to death. Later, she described what happened:

I went into his room early in the morning. I put him under the oxygen tent and tucked the plastic around him. [At the time his bed was in a high Fowler's position (patient sitting almost straight up).] He was semiconscious, and I didn't want to leave him alone, but I had to premedicate a patient who was having surgery. As I completed premedicating the other patient, a nurse ran out of his room and said, 'Stevie is on the floor.' One of the residents picked him up; Stevie was dead. The resident assured me that he must have died sitting up and then fallen. That night I had a nightmare. Stevie was in bed, and I kept trying to pull up the sidebar of his bed. The oxygen tent also kept falling off. The harder I would try to pull them up, the more resistance there was. I became frantic and repeated the action over and over until I awakened. The side of the bed was the same side as Stevie fell over.

The dreamer's thoughts about the dream were as follows:

What struck me was a feeling of helplessness, an inability to prevent the death. If the bars were up then he wouldn't have fallen out of bed and he wouldn't have died. There's just that real feeling of helplessness that there is no way of preventing the death. Having to realize that and yet make the most frantic efforts in hopes that somehow, some way I might be able to prevent it.

In a general discussion of the dream, other nurses stressed the guilt associated with being the person last in the room before a patient dies alone. As one nurse put it, "You think maybe if I had stayed, something would have been different. Ninety-nine times out of one hundred you know nothing would have been different, but because you were the last person you really have the most guilt feelings. If you would have stayed five minutes more, and those five minutes more could stretch into days and days and days, perhaps something would have changed the situation. When a patient dies alone and you could have been with him, you always wonder if your presence wouldn't have made a difference."

The second dream occurred shortly after a nurse had accompanied a dead ten-year-old boy to the hospital morgue. Although she linked the dream with that experience, this was the only dream submitted which did not portray a pediatric patient.

I and another nurse were walking towards the morgue to take count of those who died. I told the other nurse that this was the only part of evening duties I disliked. On the morgue table was a naked, dead old woman covered with a sheet from the waist down. There were shelves surrounding us with parts of bodies on them. There were no children in the morgue. As we passed, I heard a scream and turned to see the dead woman pull off the sheet and start to get off the table. I let out a terrifying cry since the woman had a determined look on her face, and I feared she was going to get me. Some pathologists heard my cry and rushed into the room. I remember feeling that because of their reaction that what was happening must be true. I woke with the sensation of running, screaming, and trying to get away.

When I spoke alone to the nurse who had the dream, her associations went quickly from the dead boy to the death during her childhood of an aged and beloved great-aunt. Interestingly, while growing up she had had at least one extremely frightening dream about this woman.

Reactions to the dream by the nurses' group revealed a number of other concerns. Some had never before been so clearly articulated. A sampling of the reactions includes one nurse who described her feelings about the hospital morgue: "You just go into this room and there are shelves. A fellow human being whom you cared about and you just kind of cart them down there and shove them in a freezer. You just consider that this person was alive and breathing a short while before. You just close the door and that's it. It's just such an empty feeling." Another girl added, "What really hit me the first time I took anyone to the morgue was that the stretcher they use doesn't have any padding on it. You suddenly realize you're no longer treating that person as a human being. It's sort of a cold, cruel, almost rejection of the patient. You close that heavy door and that's that. What I heard in the dream was sort of an angry response in a corpse coming to life and chasing you because of what you're doing to them or have done." "On the other hand," said a third nurse, "many times I watch somebody who is really suffering and I don't want to admit it to myself, but I almost pray that they will just go in peace; but, inevitably, every time I prepare a patient with a shroud I always feel this is going to happen to me some day and will I want someone to put a shroud over my face. Automatically I treat the body with more respect. I went to a Catholic nursing school and high school, and we were always taught that death was beautiful because you get to live with God. Yet when you watch a child die, you know, someone who has so much experience to live for and who leaves so many behind, well, heaven doesn't seem like much of a consolation. I do believe in God, but I have a lot of trouble believing with things like this." Yet another nurse spoke of feelings of anger and resentment. "Just after a death I have to really watch myself, my attitude toward other people. It usually doesn't go on for a long time, but without guarding myself I become very angry with everything around. In nursing school they teach you that you are the professional who can't show emotion and whom others lean on. They also teach you that sadness and grief are the standard reaction of society to death. Well, all this flying back and forth makes you mad because you must act one way when you feel the other way. I know that I spend more time with healthier patients after someone dies. I don't want to get close to someone who is really sick. I want to see healthy people. I want to see people with life in them."

Conclusions

I will confine my discussion to two aspects of these dreams. The first concerns their structure and the second their impact on and usefullness to the hospital staff.

The dreams follow the external stress of caring for a dying child, and their manifest content clearly expresses the wish fulfillment of the patient's recovery. Undoubtedly, many more of the nurses' dreams involved reactions to dying patients, but only the obvious ones are recognized and presented for study. Since the nurses state that they usually do not experience this type of simple wish-fulfillment dream, these examples are unusual. One might speculate that the more dramatic the day residue, the more likely the dream will remain undistorted. The nurses were often awakened by the dreams, and although they were seldom repeated, they have a similar quality to the repetitive dreams experienced in a traumatic neurosis. The words reported as spoken by the patients in the nurses' dreams very much support Freud's contention that speech in dreams repeats words spoken by that individual in real life and also support Isakower's suggestion that speech elements contribute a super-ego representation.

These dreams provide one more piece of evidence of the strong impact of death on the personal lives of hospital staff. Nurses generally dreamed about patients whom they knew well and who had been hospitalized for a relatively long period. In every case the nurse has been subjectively depressed about the adolescent's fatal illness.

The dreams provide invaluable material for aiding members of the staff to confront their reaction to patients' deaths. Although the associations of others may be completely different from those of the dreamer; the fact that another nurse (sometimes acknowledged; sometimes anonymously) reveals her dream invites an intimacy and frankness in the group discussion which is seldom otherwise obtained. Therefore, one individual's very personal internal experience can be used to modify and enlighten the observations and external actions of many others.

Summary

A number of nurses' dreams experienced as responses to dying adolescent patients is presented. The dreams are relatively undistorted wish fulfillments of making the patients better or bringing them back to life. A common reaction to the dreams concerns guilt at not having cared well enough for the children. These dreams have provided a valuable vehicle for group discussions of the impact of patients' deaths on the emotions and actions of ward staff.

Bibliography

1. Schowalter, J. E., Death and the pediatric house officer, *J. Pediat.*, 76 (1970), 706–710.
2. Schowalter, J. E., Death and the pediatric nurse, *J. Thanatology*, Vol. 1, pp. 81–90, 1971.
3. Freud, S., *The Interpretation of Dreams*, (1900) Standard Ed., Vols. 4 and 5, Hogarth Press, London, 1953.
4. Erikson, E. H., The dream specimen of psychoanalysis, *J. Amer. Psa. Assoc.*, 2 (1954), 2–56.
5. Isakower, O., Spoken words in dreams, *Psa. Quart.*, 23 (1954), 1–6.

The Need to Mourn

Norman L. Paul, M.D. (U.S.A.)

> *"And some cease feeling*
> *Even themselves or for themselves."*
> *(Wilfred Owen)*

Grief Recaptured

"I could put my arm around him," John H. said tearfully, observing himself on the television monitor in the hospital. He was viewing his own twenty-year belated grief reaction to his father's death recorded on videotape four months before. John is a 28-year-old, white, married father of four children, a severe narcotics addict since his discharge from the army ten years ago. He has also been consuming up to 2000 mg of barbiturates a day, has been hospitalized at least ten times, spent four years in prison, and has a younger brother who is currently in prison for narcotics addiction.

This videotape recording, taken during John's second interview—the first one with his wife—represented an experiment in grief induction. It was learned in the first interview that his father had died when John was eight years old. At the beginning of the second interview, John was withdrawn, confused, disheveled, and passive, exuding an aura of disinterested bravado; his wife was silent. It was learned that Dennis, their four-year-old son, would often place his father's tourniquet around his forearm and pop veins: John felt obliged to be open about "shooting up," often doing so in front of his terrified children.

The technique of grief induction used here began with an eight-minute audiotape playback of another couple wherein the husband breaks down in sobs recalling his belated grief over the death of his beloved Aunt Anna. John and his wife were encouraged to remember a time when either had had a similar experience.

After the playback, John was asked for his reactions. He demurred saying that he didn't want to be bothered. His attempt to distance his former grief was countered by directed persuasive questioning about his feelings. Suddenly a force intruded on his consciousness and John began to cry bitterly in a manner that evoked in the therapist the image of large, hitherto calcified chunks of pus being dislodged from his guts. He resists crying, blurting out, "Crying is for girls."

He is eight years old and he awakens one winter morning alongside his alcoholic father only to discover that his father is dead. (He begins to describe the shock and loneliness and fear, and a painful era of his life comes alive.) The final doleful viewing of his father in the casket is occasioned by his placing his prized Hop-a-Long Cassidy ring on his father's right index finger.

The above scene on videotape, observed *four months later,* generated an empathic resonance with himself living through his hitherto forgotten intense pain, something he had never shared with anyone before. Stunned with almost disbelief, he is at last aware of his repressed pain attendant to his father's death and that this has taken a tremendous toll of himself. Later he acknowledged that he missed having a father and angrily said that if his mother had been at home, perhaps she could have saved his father's life. Of interest subsequent to viewing this scene on the monitor, John was observed by the staff feeling the walls and arms of chairs experiencing different textures as if he were becoming denumbed. . . .

Briefly reconstructing this curious phenomena: John had totally forgotten his pain of grief. It was only after sanctioning his presumed grief as a normal experience for a man, through the audiotape stimulus, could his defenses (of denial and isolation) be neutralized pro tempore. Only after his grief had been induced could one infer that here was an instance where there was a need to mourn. It was obvious, post facto, that he had gone to great lengths to deaden himself to his own pain and in part had identified with his dead father. Because John had had no access to an empathic ear after his father's death, for survival purposes he had to forget that his pain existed.

Definitions

Mourning is the total sequence of responses to a major loss including both formal and spontaneous physical behavior, both private and shared grief, and other psychological processes. *Grief* refers only to the subjective state of mourning. It includes feelings such as helplessness, anger, despair, guilt, and bewilderment, as well as variable somatic distress.

Although *grief* and *mourning* can be broadly related to loss of anything valuable such as an ideal, a fantasy of being loved (or unlovable), or even bodily symptoms, here these terms are restricted to those experiences involving the death of a loved person.

Si vis me flere, dolendum est primum ipsi tibi.*

Empathy is an existential state which can be used to heal the hitherto unshared grief of the bereaved. It is an interpersonal emotional experience during which the initiator of the empathy presents himself as one who can bear the other's pain of grief: ranging from oceanic despondency to terror and rage at the deceased for the pain of being abandoned.

Cultural Perspectives

". . .the last enemy that shall be destroyed is death" (I Corinthians 15:26).

"In the midst of life we are in death" (Book of Common Prayer, Sept., 1945, pp. 332)

Part of the dilemma of the contemporary scene is that death is less often experienced at home in the heart of the family but rather in the aseptic hospital setting. In prior generations death was experienced, along with mourning, as part of home life. Without the prior frequent experience of death, there has evolved an aversion to the mourning process. That denial of mourning is rampant in our society is no better depicted than in a contemporary work by Choron [1] that points to "the need to cope with the acute awareness of our mortality" but contains no reference whatsoever to grief or mourning.

---

*"If you wish to draw tears from me, you must first feel pain yourself." (Horace, *Ars Poetica*).

Historically, there has been a polarization of belief about the mourning process. Homer, in the *Iliad*, makes it clear when he describes the death of Hektor that mourning is necessary and that an important expression of it includes recollections of the deceased. An opposite view, and probably not unconnected to the development of stoicism and to our modern aversion to mourning, is expressed by the Platonic Socrates who felt that mourning should play no part either in relation to his own death or to the occurrence of any death in the ideal state. He believed that superior individuals should neither fear death nor mourn the loss occasioned by it. Such unseemly behavior was only proper for women or inferior males.

This difference between men and women in relation to mourning may represent a critical incompatibility, especially in marriage. Plato clearly sets a premium on the ability to show restraint and self-control with respect to the external expression of grief as well as the fear of death. This and the associated thrust towards immortality are prized as masculine traits.

It is well-known that a prominent sex difference in child rearing in most cultures has to do with the suppression of sad and fearful reactions in the boy as indications of "sissiness." Shaming techniques are commonly used to encourage denial and isolate hurt feelings. Many boys suffer from this embargo and secretly envy their female companions who have sanction to express their emotional reactions to the distress of physical and psychological hurt. Such envy may later be perceived as a fear of homosexuality where the latter is equated with femininity.

The fear of death, the yearning for immortality through death, and the disregard of death have been incorporated into religious doctrine and thereby shaped the nature of western civilization. Man's helplessness in the face of his own mortality has helped to generate a counterbelief in the immortality of his soul and his eventual triumph over death. The Judeo-Christian tradition recognizes the need to grieve in a proscribed manner within a strictly defined time span. The ritualized mourning designed to purge the bereaved of his grief promotes a formalized sharing of this experience and encourages dependency on the religion.

At the core of the whole experience, there seems to be a reciprocity between the fear of being abandoned by the death of the other and the fear of one's own death. Man's search for the meaning of his existence has generally been provided for by religious belief. According to Tillich [2], an important part of man's concern about his own death has to do with his feeling of being abandoned by God.

> Man cannot stand the anticipation of death and so he represses it. But the repression does not remove his ever-present anxiety, and there are moments in the life of everyone when such repression is not even slightly effective. . . . The meaning of the anxiety of having to die is the anxiety that one will be forgotten both now and in eternity. Every living being resists being pushed into the past without a new presence... . A rather superficial view of the anxiety of death states that this anxiety is the fear of the actual process of dying which, of course, may be agonizing but which can also be very easy. No, in the depth of the anxiety of having to die is the anxiety of being eternally forgotten.

The Death of the Child

Perhaps the most difficult grief experience is associated with the death of a young child. The common pattern in parents for dealing with it is to deny the grief, try to forget the child, and perhaps seek to replace it with a new one much as they do when a child's pet dies.

A middle-aged woman, Janet, had just observed herself on the TV monitor reviewing the death of Wilma, her six-month-old baby, an event that had transpired 21 years before. The videotape had been recorded earlier that same session. "I didn't know this was so important to me," she said and sighed with relief as she scooped some cigarette ashes off the floor.

This was her second marriage. She and her first husband, Paul, were quite happy when a daughter, Wilma, was born, a year after their marriage, in 1947. One autumn afternoon she and Paul had gone to the supermarket and left their infant daughter in a car crib in the back seat of their car. When they returned, Janet looked over the front seat of the car to check and discovered that Wilma was lying prone and not breathing. In shock and bewilderment a chain reaction began: Paul wept with abandon but briefly that very day as did Janet. Preparations for the baby's cremation were made at a local funeral home but the body had to be shipped off to a larger city for this purpose. Within a week after the death, Paul had his first affaire. As time passed, the couple became increasingly estranged: nevertheless, a year later Linda was born and over the next eight years three more children arrived alive and healthy.

Within a month after Wilma's death, a canister arrived at the house containing her ashes. Janet placed it, still in the original wrappings, inside a bag on the top shelf of her bedroom closet where it remained until it was brought into the session referred to above.

Ten years later, while Janet was pregnant with her fourth child, Paul, in the course of several affaires, had made another woman pregnant. This ultimate breach of loyalty rendered divorce inevitable from Janet's point of view. She remained in the house that was awarded her and two years later married Don. Don had been married twice before but had no children of his own and Janet promised that she would give him his much wanted child. After eight fruitless years she became menopausal and Don's great disappointment and wish for a divorce prompted them to consult me. In the course of the sessions with the couple, I learned of Wilma's existence and I also found out that the oldest living child, a daughter, Linda, now 20 years old, had moved from LSD to heroin and was now addicted to these drugs. It was then that I was informed that Wilma's ashes were still in the closet.

What was videotaped was Janet's reaction to opening the bag within which was the still packaged container of ashes. She first recalled a guilt-laden dream of the previous night wherein she had caused the death of someone else and then she cut the twine and opened the container. As she did this she gave a look of horror that presumably was the reactivated fright she had felt 21 years previously when she had looked back over the front seat of the car. Crying bitterly, she then showed her present husband old snapshots of Wilma for the first time with the comment that he could see that Wilma was a normal, happy child.

From her remarks it was clear that Linda had been a substitute for Wilma. She, therefore, had to be both herself and Wilma whose existence she had never even heard of. . . .

The past is a burden for those who forget it.

Bibliography

1. Choron, J., *Modern Man and Mortality*, Macmillan, New York, 1964.
2. Tillich, P., *The Eternal Now*, Scribner, New York, 1970.

A Child's Capacity for Mourning

Robert A. Furman, M.D. (U.S.A.)

I have been asked to present here a brief summary of my thoughts about a child's capacity for mourning, the factors that can interfere with the utilization of this capacity, and the consequences for the child who fails to fulfill the requirements of the mourning task. My thoughts on this were first presented in 1964[1,2], parts of which were disputed by Wolfenstein in 1965 [3] and 1966 [4] and by Nagera in 1970 [5]. I attempted to deal with some of these criticisms in papers in 1968 [6] and 1970 [7].

I mention these differences of opinion at the outset to make certain the reader is aware that the thoughts I will present are not universally accepted and to offer the necessary references for those who might wish to pursue these questions further. In essence, I have felt a child usually has the capacity for mourning, under proper circumstances, from somewhere around age four, whereas Wolfenstein and Nagera feel that a child cannot mourn until the termination of adolescence. This would mean, to me, until young adulthood is reached. In other words, I believe a child from about age four on has the capacity for completing the requirements of the mourning task; and they believe, if I understand them correctly, that no child can complete this task.

Attempting to understand scientific disagreement can be both stimulating and helpful. I believe one of the difficulties lies in the utilization of certain manifestly grieving adults as the model for mourning. This seems unfortunate as the focus is then apt to be placed on what Spiegel [8] described as the "grieving state of mourning" as opposed to "the work of mourning (which is) the cause of that state." In *Mourning and Melancholia*, Freud's description of this work of mourning is of an adaptive or reparative response to loss that is characterized by the gradual decathexis of the internal mental representative of the lost object, the withdrawal of the feeling investment in the mental image of the lost loved one. This is accomplished through recurrent remembering of the object and then the painful acceptance of its permanent absence. In 1923 in *The Ego and the Id*, Freud [10] added that "It may be that an identification is the sole condition under which the id can give up its object." It is these psychological tasks that are to me the essence of mourning. When these are completed, feeling investments will have been freed and made available for new object relationships in the reality world of the living. The child's lack of an externally visible grief reaction similar to that of an adult has to my mind no more bearing on his internal capacity for mourning than his apparent sexual innocence would indicate the absence of his sexual feelings and fantasy life.

Many factors complicate for everyone a consideration of a child's mourning. The child's apparently helpless fragility at a time of grave loss has a poignancy that evokes from all a great depth of feeling and a recall of one's own past losses. All of us who have worked with bereaved children either directly or through their surviving parent have been so impressed with the personal emotional strain of such work that no one wants to take on more than one such case at a time. The reader should be prepared that in considering doing any supportive work in this area an emotional response of his own cannot be avoided.

In addition, at the heart of the question about mourning is that of death. This means the topic will also immediately involve us with questions of aggression and our comfort or discomfort with this aspect of our own psychological makeup. What has always been striking to me is the adult's usual need to deny the small child's ability to understand the concept of death, something the child can comprehend from somewhere around age two on. A colleague described for me the situation of coming upon a dead bird while on a walk with some friends and his children, including a two-and-a-half-year old. One of the friends was about to remove and hide the bird "so the little one won't be upset" when the little boy spied the bird himself. He came over, picked it up and said, "The poor birdie is dead. I'll put it back into the woods, O. K. Daddy?" A. Freud [11] states that adults deny the child's capability to understand death to protect themselves from the child's sadism. I doubt if she would object to the addition "that recalls for them their own conflicts over sadism."

I pursue these points at the outset because I believe the reader should be prepared for the difficulties inherent in this topic and because I want to put central the question of the work of mourning to enable us to examine the attributes a child must have acquired to manage this psychological task.

To begin with he must have the concept of death and its finality. If this is realistically taught the small child, he can readily accept it. If his parents avoid or deny the reality of death, the child will accept his parents' prohibition and denial. No prelatency child can cope with the abstractions involved in the concept of heaven and will comprehend it only as a reality place where people go and exist and hence are not dead. The explanation of death as the absence of life is best offered the child when he first encounters it with insects and animals. Without such a reality concept of the death, no child can cope with its feeling consequences.

To withdraw a feeling investment from a mental image of a lost loved one, to decathect the internal representative of the lost object, a child must first have a stable internal representative that can survive and endure after the vast majority of loving investment has been removed. Our theoretical knowledge and clinical experience would indicate to us that this is possible after the achievement of object constancy dominance and a mastery of the ambivalence conflicts of the anal sadistic phase of development. In an otherwise emotionally healthy child it is reasonable to anticipate this level of development sometime around age four. The ability to form adequately mature ego identifications is to be anticipated at about the same age.

It is in proceeding with the internal psychological work of mourning that difficulties arise for many, children and adults. There must be a healthy availability of feeling, not an unwarranted degree of suppression of feeling by neurotic defenses. There must be a fluidity, a flexibility of personality structure, not a rigid character unable to adapt to change. It is with these personality attributes that many children and adults fall short of having the capacity for successful mourning and would need psychological treatment to attain the mental health necessary successfully to complete the mourning task. In underlining a child's inability to mourn, it has seemed to me as if some have idealized adult mourning which would mean a denial of the inability of so many adults fully to master the demands of mourning.

But to do this painful work a child has some special requirements that do not exist for the adult who has attained the maturity and independence that should accompany the successful completion of his adolescent development. A child has physical and emotional needs that must be met for his survival and if his loss is that of a parent, he must be certain, before he loosens his attachment to his internal representative of the lost one, that these needs will be met. In response to his bereaved son's question as to who would take mother's place, one father said simply, "No one can ever take Mother's place, but I can see to it that all her jobs are done." This is an enormously difficult task, even in the best of circumstances, calling for the most resourceful family and often community effort. If the physical needs can be met and the child has been consistently shown that they are being met, he will then be in the position of being able to begin the decathexis of the internal representative. The child's ability to continue his psychological development in the absence of one parent will depend on two factors. First, he must decathect the image of the lost parent to free his feelings for growth through investment in new objects. Second, there must be available to him some consistently interested adult of the proper sex, grandparent or close family friend, for example, in whom these feelings can be invested sufficiently for their growth and maturation.

But a child will need even more to be able to utilize his capacity to do the mourning work. He will need the acceptance of his feelings, fears, and reality evaluations as he is able to put them into words. One little bereaved girl with whom I was working to help her accomplish, somewhat belatedly, her mourning of her mother, received a terrible setback in this work when her father and stepmother had to deny quite strongly some of her reality observations about some of her dead mother's quite human shortcomings. At times a child may need the judicious interpretation of the defenses he might employ to avoid his pain. One father replied in such a situation, "We both know Mother is not alive any more. Maybe sometimes we want to pretend it isn't so because it makes us so unhappy." Some surviving parents, in the midst of their own mourning, may need support to make such a statement. In one instance I know of it came from another sibling. A younger child was concerned that mother was cold in the grave and the father was explaining that despite the fact it was winter, the casket would keep mother from being cold. The older sister said, "But Daddy, you know Mother is dead and can't feel any more."

And yet there is one more difficulty that a child will face. The losses he endures of parents or siblings are always premature and untimely, either because of illness or accident. The manner in which these premature deaths have occurred has a tremendous potential as a trauma in and of itself. The child who has lost a sibling through illness will, for a very long time indeed, have a tremendous dread of even the most minor illnesses in himself and all others. The child who has witnessed a violent death, such as in a car accident, or has been aware of or seen the results of extensive surgical procedures, such as a mastectomy, will have these most difficult realities facing him whenever he begins to cope with his loss. Deaths of grand-parents at an advanced age are always so much easier because the unnatural and so often terrifying aspects mentioned above are absent. These potential traumata in the premature losses must be taken into account in helping a child achieve some degree of freedom from untoward anxiety before he can utilize his capacity to mourn.

I hope that by now I have sufficiently sketched why I believe a young child has the capacity to mourn as well as the factors that can readily interfere to preclude his utilization of this capacity. Specifically, I am referring to the need to present death realistically, meet a bereaved child's needs consistently, accept his feelings, support his reality testing, judiciously interpret his defenses, and assist him with mastering the inevitably terrifying reality which caused his premature loss. These are all most difficult tasks, sometimes impossible to accomplish. But this should not preclude our making the maximum effort we can for success is possible and its rewards very great indeed.

A loss in childhood that is unmourned, unmastered stays active in the personality and, through the defenses utilized to ward off its awareness, influences all aspects of dealing with feelings and the making of lasting object relationships. In addition, if the feelings stay invested and attached to a deceased parent or sibling, they are unavailable for growth and maturation and this will inevitably lead to varying degrees of arrest at that stage of development when the loss occurred. The absence of conscious awareness of such losses or their meaning is exactly what enables them silently and unimpeded to exert such influence. In this regard, Helene Deutsch's [12] 1937 paper, "Absence of Grief," remains a classic. She presents four such case examples in which the unmastered loss caused either inexplicable periods of recurrent sadness and depression or else the warding off of such feelings was accomplished only by the suppression of all feeling. Needless to remark, in part because of these difficulties with feelings, all four of her patients had serious impediments to forming meaningful adult object relationships.

The ideas presented here have been refined through two years of study with the Bereavement Research Group of the Cleveland Center for Research in Child Development headed by Mrs. Erna Furman.

Bibliography

1. Furman, R., Death and the young child: some preliminary considerations, *Psychoanalytic Study of the Child*, 19 (1964), 321–333.
2. Furman, R., Death of a six-year-old's mother during his analysis, *Psychoanalytic Study of the Child*, 19 (1964), 377–397.
3. Wolfenstein, M., Death of a parent and death of a president: children's reactions to two kinds of loss, in *Children and the Death of a President*, edited by M. Wolfenstein and G. Kliman, Eds., Doubleday, New York:, (1965), 62–79.
4. Wolfenstein, M., How is mourning possible?, *Psychoanalytic Study of the Child*, 21 (1966), 93–123.
5. Nagera, H., Children's reactions to the death of important objects: a developmental approach, *Psychoanalytic Study of the Child*, 25 (1970), 360–400.
6. Furman, R., Additional remarks on mourning and the young child, *Bulletin of the Philadelphia Association for Psychoanalysis*, 18 (1968), 51–64.
7. Furman, R., The child's reaction to death, in *Loss and Grief: Psychological Management in Medical Practice*, B. Schoenberg, A. Carr, D. Peretz, and A. Kutscher, Eds., Columbia University Press, New York, (1970), 70–86.
8. Spiegel, L., Affects in relation to self and object: a model for the derivation of desire, longing, pain, anxiety, humiliation and shame, *Psychoanalytic*

Study of the Child, 21 (1966), 69–92.

9. Freud, S., *Mourning and Melancholia,* Standard Ed., 14 (1917), Hogarth Press, London, 1957.

10. Freud, S., *The Ego and the Id,* Standard Ed., 19 (1923), 3–66, Hogarth Press, London, 1961.

11. Freud, A., see footnote in Children's reactions to death of important objects: a developmental approach, *Psychoanalytic Study of the Child,* 25 (1970), 379.

12. Deutsch, H., Absence of grief, *Psychoanalytic Quart.,* 6 (1937), 12–22.

Pathological Mourning

Marilyn Winograd, M.A. (U.S.A.)

The processes comprising mourning in childhood (or the apparent absence of mourning in childhood) have engaged the attention of clinicians over the past half-century. The reaction of the child to object loss has stirred up much controversy. At the conclusion of an article on grief and mourning in infancy, Bowlby has this to ask: "What are the conditions which influence the selection and course of responses to loss; and, in particular, what do we know of those that lead them to take a pathological turn?" [1]

The Case of Sarah

The case of Sarah is an example of pathological mourning in childhood that appears to follow a course of treatment similar to that described by Mahler [2]. Although she did not appear to be psychotic at the time of referral, as treatment progressed she developed psychotic reactions that led to a complete breakdown of ego functions and the development of a paralyzing depression.

Her breakdown occurred after she began to experience overwhelming feelings of anxiety in the safety of the residential treatment institution. In this protected setting her fears of abandonment and annihilation could no longer be denied or repressed, for, as Mahler observed, once these children are in a situation where hope is rekindled, they begin to evolve new images of a symbiotic object and to develop fears of possible loss.

As the treatment progressed, the development of a Utopian transference to the therapist came to an end when acute anxieties over reality separations from the therapist revived memories of her mother's death (When Sarah was only four), and brought about a severe regression.

As she emerged from this, she took over aspects of the behavior of other children in her group, becoming, at times, an "as-if" person. Development toward separation-individuation proceeded in relation to the therapist as the mourning processes were worked through in treatment.

Background

Sarah was referred by her father to a private social welfare agency which placed dependent and disturbed children in foster homes and residential treatment centers. At the time of referral, when she was almost ten years old, Sarah was a rebellious and demanding child, exhibiting symptoms of enuresis, stealing, and temper tantrums at home, with increasingly poor performance at school in spite of the fact that she tested within the normal range of intelligence.

She had been adopted shortly after birth by a couple who wanted to have a baby girl even though the adoptive mother was already suffering from a terminal illness. Sarah then became the recipient of those mixed parental feelings until the mother died four years later. After the mother's death, Sarah would run up to strangers and call them "Mommy." The relatives felt very sorry for her and her father told her to be a good girl.

A year and half later he married again. The new mother was a self-centered schizoid young woman who made it clear that she considered her husband's adopted daughter an unnecessary burden on the marriage. From the outset, she openly rejected Sarah, and within three years she and the father had two babies of their own. As one might expect, the stepsiblings demanded and received all of the maternal and most of the paternal attention available in the family. Moreover, Sarah had become the object of the stepmother's primitive infantile projections. "When I look at Sarah," she told the social worker during the intake study, "I see an ugly, smelly ape who lays in bed in a stupor sucking her thumb. She makes me sick."

Sarah's father felt helpless in the face of this overwhelming rejection on the part of his wife. In order to save the marriage he felt that he had to get his daughter out of the home and, hopefully, into a more benign setting.

Thus, with considerable guilt for all that had happened, Sarah's father approached the agency for placement. He agreed to cooperate in whatever visiting arrangements were planned and to begin casework treatment for himself.

Diagnostic assessment

During the diagnostic evaluation, the psychologist described Sarah's reactions as those characteristic of a "burnt child." His findings indicated that she could not invest herself in anybody or anything because of unconscious fears of rejection. Strong depressive features were present centering on unresolved dependency gratifications and on general feelings that she belonged to no one. When her defenses failed her, she was liable to act out in an extremely infantile and impulsive manner. The psychologist, however, felt she would be quite accessible to a psychotherapeutic approach.

The psychiatrist, in his interview, found Sarah to be an anaclitically depressed child who was unable to learn and used denial as a primary mechanism of defense. He found no evidence of psychotic processes and felt her condition had resulted from early parent loss. Her defenses included withdrawal, regression, identification with the aggressor, and projection.

Recommendation was made for her placement in one of the agency's small girls' residential treatment institutions where she would be in a therapeutic milieu, attend the special school (also under the supervision of the agency), and have individual psychotherapy with the author.

Preliminary Contact

I met Sarah for the first time when her father brought her to meet me. She was tall with dark curly hair and a dark complexion. When I invited her to come with me to my room she looked at her father as if to say, "Do I have to?" He urged her to go along and she then came readily. In the office she soon told me how her stepmother would make her ride in the back of the car and would sometimes get so mad at her that she would hide under the seat. I told her that I knew things had been very difficult for her at home and that was why her father had come to us, to see if we could find a place for her to live where she could get the care she needed. I then told her a little about the institution that consisted of two groups of six girls living on separate floors of an apartment house in a residential neighborhood with one resident counselor to each apartment. At the end of my discussion she spontaneously told me a story about two little boys who were outside on the school playground. They found a baby bat, she said, that had fallen out of its nest and been hurt. The boys yelled up to the teacher to ask what they should do with it. The teacher told the boys to bring it up to the schoolroom where it would be taken care of.

I had no trouble in connecting this little story to her own situation and when the interview ended, I was left with a feeling of optimism about her future in therapy.

We arranged two preplacement visits to the institution and on those visits Sarah was appropriately shy and curious. The counselors found her to be an appealing child and from the beginning everybody was motivated to reach out to her.

The treatment lasted 19 months and was divisible roughly into four phases: utopian, regressive, convalescent, and recovery.

Treatment

THE UTOPIAN PHASE

In the first phase of therapy, lasting about nine months, Sarah developed themes making use of two soft hand puppets, a tiger and a monkey, one she placed on her own hand and the other on mine. The tiger and monkey were playful; they hugged and kissed, rolled around together, swam in a swimming pool and ate "German chocolate candy." The candy was actual candy on my desk and Sarah labeled it "German chocolate candy," because her major counselor was Wilma who was born in Germany. In this fantasy, Wilma, the counselor, and I, the therapist, had become fused into the good candy-giving mother. Then Sarah had the puppets bring some abandoned babies home to the place with the swimming pool (a section of my desk) to live there. They swam in the pool and took sun baths afterwards. She was creating a Utopian institution for rejected children.

While this play was being enacted in therapy, Sarah was, in reality, beginning to soak up the warm atmosphere of the institution. She ate voraciously, became babyish with Wilma, and demanded more and more individual attention. Any change in the routine, however, was perceived by her as a loss and she would become disorganized. Unexpected shopping trips, for instance, were frightening even though the counselor was at her side. After she returned from a summer camping trip with the whole group, she behaved as if she did not know who she was, a little girl or a big one. When she came for her session to the therapy room she almost collapsed as if wanting me to carry her bodily.

In her early years, if seems that she had held herself together rather than express the fear and rage she must have experienced as a result of the mother's unpredictable, repeated withdrawals due to illness. Her ability to function at all was probably at the expense of real libidinal identifications. Furthermore, one would expect that a child who is adopted to fill the last years of a dying parent's life must surely have an ambivalent internal picture of her own worth and lovableness.

Her developmental history was reported as being fairly normal with the exception of unsuccessful toilet training. The symptoms which precipitated the father's request for placement did not become acute until after the second marriage. Our hypothesis was that in the second mother she had at last found a bad object against whom she could direct the hostility she had not dared to express earlier. In Sarah's eyes, then, no matter how hard she might try to be good, it would not matter for the cruel stepmother hated her and wanted her out of the house. Thus she might as well express her badness and get the punishment she felt she deserved.

Then she entered our institution. Her reality testing was intact and she quickly perceived that here were other girls who were not behaving "correctly" (actually, a majority were psychotic in some form), but no one was mean to them or asked for them to be removed when they misbehaved. In addition, Sarah seemed to sense that here one's dependency needs would be met to a degree of fulfillment she had long since renounced. So she allowed herself some hope. The institution offered the expectation that, no matter what, there would be people here to care for her. With these feelings she could afford to give up the "Scotch-tape" defenses that had held her together for so long. This phenomenon is not different from that of adults who have maintained themselves under extreme situations such as war or Concentration Camp internment, only to break down afterwards when, at last, they feel safe.

The signs of the breakdown of Sarah's defenses were observed first in the institution and later in therapy. While the Utopian chocolate-candy fantasies were still playfully enacted in the therapy sessions, Sarah began to experience discomfort and depression in the institution. She started to have night terrors, to run wildly out of the schoolroom and to react with intense sibling jealousy when she had to share Wilma with others. Her rage against the counselors appeared at times to be totally irrational. As her ego functions slowly disintegrated, all the regressive characteristics of a full-blown anaclitic depression, with psychotic features, gradually appeared.

THE REGRESSIVE PHASE

The phase of acute regression lasted about three months. In our therapy sessions, just prior to the onset of the regression, Sarah had stopped playing with the tiger and monkey puppets. Instead, she would sit dejectedly twiddling an ash tray or doing nothing but sucking her thumb and twirling her hair. Her wordless depression filled the room. The paradise she had created with the puppets had gone; paradise won had become paradise lost.

The fantasies that she brought up now were related to confused memories about her past. In one story, for example, her mother went into the hospital to die or to have babies. It was not clear. She had obviously condensed the repeated hospitalizations of the sick mother with the stepmother's obstetrical trips to the hospital. In other fragmentary memories, aspects of the mother's funeral were recalled fearfully in connection with that of a grandfather.

The anxieties stimulated by the recovery of these memories could not be contained in the office. They spread to all areas of Sarah's life and so overwhelmed her that eventually there was no recourse except angry irrational behavior or withdrawal. She literally did not want to get out of bed in the morning and we decided, after struggling unsuccessfully to maintain her in limited areas of functioning, that we would accept this regression as a stage of treatment. Our hypothesis was that since she had once reached a considerably higher level of ego functioning, with the appropriate therapeutic management, she would be able to regain the earlier level of integration, perhaps this time with more appropriate libidinal identifications.

Accordingly, we reformulated the therapeutic plan to support her regression. We withdrew all demands on her to participate in any activity except eating in the dining room with the others. (Thankfully, she never gave up her interest in food. Indeed, she was growing chubbier all the time, even in this regressed stage.) It was decided that I would go to the institution and see her there in whatever manner was most comfortable for her. A mild sedative was prescribed for the night time so that she (and the counselors) would be able to get some rest. Above all, she was not encouraged to tell us her memories or her dreams. We wanted her to repress feelings associated with the grief, mourning, and fears of abandonment that had come to consciousness before she had gained sufficient ego strength to deal with them.

THE CONVALESCENT PHASE

The staff was very relieved when she once again began to show a tenuous interest in the world about her. At first when I arrived at the institution to see her, I would find her curled up in bed, silent. I sat with her, as one does with a hospitalized patient. Within a few weeks I arrived to find her curled up in a big soft chair near the television set, sucking her thumb, watching a childish daytime TV program. For many weeks I sat near her commenting on the program since any comment about herself only produced anger or further withdrawal. It was safer for me to discuss the program, "The Beverly Hillbillies," than to draw attention to herself and her feelings. Her psyche was still too raw.

After a few more weeks, she was able to move from the safety of the living room to a therapy office on another floor of the institution. Wearing a counselor's big old shirt, like a transitional object, she stayed with me for half the session in the downstairs office and then ran upstairs to show Wilma where she was. This stage of therapy, which we have called the convalescent, stretched over three or four months before Sarah was able to go outside the institution with a counselor, and then, eventually to come downtown to have

therapy sessions once more in my office. Five months after the onset of the depression she returned to school, at first for an hour a
day; later, with increased time.

During the convalescent stage I followed Sarah's lead in doing
whatever she wanted to do in her sessions with me. The first attempt she made toward an activity was in the area of painting-by-
number. She wanted to paint a head of a horse according to a num-
bered outline. I had to help her. Repeatedly, we painted other
figures working patiently and carefully until each figure was finished. I felt that Sarah was coming back into the world fortressed
by compulsive, rigid lines that bound her anxieties and made it safe
for her to look outward. After completing many such paintings
Sarah asked for blank paper and when I gave it to her, she painted
tiny colored lines in each corner, leaving the rest totally blank. She
seemed to be wiping the slate clean in order to proceed further.

THE RECOVERY PHASE

The staff dated the beginning of Sarah's return to more adequate
functioning when she started one day to imitate two of the members in her group. Both were "groovy," "cool" teenagers enam-
ored with the Beatles and the Monkees and Sarah behaved in exact
imitation of their "hysterical" teen-age enthusiasm for the pop
world. Renouncing her narcissistic, infantile wishes but not quite
knowing who she was, Sarah began a phase which we called the "as-
if" period. Although the behavioristic mannerisms of the teen-agers
didn't quite suit Sarah, we interpreted her wish to be like them as
an assertive desire to grow up. For our therapy sessions I had to
bring her pictures of each of the four Beatles to paint-by-number
and I listened to her exaggerated distress when one of the Beatles
got married. She acted as if she had been left at the altar, along
with millions of other normal teen-age girls! The crucial fact was
that Sarah was talking to me again, even about abandonment, the
abandonment of teen-agers by a member of the Beatles. No one, in
this case, was destroyed by despair although a lot of girls had screaming fits whenever the Beatles appeared.

Slowly, then, Sarah was able to focus her talk to the frightening
past and renew her questions about the adoption, the illness of the
first mother, and why she did not have babies; about the father and
the grandfather, and a best friend next door to whom she still wrote.

She was now able to contain the anxieties within the therapy sessions. Even when the sessions ended she could leave the office without attempts to prolong the hour or to appear to lose all functions as she walked away from me.

In the institution she began to write notes to me when she was frustrated. She would go to her room and draw endless connected circles, like embryos tied to each other. She wrote me letters on the backs of the drawings telling me why she was unhappy. When a holiday canceled one of our appointments, she sent me a note asking for a make-up session. This material suggests that Sarah had begun to internalize me, to function without my immediate presence and to develop an ability to postpone gratification.

During this period, she had two supervised visits with the father planned therapeutically to allow her to ask him some of the questions she had been asking me about her past. It should be noted that in spite of the father's apparent weak and ineffectual relationships with his wives, he had remained, in his own way, consistently concerned about Sarah. His caseworker had prepared him for the first visit with his daughter. It took place right after the death and televised funeral of Martin Luther King. Sarah had watched the funeral with the other girls in the institution. We had been afraid it would revive frightening memories but were pleased to observe that it did not do so. Then when the father, Sarah, and I met for the visit, Sarah and he discussed Mrs. King and the three King children. The father turned to her and said with genuine warmth, "You know, although Dr. King was a great man to the world, he was the husband and father of his children and they will miss him more than anyone else." I felt that the father and Sarah were talking with emotion about the death of the mother for the first time.

Having received the father's and my permission to express grief for her mother, Sarah could begin to work through the fantasies of an all-giving or an all-punishing mother. It was now possible for her to sort out the reality from her distorted memories of it. In the next several months she developed an active curiosity about her family, her other relatives, the stepmother, and the siblings. Learning took on new meaning in school and she came to the office eager to show me her papers in science and math.

Along with this development Sarah began to perceive me as a real person who treated other children. Her rivalry with another patient of mine, also living in the institution, was expressed by Sarah's attempt to imitate this girl's behavior which I interpreted as Sarah's way of thinking that this was how she could get me to like her more. I encouraged expressions of Sarah's own wishes and separateness.

In the nineteenth month after therapy had begun, I told Sarah of my forthcoming resignation from the agency and work began on the termination phase. At first she was angry about this but cried with Wilma when she got home. In the second session she became more clinging and sad and would not hear of another therapist for her. Then she was able to say that she was afraid the next therapist would be cruel like the stepmother. In this same session she burst out with an angry response to a benign statement of mine about her growing up. "I did not grow up to go to my three mothers' funerals!" she cried.

During the last two weeks of our work Sarah repeated in condensed fashion much of the behavior observed in the whole course of treatment but in less intense form. The tiger and monkey puppets now were teen-agers and were brought out and prepared to be moved to the new therapist's office. I was also directed to tell the new therapist all about her past.

In the last hour she brought a greeting card she had purchased for me. Printed on the card was the line, "you're in my thoughts!" To this she added in her own writing, "and always will be, and I'll write to you every day even though you'll be far away. Love, Sarah." On the other side of the card she wrote, "I'll miss you very very very very very very much," and she drew four drops, labeled "tear drops."

Discussion

We have seen how a ten-year-old girl whose development had been arrested before the age of four achieved a new level of object constancy as she worked through the mourning processes. After the first stage of treatment the weak underpinnings of her ego dissolved and she regressed to an infantile position. One might speculate that Sarah's not wanting to get out of bed also might have represented an unconscious identification with the sick mother.

Nevertheless, the course of treatment appeared to follow Bowlby's conceptualization of the phases of mourning: protest, despair, and disorganization of the personality, and "finally, a phase of recovery during which reorganization takes place partly in connection with a new object or objects." The clinical material from the termination phase suggests that Sarah had reached this stage.

We also saw that this child utilized transitional objects (wearing the counselor's old shirt) and transitional object relationships (the "as-if" person) as she emerged from the regression trying, as it were, to connect herself to the people around her before she had achieved the identity of a separate self. Then, as it became possible for her to perceive the therapist as a real person, she could accept the frustrations and separations of this relationship without recurrence of the earlier feelings of overwhelming anxiety.

Bolstered by a growing sense of self-esteem and self-worth, Sarah was able to find gratification in more age-appropriate activities. The mourning processes could now be completed because the losses were no longer irretrievable.

Bibliography

1. Bowlby, J., Grief and mourning in infancy, *Psychoanalytic Study of the Child*, 15 (1960), 9.
2. Mahler, M., On sadness and grief in infancy and childhood: loss and restoration of the symbiotic love object, *Psychoanalytic Study of the Child*, 16 (1961), 332.

Who Mourns When a Child Dies?

Albert J. Solnit, M.D. (U.S.A.)

Wanting live things in their pride to remain is painfully challenged in a shattering manner when a child is dying. This article is based mainly on observations in hospitals of children dying of a fatal illness.

Some Principles in Management

There are some principles that can guide us in understanding children with a fatal illness and in understanding their family, their fellow patients, and the adults who are responsible for the care the children receive. These principles can be represented in the following questions:

1. What are the advantages of privacy in the dying process and who should share in that privacy?
2. In old age there can be a fullness to the cycle of life that enables the adult to prepare for death and in which dying is a developmental process with which the individual can cope. Can a child, whose life has only begun, be prepared for death when dying is an absolute obstacle to all further development?
3. Can a child be helped to come to grips with the dying process if his parents, doctors, nurses, and others who care for

him have not been able to deal with their own feelings and attitudes about it?

Although I do not think we shall ever be able to answer these questions fully, they are indicators of ageless concerns about man's inevitable dilemma to which he regularly seeks absolute answers. There are no absolute answers—there are answers that serve today and that will need to change tomorrow—there are answers that help but do not resolve the dilemma in any final way except as they are woven into the fabric of each survivor's life. We must seek useful answers, one at a time, for one child and the people with whom he lives and whom he shall leave when he dies. That child and the people with whom he lives have a unique history of alliances and conflicts, and that unique history of alliances and conflicts reflects not only the biological and psychological realities for that group but also the social and technological realities of their epoch. For example, over 20 years ago, as health professionals trying to help a child who was dying of glomerulonephritis in a hospital, and trying with the aid of nurses, social workers, and others to help the parents and grandparents of that child, we were not able to think of peritoneal dialysis and a kidney transplant as one possible alternative. Also, we were not able to think of remissions of three to five years for children receiving treatment for leukemia. Now we must include in our thinking and planning the consideration of such possibilities that may be a viable alternative or tormenting doubts.

The care of the child with a fatal illness, especially in the hospital, may include a significant amount of uncertainty and ambiguity until we know that child and his family and until we have formed an alliance with them to approach this cruel problem in such a way as to give that particular child and his parents an active role in dealing with the dying process. To some extent this reflects the necessary and unnecessary discontinuity of care between out-patient and hospital care of patients. The reduction of somatic discomfort and the provision of support to reduce the psychological pain of loneliness and uncertainty in a manner that is appropriate and useful to that child and his family are crucial components of care that promote alliances.

Certainly, in helping children, we must bring our point of view into line with what is acceptable to parents as well as to ourselves.

We seek an approach that respects each child's unique combination of knowing and not knowing, of seeking answers to partial questions without question marks, as well as to finding the useful level at which to be able to communicate helpfully with patients in the hospital. There is a tendency to overlook the needs, questions, and wishes to help on the part of the fellow patients and their parents in this small community that we call the hospital ward.

The Questions of Secrecy, Privacy, and Peace

In our own culture and in this generation, death as a universal event seems to have been banished; it has replaced sex as our most prohibited biological subject. The Victorian child had death in his prayers and his precepts; modern children are more likely to be taught about their origin than about their departure from this world. Doctors are unwittingly as bad as other groups in prohibiting talk of death.

Along this line, it will be pertinent to take up another matter of privacy. If we aim to help the child die in peace and if death must or should occur in a hospital, we should hope that there is the option of a private room for the dying child and his family, not only for their own privacy and closeness but also so that the other children and their families may realize that death is a sad but solemn and dignified event. In order to create the atmosphere that permits this approach to dying, we must avoid the whispering and scuffling behind screens, the furtive secrecy and pretense that nothing is happening. The so-called "secret" is known by every child on the ward and we do well with them and ourselves to show that we are sad, to answer questions to the point that they are asked and answerable, and to have the time to help children absorb the facts and talk about them openly. The secretive, furtive behavior promotes and encourages endless frightening unlimited fantasies and deprives children of the opportunity to talk about their fears, to be active in coming to grips with the reality with which we wish to help them recognize and cope!

Such principal considerations also will help us avoid the tendency to not allow anyone to die without being "cured" by last minute, hopeless, desperate measures. In that vein, perhaps we in the healing professions can then give the parents the opportunity to choose whether they want their child to die at home rather than in a hospital.

The Needs of Parents and Professionals

The parents of a child with a fatal illness need to feel sympathy and understanding in the hospital environment; and above all, in order to be able to perceive this sympathy and understanding, they should be able to feel confident that their child is being well cared for and that he is in competent hands. In this respect, judicious expert consultation, the benefit of a second opinion, is often quite appropriate and useful for all.

The parents and other members of the family will often react with anticipatory mourning reactions which represent their preparation for the inevitable loss to themselves and their family. Mourning is the repetitive and intense mental and emotional review in feelings and thoughts of past and present relationships to the child accompanied by bitter and resentful emotional reactions to the tragedy of a child dying before his life has unfolded. Such reactions refer not only to the loss of the child, but to the impact of this loss on family relationships and atmosphere. For many parents, the death of the child represents a permanent severing of one line that they have put out to immortality.

Health workers who decide to specialize in the care of children often are motivated by their fascination with children because of their vigorous, colorful, and changing characteristics. In the care of a chronically or fatally ill child, we may be confronted with what we expected to avoid by electing to become interested in children, namely, death, chronic physical illness, and the end of a life rather than the beginning of one. Usually, the child who is chronically ill or dying will indicate rather clearly his fear of pain, his disappointment in not feeling well, and his resentment and anxiety when he feels separated or the threat of separation implied by hospital care and the course of his illness. The sense of helplessness experienced by a chronically ill or dying child often represents a composite feeling caused by the effects of the physical illness and its treatment as well as by the impact of the anticipatory mourning reactions and depressed expectations of the parents and medical and nursing staff involved in his care.

The pediatric staff in facing these issues in the care of a particular child and his family is confronted by a growing and somewhat contradictory literature. The apparent contradictions reflect the tendency of individual reports to categorize the recommendations of how to conduct the psychological care of such patients and their families rather than to particularize the psychological treatment according to the child and family's tolerances and capacities. Our knowledge does indicate critical guidelines available to the pediatric staff which can be adapted in their own way to the individual situation.

The physician, who is responsible for the care of the dying or chronically (incurably) ill child is in the most advantageous relationship to the child, his parents, and siblings to accept their fears and resentments, to provide explanations, and to facilitate the mourning reaction as a crucial psychological preparation for what lies ahead. In the case of the incurably chronically ill child, it is the parents' adaptation to the loss of a healthy child and the acceptance of a handicapped or defective child that the family faces with the assistance of physicians, nurses, social workers, friends, and often the support of their religious leader. In the instance of the fatally ill child, the anticipatory grieving reactions are a preparation for the devastating loss of the beloved child.

In relieving pain with analgesics and sedatives, in reducing the fears of loneliness through living-in arrangements or a liberal visiting schedule, and in providing an opportunity for the child and his parents to talk to and question them, the staff have extended their understanding in a therapeutic manner. Of course, where they can answer the questions of the child and his parents, using tact to match the tenor and extensiveness of the questions and the tolerances of all concerned, the doctor can further the symptomatic relief by mitigating the excruciatingly fearful pain of the unknown.

In coping with the dying process, denial of painful sensations, somatic and emotional, and of the knowledge of what lies ahead is often a necessary and effective coping device. However, this does not imply that the staff should encourage denial to the point where the patient and his family, who would feel strengthened by knowing, gain the impression that they are naughty or lacking in judgment if they ask questions or in some other way indicate that they want to understand what is happening. The staff will gain an impression of how to be most helpful to a particular child and his parents by gauging the tolerances and preferred ways of coping with life expressed by the child and his family as well as by understanding the significance of the customs and social values transmitted to them by their cultural and religious beliefs.

The Needs of the Dying Child

The child who is dying, depending on his age and the nature of his illness and its treatment, usually selectively denies his sense of the death process. He may sense his fatal illness through the combination of his physical feelings and the perception of the grieving moods and depressed emotional communications by his parents and others who care for him (including physicians, nurses, et al.). The child may feel sad and frightened without being able to account for his reactions. If the patient is *a young child under four*, only the closeness of his mother and father and the absence or reduction of pain will relieve him. Often his anxiousness will manifest itself by a great deal of motor activity. For the younger child, intolerable tension is often expressed through restlessness and motor discharge. If the child is over six, he can find additional relief by having his questions answered in an appropriate and tactful way.

In *older children*, the closeness of death may be accompanied by the fearsome and intolerable psychic pain of anxiety, sadness, and a sense of helplessness. The latter is particularly depressing in a school-aged child or young adolescent who has experienced the satisfactions of independent strivings and the mastery of social and intellectual competence. Anxiety, sadness, and the fearsome sense of helplessness can be relieved by appropriate opportunities for the patient to talk about and understand what he senses up to the point of his own tolerances.

There are many levels and kinds of truth that are ethically sound and medically correct in meeting the questions, anxiety, and need to feel understood by the patient and his family. The physicians and nurses listen carefully to the patient and his parents and observe what their behavior communicates in order to use that level of concept and explanation that provides relief and support. One cannot advise that all leukemic children should be told they have a fatal illness or that no child with leukemia should be told what is wrong with him. A young child may suffer more from the painful fear of being alone (psychic pain) than from the pain caused by metastases (somatic pain), though the parentheses are an artificial device to enable us to consider components of pain that are often indivisible.

The child with a fatal illness may suffer significantly from the adults' prohibitions against telling what he knows of his illness and against asking more about it. Children have often indicated, "I'm not supposed to know." Many, perhaps most, children cannot bear knowing about their fatal illness and its consequences; however, they also cannot tolerate a complete denial of the illness and its treatment. Depending on their age and the illness, most children benefit from explanations about what is being done to them and why. They are relieved by being told directly that they will be given medicine for pain and will not be left alone for long. The age and past experiences of the child and his family, how the doctor communicates most effectively, and the conditions of human life in that particular environment are critical guides for the physician on how to listen and talk to the dying child and his family.

Therapeutic Alliance with the Dying and Surviving

The physician, the nurse, and the social worker have the same responsibilities to an individual who is dying as they have to the patient who is expected to live. These responsibilities include relieving somatic and psychological pain, familiarizing the patient with his own resources, and helping him to find and derive benefit from medical resources. The dying patient's resources that are challenged include the capacity to tolerate pain and to accept comfort, to live with sadness, and to review and experience crucial human ties as a preparation for giving them up. Knowledge of the illness, its treatment, and what lies ahead may be a source of strength for certain patients and their families.

Thus, the staff's responsibilities and capabilities include forming a therapeutic alliance with those who are dying of their illness as well as with those who survive. Reports of studies of the dying child can be helpful if they are not imbibed as a prescription. By using them to catalyze his own clinical knowledge, including self-understanding, the physician can develop an effective style and competence in helping patients medically with their problems of dying.

As a protector of the child's health and development, the doctor can also provide crucial assistance to children and their families when a member of the family, especially a parent, dies. Through standing by, offering opportunities for questioning and expressions of sorrow, fear, and resentment, the physician provides one of the major supports for the bereaved who are in need of experiencing their loss as a preparation for life today and in the future. The influence of the past, especially a death in the family, can be inappropriate and disproportionate or it can provide a perspective that is strengthening and supportive. Mourning for those who have died is appropriate and necessary. When mourning and understanding what has happened are significantly limited or not available, the past may live on in the present in attitudes, moods, and restrictions that are inappropriate and that may stunt a child's capacity for emotional attachments and intellectual development.

ILLUSTRATION

A pediatrician who was keenly interested in such matters was making a house call on a bleak November day when his car radio program was interrupted by the news of the tragic death of a young lineman who had been electrocuted accidentally. The lineman was the father of three children who were patients of the physician. After completing his house call, the doctor proceeded to the home of the bereft family where he quietly expressed his sympathy to the wife and asked if he could be helpful. She tearfully asked how to break the news to the children, and he agreed to stand by and help as she explained to the children what had happened. The three-year-old boy sat in his mother's lap tearfully telling her not to cry, alternately clinging and running about to bring his favorite toys into the room as though to distract everyone. The pediatrician played a simple game with him while the mother tried to answer the six-year-old daughter's and the nine-year-old son's questions. The daughter asked how it happened and, without listening, tearfully asked if they would have enough food and if they'd have to move away from their nice house. The oldest child asked why it happened and listened carefully when the accidental aspect of the event was described. As the mother further explained she didn't know all of what had happened, the nine-year-old boy began to provide explanations, suggesting that his father was hurt but not dead and explaining away the finality of death. The pediatrician helped the mother explain that there would be enough food, that the grandparents, neighbors, and others like the doctor could help them and that if they could find out more about what happened to daddy, they would explain it to the children.

After the acute phase of the numbing overwhelming reactions to the father's death, the children had further opportunities to talk to and to question the pediatrician. It was clear several months later that the most important help for the children had, of course, been provided by the mother. She had been able to lean on her children's physician while she explained initially what had happened, continued with help to manage her household and family, and had been enabled to express her grief without overwhelming the children as relatives, friends, and the pediatrician continued to stand by. The physician's guidance was available to the mother as each aspect of this tragic loss was encountered and reacted to by the children in the next few years. The acute and accidental characteristics of this death indicated to the pediatrician that the lack of preparation would have to be overcome gradually, each member of the family approaching the complex event according to his developmental capacities and to his individual relationship with the father and husband.

Conclusion

It is ironic that man's search for certainty is most discomforting when facing the end of life, especially from illness. The child who is dying of a fatal illness arouses in himself and his family, as well as in the physician and others who care for him, the most fearful and resentful awareness of uncertainty and loss. Recent literature on the management of the dying child [2, 3, 4, 5, 6] has examined various facets of this tragic, inevitable experience of human destruction and loss—a life snuffed out before it has unfolded. Each author reports finding an approach that should enlist the active interest of other professionals in this area. Most of these studies have concentrated on the differing reactions of those who survive the dying patient, but a few have also approached the reactions of the patient himself[1,4].

These studies in economically privileged countries may be mobilized now in part because of our improved prenatal services, antibiotics, immunizations, and agents that decelerate malignant changes. The center of the hospital stage is more frequently occupied by chronic fatal illnesses and their prolonged, repeated, and often terribly painful treatments and reactions to treatment, e.g., peritoneal dialysis, transfusions, or cytotoxic drugs. Children suffering from malignancies and the failure of vital organ systems, such as the kidneys, are typical examples of the conditions we are attempting to understand, relieve, cure, and prevent. In explicitly studying the psychology of the dying child and his family, we are painfully acknowledging one line of endeavor to conserve and protect our most important human resource, the lives and development of our children.

Bibliography

1. Nagy, M. H., Natterson, J. M., and Knudson, Jr., A. G., Observations concerning fear of death in fatally ill children and their mothers, *Psychosom. Med.*, 22 (1960), 456.
2. Richmond, J. B., and Waisman, H. A., Psychologic aspects of management of children with malignant disease, *Amer. J. Dis. Child.*, 89 (1955), 42.
3. Solnit, A. J. and Green, M., Psychologic considerations in the management of deaths on pediatric hospital services., I. The doctor and the child's family, *Pediatrics,* 24 (1959), 106.
4. Solnit, A. J., Pediatric Management of the Dying Child. II. A Study of the Child's Reaction to the Fear of Dying, in *Modern Perspectives in Child Development,* International Universities Press, New York, 1963, 217.
5. Toch, R. et al., Management of the child with a fatal disease, *Clin. Pediat.,* 3 (1964), 418.
6. Vernick, J. and Karon, M., Who's afraid of death on a leukemia ward?, *Amer. J. Dis. Child.*, 109 (1965), 393.

Mourning and Psychic Loss
of the Parent*

E. James Anthony, M.D. (U.S.A.)

The internal representation of the parent undergoes many vicissitudes during the course of development. With each successive stage, some new aspect of the parental function is assimilated so that the image within is elaborated and modified and accommodated (to use Piaget's terminology) to the current external reality. Thus, the representation is constantly nourished by the experience of the nutritional mother, the training mother, the Oedipal mother, the mother of latency, and the mother of adolescence, any one of whom may act, react and interact quite differently. Nevertheless, under the average conditions of a fairly predictable existence, a sense of continuity and constancy is established and a sufficient measure of security thereby achieved. This is because there seems to be, underlying the transient changes of good-bad, loving-punishing, accepting-rejecting, indulging-frustrating, and giving-depriving, a basic core of goodness stemming from all the positive transactions that the child has experienced with the parent. When the parent is lost, this essential core is magnified so that an idealized picture emerges. When the parent is dead, there is no further opportunity to correct any

*Supported by U. S. P. H. S. M. H. 12043 and M. H. 14052.

dissonance between the actual and idealized image; when the parent is divorced, the separated parent may attempt, during visitations, to live up to the idealized image; when, however, the parent becomes psychotic, the child not only experiences psychic loss but may be constantly confronted by the marked discrepancy between the actual and idealized images.

The total internal system representing the parent is a surprisingly accommodating one that adjusts to the various stresses and strains of parent-child life without distortion or disruption to the core structure. In practice, the clinician is repeatedly confronted by the surprising faith of a child in a relationship with a parent that seemingly has no goodness whatsoever in it from the external point of view. In this same context, Mahler has called attention to the capacity for children, in their efforts to survive psychologically, to extract emotional nourishment from the most ungiving and neglectful mothers. Psychosis in a parent can place an unusual tax on the resilience of the inner representation so that the core of goodness, reliability, protectiveness and confidence may be shattered with resulting discontinuity in the internal experience of the parent.

The Psychotic Break

This presentation, therefore, is concerned with the radical change that takes place in an individual as an effect of psychotic illness and the experience of this change by a child. I have previously illustrated some of the dynamics of change provoked by psychosis [1] but here the focus will be on psychic loss. There are a number of different factors that determine the characteristics of this disjunctive crisis. The discontinuity, both in the internal and external experience of the parent, may give rise to two separate psychological reactions:

1. A sense of alienation amounting at times to severe stranger anxiety and provoking avoidance behavior in the child. The parent has become a different person with bizarre qualities that are disturbingly unfamiliar.

2. A sense of abandonment associated at times with strong separation anxiety. The parent has become withdrawn, remote, inaccessible and unresponsive. The change provokes approach behavior on the part of the child but this is

frequently frustrated.

In the first instance, the gap is instituted by the child but not intentionally. His wishes, as manifested in dreams and fantasies, are for the recovery of the parent and the resumption of normal relations. In the second situation, the parent, as it were, separates from the child but the wish, again, is for reunion with the parent. Both alienation and abandonment, therefore, are examples of psychic loss. The former is predominantly associated with perplexity, mystification, and uncanny feelings of difference whilst the latter has as its principal component unutterable feelings of grief for the parent "who is there but not there."

There are three important factors that determine whether the child's reaction will be one of alienation or abandonment. Firstly, there is the nature of the premorbid personality. When the parent has previously been schizoid, paranoid, or peculiar, with an abnormal adaptation to life, the subsequent decompensation into frank psychosis does not appear to give the child an experience of great change and discontinuity. The difference between the internal representation and the external presentation may be minimal. On the other hand, the traumatic aspect of change and the sense of loss may be considerable when the premorbid personality has been within fairly normal limits. Secondly, the nature of the psychotic behavior, as seen from the child's point of view, is often critical in determining his reaction. In the *involving* psychosis (that is, psychotic behavior that invades and envelops the child's life so that he is forced to play an integral part in the chaotic sexual, aggressive, delusional and hallucinatory systems of the parent), the sense of alienation may be extreme and avoidance behavior marked. In the *noninvolving* psychosis, on the other hand (where autistic withdrawal is the most significant feature), the sense of abandonment is very evident and the efforts to recover the lost parent may be frenetic and pitiful. Finally, the quality of the preexisting parent-child relationship is a third and equally important factor governing the child's response to the psychotic break. When the tie is strong and even, as in many cases, symbiotic, the sense of abandonment may predominate even when the psychosis has been accompanied by a bizarre change in personality. Here the two elements of abandonment and alienation may coexist and grossly aggravate the child's predicament.

His confusion may be extreme. He is both bewildered and heart-broken and is torn by conflicting impulses to approach and avoid the parent. Where the child has been closely identified with the parent and involved in his sickness, he may compensate for loss by an "identification with the crazy one" so that the gap between him and the parent is bridged by a *folie à deux* or a Ganser reaction. The internal argument here is that if craziness in the parent has caused the loss, craziness in the child might well reduce the loss. Psychosis fantasies, like death fantasies, are based on ideas of reunion.

The nonspecific factors that are also important in deciding the nature of the child's response are the age of the child, his phase of development, his sex in terms of the sex of the psychotic parent, the support offered by the nonpsychotic parent, and the quality and acceptance of surrogation. Whilst the sense of abandonment generally diminishes with age, the sense of alienation tends to increase. I have also described elsewhere the impact of psychosis on a child during the vulnerable, animistic, magical period between four and seven in terms of the way in which the parent's psychotic system and the child's developmental phase may reinforce each other [2].

ILLUSTRATIONS OF PSYCHIC LOSS

An adolescent girl said: "You can't believe what it's like to wake up one morning and find your mother talking gibberish."

A ten-year-old boy remarked: "I wake up dreaming or maybe just day-dreaming, I don't know what, but her face is coming toward me and she looks good, and then suddenly her face begins to change and look mean and horrible like a monster."

A seven-year-old girl said: "Everything goes upside down and we go upside-down with it. When Mom goes mental, I go mental also. It's worse if I try to stay the same. Then she really hollers at me."

A ten-year-old boy had this to say: "She's quite a nice mother really. She doesn't do anything bad. She doesn't hit or anything. She just sits. She's like a kid mostly. When I give her a lot of candy, she just sucks it all up like a vacuum cleaner. She doesn't comb her hair and her dress has spots on it. Sometimes she laughs at me and I'm not making any jokes. I say: 'Mom, why are you laughing at me?' and she just laughs more. I don't like it when she laughs like that. It's not like real laughing. She never used to be like this when I was little. She was just ordinary."

A twelve-year-old boy said: "I was sitting at the table just eating my cereal, and as I was pouring out the milk my hand hit his cup and went over his lap and he jumped up and shouted at me and said I did it on purpose and that I was trying to burn him. I wasn't trying to burn him at all but he said I was trying to kill him and that he knew I hated him. Then he hit me on the head and said I had plans and he knew about them and he'd get me first, and I said it was an accident but he just wouldn't listen to me. He wasn't so grouchy last year. He has become so mean."

A teen-age girl gave this comment: "She does nothing all day, just sits about upstairs and looks at the wall and never says anything. It's just as if she were dead. I can't help crying whenever I go into the room. But when I give her a hug and say 'Hi Mom,' she doesn't even look at me and I feel I want to die."

In all these illustrations, the child is talking about the tragic loss of the parent he once knew. She looks good and then quite suddenly she becomes monstrous; she was ordinary and then she becomes peculiar, like a kid; he was nice but now he has become grouchy and mean and thinks I am trying to kill him; she was just being a mother and now she is like a zombie and dead.

The reaction to the first psychotic episode is nearly always different from the subsequent attacks. Later the child's defensive and coping mechanisms have begun to operate and he no longer appears so pathetically vulnerable. This, however, is not always the case. For example, a child had experienced a sixth psychotic recurrence. When she was small, she had shown no apparent reaction except some tendency to hyperactivity but now, at adolescence, she seemed quite depressed. She said that she wept almost every night "for my poor crazy father." Incidentally, she had manifested a strong oedipal attachment to him during her preschool years.

Loss Through Psychosis

There is no doubt that grief, sometimes frantic, occurs with loss through psychosis but, for the most part, these cases tend to exhibit pathological variants of mourning which means that the children replace the mourning process by a wide range of symptoms that they themselves do not directly associate with the psychotic break. They behave badly, sadly, angrily, frustratedly, emotionally, and hypomanically to the consternation of those around them. To understand some of these pathological responses, one must take note of the peculiar symbiotic attachment of these children to the prepsychotic parent and the often total submergence in the parent's distorted mode of living. Nevertheless, the wish of the child to escape from this bondage may be intense and linked to a high degree of ambivalence.

The Bowlby model of protest-despair-detachment may undergo subtle variations determined by the nature of the psychosis, the number of psychotic breaks that the child has experienced and, of course, the age of the child. With a strong premorbid tie and a first attack, protest is often marked in the younger child and he may rage at the forces that have engineered, in his mind, the removal of the parent. With some of the bizarre psychoses, the child is perplexed and frightened but rapidly detaches himself from the situation and tries to lead his own independent life. With the withdrawn parent, the child may react with frustration at first but in the face of inaccessibility, he may settle into a state of quiet desperation. The mixture, therefore, of these three ingredients—protest, despair, detachment—varies with the type of psychosis. The amount of rage sometimes occasioned by psychosis is considerable, especially when parental behavior has taken the form of irrational demands, unpredictable attacks and chaotic interchanges. The rage is frequently followed by strong feelings of guilt, especially when the child is told, over and over again, that the parent cannot help his unpleasant behavior and that he is sick and not angry or sad or preoccupied or worried in the ordinary human way. The child may be encouraged to feel compassion when he is actually experiencing dread and dislike. The situation is, therefore, much more complicated than with death. The child's feelings are hardly ever in keeping with the situation and this is further aggravated by demands that he should feel what he does not feel and not feel what he does feel. The conventional expectations are not so clearly defined as in the case of death and the cues for appropriate behavior may not be forthcoming from other adults who may be as bewildered as the child. The information given is even more false than is the case with death. The explanations offered may intensify the mystification and lend themselves to the elaboration of strange theories to account for the behavioral changes observed and the adults' reactions to them. If the family as a whole shares in a theory, however erroneous, the disturbance in the child is inclined to subside.

In the initial phases, he will make clinging demands on the

withdrawing parent and disengaging attempts in the case of the attacking parent. He is confused by the unfamiliar, frightened by the unpredictable and resentful at all the changes being forced upon him. At times he gives the impression of almost trying to shake his parent back into reality and when his efforts fail, he may cling hopelessly and helplessly to the well parent or surrogate. With repeated attacks, the detachment, the distancing and the objectivity enter the picture. Before reaching this point, however, he may undertake a complete repertoire of recapturing behavior—frenetic searching, attaching, clinging to, finding and losing, substituting, and detaching.

There is a great longing for the parent as he used to be; a great longing for reestablishing contact with the earlier image of the parent. "When Dad's well again, we'll be able to go to the ball game as we used to do." There may be a strong denial of the fact that the parent is no longer what he used to be in spite of all evidence to the contrary. When the parent remits and returns home, the child who has confessed to missing him may surprisingly react with great hostility and make homecoming extremely painful for the returning psychotic. "He acts as if he wants to drive me back into the hospital again," complained a mother. These "psychosis wishes" are similar to "death wishes," both having a common ambivalent basis in a hostile rejection of the parent and a wish for reunion.

Thus at one extreme, the children may refuse to accept the parent as different in any way and at the other, they may look upon him "as good as dead." In order to bridge the gap brought about by psychotic alienation, the children may attempt several classical devices. One is to become sick like the sick parent (folie à deux), a second is to remain symbiotically fused with her, and a third is to behave "crazy" and thus magically to remove the psychosis from the parent. These mechanisms of sharing and sparing are quite effective in dealing with loss since these children show little of the misery that characterizes children who do not develop pseudopsychosis. The children lacking such mechanisms may succumb to grief or resort to acting out. Their dreams often have to do with the death of the parent, his going away and, in one case, his changing into an animal, which then had to be shot for developing rabies. This would seem to support the thesis that the psychic change is looked upon as psychic loss comparable to the losses by desertion and bereavement. There are, nevertheless, differences. The parent is there but not there. He looks the same but he is not the same. As one child said: "I've got no mother. She is not my mother. She's just a witch!"

The two hypotheses (III and IV) put forward by Pinderhughes [3] in relation to psychic loss might be specially relevant to the condition of psychic loss through psychosis. For example, nonpathological paranoid mechanisms may be observed in the child in his efforts to resolve ambivalence. Frequently, he develops an aggressive response to the psychotic parent who is devalued and an intensification of the attachment to the nonpsychotic parent who is idealized or aggrandized. The family itself may show, as a group, paranoid reactions in an effort to reduce the impact of psychic loss. The strength of the dependent and affectionate bonds within the family as compared with the mistrustfulness shown to outsiders amounts almost to xenophobia.

The earlier reactions of the children to loss, such as the separations relating to sibling birth, weaning, hospitalization, going off to school, etc., may give some indication as to how the child will react to the psychic loss through psychosis. If he has manifested equanimity in the face of crisis, he will show less sense of abandonment, adjusting himself to everyday activities and paying little heed to what is taking place in the parent. There is a defensive splitting of the ego and a denial of affects and perceptions. These self-protective mechanisms seem to be essential for the continued functioning of the child. The child's major struggle is around the process of identification. He struggles constantly to identify with the lost parent and as constantly against identification with the terrifying image of the parent's illness. He is guilty that it is his badness that has driven the parent crazy and yet there is a deep wish at times to drive the parent crazy. These crosscurrents of feeling may drive the child to religion, to overactivity, to substitute relationships, to promiscuity, and, in a few cases, to genuine creativity.

As in the case of death, the children never really recover the original parent. His personality and behavior are always a little tarnished, a little suspect and when he is on drugs, as he often is, his behavior is still perplexingly different. It is difficult under these conditions to recathect the old image. The involvement with the new psychotic image may remain so intense that the continuity with the past representation is tenuous and extremely vulnerable to the next psychotic break. The loss brought about by psychosis may be, in many respects, more difficult to deal with than the loss occasioned by death.

Conclusion

The problem of psychic loss through psychosis is that, like divorce or desertion, it is incomplete. The promise of recovery is always there and may postpone grief, mourning or attempts at successful decathexis of the representation of the lost object. The confusion of affects (anger, anxiety, sadness, grief, guilt, shame, and helplessness) may become subterranean through denial and repression but recovery and reunion fantasies remain in the offing and hopefully resurrected by the first remission. Where psychosis becomes chronic, the object is given up almost bit by bit, reluctantly, and resignation ensues as with bereavement. The loss of self-esteem accompanies the piecemeal dismemberment of the psychotic object but the process is not complete until adolescence when depression is observed but seldom in relation to the psychotic illness. Restitution fantasies may make their appearance at this time. An adolescent boy, for example, whose family had been scattered into various homes and foster homes across the state as a result of a process psychosis in the mother elaborated a complex fantasy in which the family as a whole was brought back together in the operation of a family-owned railway. Each member was given a role as befitted his capacities, and the mother was brought out from her back ward to clean the floors and walls of the train since this is what she did on the ward.

There is some suggestion, from our research, that the abreaction of feeling and the "demystification" of mysterious psychotic phenomena may help to mitigate the sense of abandonment and alienation occasioned by psychic loss through psychosis.

Bibliography

1. Anthony, E. J., The mutative impact on family life of serious mental and physical illness in a parent, *Canad. Psychiat. Ass. J.*, 14 (1969), 433–453.
2. Anthony, E. J., The Influence of Maternal Psychosis on Children – Folie à

Deux, in *Parenthood – Its Psychology and Psychopathology*, E. J. Anthony and T. Benedek, Eds., Little, Brown and Company, Boston, 1970.
3. Pinderhughes, C. A., Somatic, psychic and social sequelae of loss, *J. Amer. Psychoanalyt. Ass.*, 19 (1971), 670–696.

SUICIDE, HOMICIDE, AND PARRICIDE

Editorial Comment

Unwanted infants, said Ferenczi, become children and adults with only a tenuous hold on life that can be severed at any point for what might appear externally to be trivial reasons. They have been called "expendable" children without a sense of belongingness whose parents have covertly or openly let them know that they could easily do without them. When they are products of an undesired pregnancy, many unsuccessful attempts may have already been made prior to birth to terminate their lives. Once born, the unwanted child soon becomes the rejected or scapegoated child and learns to reciprocate in kind by rejecting those who have rejected him, but in the process, he learns to reject himself as someone who must be bad to be unwanted. This is the first step on the road to self-destructiveness.

The family that generates self-destructiveness has been described as one in which there is little emotional contact, poor communication, uncaring parents, and interactions of a mainly negative kind. Two crucial reciprocities become more manifest as the child develops: first, the death wishes of the parents toward him are matched by his growing death wishes toward them; second, his death wishes toward himself are matched by his death wishes toward others so that his deeper ideation is sometimes parricidal, sometimes suicidal and sometimes homicidal. Within this setting, the child fluctuates between hopefulness, stemming from all the positive feelings that he has been able to extract from his environment, and hopelessness induced by the accumulation of bad feelings directed at him by a rejecting environment.

The role of hopelessness in the psychodynamics of suicide has lately been receiving as much prominence as the Freudian tenet of hostility and aggression turned inward. Stotland's [4] work on the psychology of hope strongly suggests that it plays a major role in motivation and action. The individual's ability to cope with the present is dependent on what he expects of the future and when the future is black or blank, the holding power of the present is reduced. Stotland has developed a theory and therapy of hope focusing on the probability of achieving some significant goal relating hopefulness to such intermediate factors as success and failure, persistence and defeatism, conflict and communication, and aggression and anxiety. This systematic exploration of the nature of hope has led to further understanding of the development of hopelessness and its culmination in self-destruction.

A single formula, whether it postulates a feeling of unwantedness, a failure of hope, or an inward turning of aggression, seems not to cover the large number of variables that investigations have associated with suicide although, admittedly, some of these are proximal and others more distal to the problem. Certain environments appear more productive of suicide than others and this is also true of certain periods in the life cycle, certain seasons of the year, and certain phases of the menstrual cycle. Children rarely resort to suicide but may be caught up unwittingly in suicidal activities by rash, impulsive, defiant behavior or experimentation. By adolescence, self-destruction becomes intentional and planned. Black adolescents are more suicidal and homicidal than white adolescents although by middle life, suicide has become largely a white problem. According to Hendin [3], suicide becomes a problem for the black youth because of the sense of despair, the feeling that life will never be satisfying, that possesses the black person very early on in life. Frustration, rage, and self-hatred are an integral part of the black family situation and are inseparable from the rage and self-hatred stemming from racial discrimination in a world that blocks fulfillment. This is akin to the "fatalistic" type of suicide described by Durkheim [1]. Epidemiological and sociological studies help with the understanding of some cases but others are too complex for just "external" consideration. For example, how would one classify the case of a seventeen-year-old girl, reported by Glaser [2], who had given bone marrow for her sister who was dying of leukemia. She had witnessed the last phase of the latter's tragic and prolonged suffering but was whisked away before death in order to spare her the emotional upset. Her previous relationship with her sister had been governed by jealousy and death wishes that she had been totally unable to express. When her marrow did not succeed in saving her sister, she felt responsible for the death and shortly after she made a suicidal attempt.

The life history is too curtailed to include all the developmental and transactional factors entering the suicidal attempt and the traumatic factors are consequently overemphasized. The behavior gets attributed to a central conflict over wishing to kill and at the same time wishing to keep her sister alive. The conflict is not resolved inwardly but outwardly; the matter is taken out of her hands and the sister dies. In an omnipotent, animistic sense, her marrow could save or destroy her sister, but her marrow, influenced by the death wish, decides not to save the sister and this makes her, therefore, completely responsible. Even in this brief clinical vignette, it is possible to assess the level of affective interchange within this family as somewhat low since she is not even permitted to become genuinely upset by her sister's death.

Rejection and favoritism breed hostility that in turn breeds death wishes toward the favored and rejecting ones. Unwantedness and neglect breed loss of self-esteem and diminution in self-preservative drive with death wishes directed toward the self. Both may conduce to suicidal ideation early in life, and the study by Adam offers us an important pointer in the genesis of suicide that could help in the diagnosis of vulnerability. The life history of an individual at suicidal risk might therefore disclose, among other still to be discovered factors, a loss of a significant figure in early life, depressive and suicidal ideation throughout childhood and adolescence, a chronically defeatist attitude in the face of problems, a preoccupation with death wishes with respect to self and others, a gradual diminution in hopefulness, a rise in aggressive feelings directed towards the self, an increased proneness to accidents, a devastating linkage of guilt with worthlessness, nothing but somber memories of the past, and an attitude to death not as death that borders on the unrealistic. Death is not a finality but another move in the game of hostility and counter-hostility as expressed in such ideas as "They'll be sorry when I'm gone"; "I'd like to see their faces when they hear what has happened."

Depending on their stage of development, children react to a parent's suicide with varying degrees of disbelief, of acceptance, and of ambivalence. From the child's point of view, suicide is an act of desertion that, like adoption, can never be satisfactorily accounted for, only rationalized. In some ways they are far better off with a particular parent dead than alive and yet his deadness itself may constitute a threat in making previously impossible wishes possible. The child's reaction is therefore dictated by the balance of his life and death wishes at the time of the act and his grasp of inner and outer reality. The chapter by Ilan helps to clarify both the manifest and latent struggles released by a father's death with the added complication that suicide intensifies and is often meant to intensify the guilt and self-reproach of those who survive. Suicide is an act that continues its aggressive impact over long periods of time on the lives of people. Hence its peculiar appeal for some individuals.

The killing of parents, like incest with parents, is almost universally regarded as a "primal" crime, and the two are often interlinked as in the original Oedipus drama. The parricide is generally an adolescent. Two of the cases reported by Anthony and Rizzo and two communicated to us by Lebovici have to do with thirteen year olds who set out to kill or actually killed their fathers. In the first of the cases, reported by Ochonisky and discussed by Lebovici, the boy belonged to a foreign family (that is, non-French) that was finding it difficult to make an adequate living in its adopted country. The father reacted to his precarious employment situation by indulging in petty dishonesties and by treating his wife and children brutally. His viciousness augmented with his general deterioration. The boy did well at school but his parents showed negligible interest in this. He became more and more conscious of the happier lot of his fellow students in their apparently stable families as compared with his own unhappy circumstance. On the day of the crime, the father pawned a rug not belonging to him to meet a pressing debt. The boy was shocked and reproached him. The latter's angry response was to inform his son that he was to be taken away from a school that had failed to teach him respect for his parents. A few hours later, the boy shot the father with the latter's own revolver and then gave himself up. The crime was not hard to understand, as Lebovici points out, either in terms of the child's protective love for his mother or of his disappointment and disillusionment in his father. It seems that he had threatened earlier to kill himself but the father had responded indifferently to the threat. He had also often borne the brunt of his father's brutal attacks on his younger brother, but it emerged in the later psychological interviews that this was done to gratify a masochistic fantasy. The interviews also disclosed a considerable erotic fixation on the father whom he chose to kill when it seemed that his own developing ego ideal was at stake. The act did not stir up the usual measure of horror accorded to parricide by the public and the case was discharged because the crime was felt to be justifiable. A follow-up interview, many years later, disclosed that the boy had become a law-abiding and well-adjusted citizen performing very adequately as a teacher.

In contrast, Lebovici mentions another case of Ochonisky's, also a thirteen-year-old boy, who stated that he had killed his father because he was afraid he would beat him for not doing adequately at school. He was the only son of a well-to-do, well-adjusted family in which both parents behaved with conventional normality toward the children. Prior to the murder, the boy had attempted to run away and to commit suicide (by swallowing phosphorous) giving the same reason that he was afraid of his father. In the subsequent follow-up study, it was found that as a young man he had murdered his mistress after a somewhat bizarre interchange with her husband. He had sent the latter an anonymous letter denouncing his own liaison with the wife and setting up a meeting between all three in order to reconcile the marital partners. After the woman's murder, he had been sent to prison and then transferred to a mental hospital because of his violent paranoid tendencies. Eighteen years after the murder of his father, he committed suicide. The complete incomprehensibility of this second act of parricide at once suggests the diagnosis of psychosis. Lebovici, however, points out that the public reaction cannot be excluded from a consideration of the further development of the two murderers. The first boy was considered an auxiliary of justice while the second was branded with horror as inhuman. The first boy might exclaim, as Dimitri Karamazov did with respect to his father, "Why is such a man alive? Tell me, can one allow him to shame the earth with his vices?" And the public would concur. The second boy would increasingly expand his delusional projections out of all proportion to reality creating a huge discrepancy between his picture of the father and the way the public viewed him. The reactions of society toward crime must, to some extent, determine the fate of the criminal after the crime, particularly in the context of his rehabilitation.

Lebovici has also dealt with the subject of abnormal sadism in children in his usual masterly fashion including biological, cultural, and psychodynamic factors in a complex interplay. There are many built-in gratifications to sadism. It may provide a reassurance against the fears of being hurt oneself, of doing to others what one fears they might do to oneself, of being active rather than passive, and of being powerful rather than impotent. In many cases, the idea of avoiding a terrifying passive experience by actively perpetrating it on others and thereby establishing a mystical union with the victim seems to be the main determinant. The case has been made for a constitutional factor that is enhanced as the child passes through oral, anal, and phallic stages of sadism. In his study, "A Child is Being Beaten," Freud investigated the development of sadomasochistic fantasies in childhood and demonstrated that they involved conflicts around the Oedipus complex. However, beating fantasies lead to neurotic developments rather than to sadism, whereas children who have been treated sadistically may develop sadistically. The beaten child may also become the beating adult.

The child who beats, who tortures, who kills, who kills his parents, and who kills himself are all variations in the vicissitude of the aggressive impulse in human development about which we still know too little. Our psychodynamic theories sound more powerfully explanatory than they really are in practice. In the evolution of his theory, Freud began to conceive of libido and aggressivity as indissolubly bound together, one reason being the constant frustration of infantile sexual wishes generates aggression and another that the guilty reactions released by aggression bring about a cycle of self-punishment and masochism. Furthermore, the realization of any wish implies, to a certain extent, the destruction of the wished for object. Later Abraham described sadistic phases of development suggesting that sadism ran a normal course, mainly during the pre-oedipal stage. Lebovici has tried to separate sadism as a perversion from sadism as a partial instinct in healthy development. Ideally, the two should be subsumed under the same general theory but the life and death instinct theory has not been enough. After 1920, in order to explain repetition compulsion, Freud postulated the existence of a death instinct or deep-seated masochism that could be deflected and thereby become the main source of aggression. He also linked aggression with anxiety when it threatened the loss of the loved object. The further elaboration of a two instinct theory came to a standstill more or less with Freud's death (although Klein made a major effort to further it); certainly the development of aggression cannot compare with the detailed theoretical development accorded to libido. For many analysts, it still remains a by-product of libido theory. Even if given a developmental history of its own, there are problems regarding its place in ego psychology. Nor is its relationship to narcissism and to object relationship too well defined. Ethologists, like Lorenz, have spoken of aggression in the animal world as a "necessary evil," but this really begs so many questions that from a clinical and psychodynamic point of view it is hardly a useful contribution. The chapters in this section make very clear some of the theoretical weaknesses involved and the need for further careful and systematic investigations.

E. James Anthony

Bibliography

1. Durkheim, E., *Suicide*, New York, Free Press of Glencoe, 1951.
2. Glaser, K., Suicide in children and adolescents, in *Acting Out: Theoretical and Clinical Aspects*, L. Apt, Ed., Grune, New York, 1965.
3. Hendin, H., *Black Suicide*, Basic Books, New York, 1969.
4. Stotland, E., *The Psychology of Hope*, Jossey-Bass, San Francisco, 1969.

Childhood Parental Loss, Suicidal Ideation, and Suicidal Behavior

Kenneth S. Adam, M.D. (Canada)

Introduction

The purpose of this paper is to describe an hypothesis concerning the relationship between early parental loss and the development of suicidal ideas and behavior. It will include a review of the relevant literature on the subject and will report on some preliminary research findings of a project which has been specifically designed to test some aspects of the hypothesis. In addition, an attempt will be made to bring this hypothesis into the perspective of known theory concerning the importance of early object relationships in the development of psychopathology generally.

Review

Since the early papers by Freud and Zilboorg which related loss of a loved object to depression and suicide, there has been considerable interest in the relationship between parental loss in childhood and later suicidal behavior. A number of retrospective studies have examined samples of suicides and attempted suicides with the repeated finding of a high incidence of childhood loss of parents. Considerable controversy has arisen out of whether this relationship, though real, is causal and, if so, which factors in the experience are pathogenic.

RETROSPECTIVE STUDIES

Batchelor and Napier [3] examined 200 consecutive attempted suicides for the presence of a broken home in childhood and found that 58% of their sample had been "deprived of a normal life with their parents" for a period of greater than six months.

Moss and Hamilton [29] compared 50 adults judged to be seriously suicidal to identical numbers of potentially suicidal and nonsuicidal subjects. They found 98% of the suicidal subjects had a "death trend" in their histories which they defined as the death or loss of closely related persons under "dramatic" conditions. Sixty percent of these subjects had experienced the loss in early life, 75% of these before the end of adolescence. Loss of the father was in excess of maternal loss and in 25% of the cases, a later loss was felt to have precipitated the subject's illness. A history of suicide in the immediate family was noted in 25% of cases.

Dorpat et al. [9] compared a group of 114 unselected and consecutive completed suicides to 121 subjects who had attempted suicide and reported some striking findings. Fifty percent of the completed suicide group and 64% of the attempted suicide group came from broken homes. Nearly half of the completed suicides had lost both parents as had two-thirds of the attempted suicides. Whereas loss of parents through death was commonest in the completed suicides, loss through divorce was commonest among the attempted suicides. A large number of subjects in both groups had suffered a real or threatened loss of some significant person a short time prior to their suicidal behavior. Dorpat hypothesized that unresolved object loss in childhood leads to an inability to sustain object losses later in life, and that the severity of the early loss was related to the intensity of the suicidal tendencies.

Greer [14, 15, 16, 17] has published several papers on two carefully controlled studies of attempted suicide in which he examined for parental loss. In both of his studies he found a significantly higher incidence of parental loss before the age of 15 in the suicidal group, and in one of his studies loss before the age of five was commoner. The sex of the parent lost did not seem to be correlated with attempted suicide, although loss of both parents was felt to be particularly important as was permanent rather than temporary separation. A higher percentage of attempted suicides than controls had experienced recent disruptions of close interpersonal relationships. Koller [25] and Kearney [22] have replicated Greer's studies using different samples and different control groups with essentially the same findings regarding the higher incidence of early parental loss in the study group.

This series of studies is particularly valuable because of the methodological care taken in defining criteria for selection of study patients and in the matching of controls. The use of the same methodology with different samples by other workers with confirmation of the original findings adds considerable weight to their conclusions. A number of other studies on psychiatric out-patients who have attempted suicide and depressed patients with suicidal trends have reached similar conclusions regarding the suicide proneness of subjects with childhood parental loss [4, 26, 35, 19].

Many of these studies have focused on specific questions related to the type of loss, its timing, the sex of the parent lost, and the age period during which the loss occurred, but without conclusive results. There is a trend in the findings suggesting that earlier losses are more pathogenic than later ones and that paternal loss may be more directly relevant to suicidal behavior than maternal. It also seems that such losses may be more relevant in the suicidal behavior of younger persons than older ones, and corroborating evidence for this can be found in studies on suicidal children, suicidal adolescents, and university students [28, 2, 32, 31]. It may be that certain groups of suicidal individuals, or specific suicidal syndromes, are more strongly related to parental loss than others, and there is at least one study which suggests this is so [34].

Criticism has been leveled at these studies from several points of view [18, 30, 27]. To begin with there is no consistency among the studies concerning the criteria for what is called a "broken home," parental deprivation, or "parental loss," nor is there a consistent definition of the duration of the separation or the age prior to which it must have occurred. Similarly there is uneven definition as to what is considered suicidal behavior. Completed suicide, the simplest to define, has been least studied and the definition of a suicidal attempt includes the threat of suicide in some samples. Many of the studies lack comparison with control samples and many draw their data from case records and other material not primarily collected for research purposes. A major fault in methodology has been the failure to place both study and control populations within the perspective of normal bereavement rates. All studies are retrospective and, therefore, open to the criticism that the mere existence of a statistical connection does not prove causality, and that intervening variables as yet unknown may be more relevant.

In spite of these valid criticisms, it is striking that all of the studies point toward the significance of early parental loss as a pathogenic factor in suicidal behavior and none argues directly against it. There seems general agreement among authorities at present that of all the sequelae attributed to early childhood loss the evidence with regard to suicidal behavior is among the strongest [5, 13, 30].

PSYCHOANALYTIC STUDIES

Although considerable attention has been given in the above studies to the possible importance of various factors surrounding the experience of loss and the conditions following upon it, there has been little recent attention given to the question of the mechanisms involved which might link this experience to later suicidal behavior. Most of the speculation relevant to these issues is found in the psychoanalytic literature which stems directly from Freud's early paper "Mourning and Melancholia" [10].

In this paper, Freud describes the processes whereby the melancholic attempts to deal with the real or imagined loss of a significant loved object. According to this formulation the melancholic seeks to avoid the pain inherent in the loss by regressing from a level of narcissistic object choice to original narcissism utilizing the mechanism of identification to incorporate the lost object within the ego. This protective mechanism, though preserving the object, fails in its task of dealing with the pain when the ambivalence felt toward the original object becomes heightened and redirected toward the now internalized representation of the object. The result is a split in the ego with one part directed against the other which is consciously expressed in self-reproaches, guilt, and delusions of punishment. Suicide, in this formulation, is a result of the ego's punitive and sadistic attack upon itself being carried to the extent that the hated internalized object is destroyed and with it the ego itself.

Klein [24], writing later about manic-depressive states, also emphasized the importance of introjected objects in suicide but did not feel this necessarily implied only the murder of bad objects but also in some cases the preservation of good ones.

In some cases the phantasies underlying suicide aim at preserving the internalized good objects and that part of the ego which is identified with good objects, and also at destroying the other part of the ego which is identified with bad objects and the ego. Thus the ego is enabled to become united with its loved objects [24].

Although both Freud and Klein speak of the identification with a lost object as important to the mechanism of suicide, neither speaks of conditions which differentiate the suicidal melancholic from the nonsuicidal, and neither speaks specifically of a *childhood* experience of loss as being a critical factor in determining a suicidal outcome. This particular association was first suggested by Zilboorg who was impressed by the fact that other dynamic constellations than the depressive can lead to suicidal behavior [36].

In his paper, "Considerations on Suicide With Particular Reference to that of the Young" [37], he related an account of a young woman who committed suicide on the anniversary of her mother's death. While agreeing that the mechanism of incorporation of the object was important in the dynamics of this case, he argued that the crucial factor determining the suicidal outcome was that the identification was with a person already dead and that this identification took place in childhood.

It discloses that the classical type of killing an incorporated object is not the only type, and that incorporation of an object is in itself not the true cause of suicide; only those individuals who appear to have identified themselves with a dead person and in whom the process of identification took place during childhood or adolescence, at a time when the incorporated person was already actually dead, are most probably the truly suicidal individuals.

Other analytic writers, following Zilboorg, have described suicidal cases where the principal dynamics were associated with pleasurable rather than hostile fantasies and where the unconscious wishes in the suicidal behavior were directed more toward reuniting with the lost object than attacking it [12, 21].

Hendricks [21] described one such case in detail where a young schizophrenic woman made two serious suicidal attempts which were seen to be the acting out of her strong unconscious wish to identify through death with her deceased brother whom she had admired and loved in childhood. He notes several differences between the mechanisms of suicide in this case and that observed in depressions with particular emphasis on the different role played by identification in the two.

> In depression, moreover, the effort to die is a consequence of an identification, while here identification is the purpose (the goal) of dying, that goal which satisfies all impulses, libidinal and destructive.

> The suicidal act of this patient is the fulfillment and not a consequence of the identification.

Common to all these studies is the central position given to identification as the mechanism, whereby the lost object continues to exert its influence within the personality with suicide being seen not as deliberate conscious destruction of the ego but rather as an objective consequence of the ego's attempt to maintain its relation to the object.

While Bowlby does not specifically deal with the problem of suicide, his extensive writings on childhood separation and pathological mourning are of great relevance to it. While agreeing with other analytic theorists about the importance of defensive processes such as repression, splitting, and denial in the development of pathological outcomes to childhood mourning, Bowlby is cautious in drawing upon explanatory hypotheses utilizing the mechanism of identification. He prefers first to focus on that which is more readily observed in children who form the subjects of his studies, namely, behavior. The behavioral reaction to separation from the maternal object which begs explanation, according to Bowlby, is the continuing yearning for and the angry reproaches which are directed against the lost object. These he sees as a result simply of the strong desire in the child to renew and maintain a relationship vital for biological survival, and the intense protest which ensues when this relationship is threatened [6, 7, 8].

> Could it not be due simply and solely to the rupture of a key relationship and the consequent intense pain of yearning occurring in a young child [7].

He sees the child's angry striving for the lost object as a means of coercing it to return, and the child's later reproaches against the object as a means of ensuring it will not leave again.

Precisely how these intense urges to recover and reproach the lost object are carried over into later life is not spelled out by Bowlby except to say that they become "split off and repressed" and continue as "active systems" within the personality influencing feeling and behavior [5].

I believe that the "active systems" which Bowlby refers to are what other analytic writers would call unconscious fantasies and that it is these persistent fantasies that are of importance in suicidal behavior.

That suicidal behavior is often related to current object loss and the dynamic themes mentioned above can be seen in countless descriptions of suicidal attempts and suicides although the association of these to previous loss experiences has seldom been looked for. It is well-known, for example, that suicidal behavior often occurs in response to rejection in one form or another from a significant person, and that an important motivation of many suicidal attempts is its "appeal function" to other persons [33]. The suicidal attempt frequently represents a reproach against the rejecting person, and this reproach can often be seen to carry with it a strong implied injunction against future rejections.

The precise content of the unconscious fantasies behind suicidal attempts is difficult to determine because of the disorganized and often dissociated state in which such behavior occurs, and as a result most accounts of such fantasies come from posthoc reconstructions or studies of suicide notes. Hendin [20], however, using special techniques including hypnosis to facilitate recovery of fantasies and dreams in subjects having recently made a serious suicide attempt, found many of the dynamic themes to be object related with precipitating factors associated with actual or symbolic losses.

In addition, direct observations of children's responses to the death of a parent, though few in number, have reported preoccupations with ideas of death and suicide including fantasies, dreams, and hallucinations of reunion with the dead parent.

Freud and Burlingham [11] noted such phenomena among children in a wartime nursery remarking that where a father had died the child often continued to talk of him as if he were alive, often insisting he had actual visits from him. Keeler [23] reported similar vivid fantasies in 11 children brought to psychiatric attention following a parental death, six of whom as well were preoccupied with suicide, some making actual attempts.

When taken together these data would suggest that early experiences of loss and later suicidal behavior are connected not only by statistical association but by common themes. Furthermore, it seems that one of the direct outcomes of childhood parental loss, at least in some cases, may be a preoccupation in the mental life with ideas of death, suicide, and the lost parent and that such ideas may persist in later life becoming themes around which later suicidal behavior may be enacted.

Research

THE RESEARCH PROBLEM

The research* I wish to describe has been designed to test some aspects of a larger hypothesis about the role of childhood parental loss and suicidal behavior which has evolved out of a long-standing interest in the general problem of suicide [1]. This hypothesis in its simplest form can be stated as follows:

> Loss or separation from parental figures at some critical period or circumstance in childhood may result in the development of pathological suicidal ideas which may persist in an unconscious form throughout life. Such ideas might later be activated by specific triggering events, such as the current rejection by a significant person or by more general factors impairing ego functioning which favor the emergence of unconscious impulses and ideas. This in turn could lead to suicidal behavior.

This hypothesis is summarized in Figure 1.

Such an hypothesis is economical in that it unifies a number of variables known to be relevant to suicidal behavior, and in linking genetic events in childhood to later events is consistent with a considerable body of developmental and psychodynamic literature.

Our project has been designed to test only a portion of this larger hypothesis, namely the relationship of early loss of parental figures to the development of significant suicidal ideation with the ultimate aim of providing clues as to which factors surrounding

*This investigation is being carried out in conjunction with Dr. J. G. Lohrenz and Mrs. Dorothy Harper, M. A., at the McGill University Health Service. It was supported initially by a grant from the Medical Research Council of Canada and is currently supported by the Laidlaw Foundation of Toronto, Canada. The results presented here represent data collected over a four-year period from January, 1968 to January, 1971. The study will continue for one more year.

Figure 1

Predisposing Factors		Contributing Factors	Precipitating Factors	
Disturbance in Early Object Relations through Parental Loss or Separation	Pathological Suicidal Ideation (Unconscious)	Interference with higher ego controls	Disturbance in Current Object Relations	Suicidal Attempt
		1. Intoxication	1. Current Loss	Activation of Suicidal Ideation (Conscious)
		2. Organic Brain Disease	2. Current Rejection	
		3. Physical Debility	3. Symbolic Loss	
		4. Personality Disorder (Impulsivity)		
		5. Personality Fragmentation (Schizophrenia)		Suicide

such experiences might be most pathogenic. The main methodological consideration in planning the study has been that it be prospective, taking at its starting point the fact of an early object loss
and then examining for the dependent variable, namely, suicidal
ideation. A second major consideration has been that the study be
controlled, allowing for comparison of subjects with a history of
parental loss to those from intact homes. The primary focus on
suicidal ideation rather than behavior is important as well inasmuch
as suicidal behavior is a rarer event than the former and because of
the dramatic circumstances which usually follow upon it, less accessible to the application of a sound methodology.

THE RESEARCH DESIGN

The sample being studied consists of three groups of university
students who came to a student mental health service over a period
of four years. One group consisted of students who had lost one
or both parents prior to the age of 16 through death, and a second
group consisted of students who had lost one or both parents prior
to the same age because of divorce or permanent separation. These
groups were compared to a matched control group of subjects all of
whom had both parents alive and continuously living together. Because of variations in bereavement rates from decade to decade all
subjects were within an age range of 17 to 27 at the time of their
interview. It is felt that the subjects studied represent an unusually
homogenous group for research purposes.

METHODOLOGY

Once selected, subjects were randomly assigned to a primary interviewer who conducted a semistructured clinical interview covering a variety of areas, namely, general adaptation, medical history,
accident proneness, depressive trends, suicidal ideas and behavior,
and attitudes toward death and dying. Key items were scored during
the interview according to pre-established criteria validated in pilot
studies and cross validated by a second independent rater using a
tape recording of the interview. Detailed enquiry was made following this into the subjects' early background and a careful documenta-
tion was made into the circumstances surrounding parental deaths,
divorces, and separations.

Every attempt was made to maintain blindness to the family
status of the subject until after the scoring procedure. This proved

to be impossible in some cases but statistical tests have subsequently shown that failure of blindness did not influence scoring.

The results presented here represent a preliminary analysis of the data relating to the primary hypothesis being tested, namely, that the two study groups with early parental loss would differ in a significant way regarding items relating to suicidal ideas and behavior from those of the control group.

A more detailed description of the sample, the methodology, and the results of other items will be published at a later time when data collection is complete.

Scoring of Suicidal Ideation

During the course of the interview specific exploration was made for the presence of suicidal ideas and where these were reported, the subject was asked to give as many details as possible about their onset, frequency, intensity, duration, and content. Responses were scored as *significant* or *not significant* according to operational criteria defining three parameters of frequency, intensity, and duration as being either of high, moderate, or low order. Subjects with two or more of the parameters of moderate to high intensity were scored as *significant* with all others scored as *not significant*. Subjects reporting a suicidal attempt of any description were also scored as *significant*. Where any doubt existed as to which category the ideation belonged it was scored conservatively as *not significant*.

Table 1 Suicidal Ideation ($n = 114$, $x^2 = 17.11$, $p < 0.001$

	Significant	Not Significant	Total
Control Subjects (Group I)	5	45	50
Parental death (Group II)	17	18	35
Parental divorce and separation (Group III)	12	17	29
	34	80	114

Table 2 Suicidal Ideation (Groups II and III Combined)
($n = 114$, $x^2 = 15.07$, $p < 0.001$)

	Significant	Not Significant	Total
Control subjects (Group I)	5	45	50
Parental death, divorce, and separated (Groups II and III combined)	29	35	64
	34	80	114

As can be seen from Tables 1 and 2, a highly significant relationship was found between the parental loss groups and the presence of *significant* suicidal ideation when compared to the control group. The relationship holds equally strongly whether the two parental loss groups are treated separately or together with no obvious differences between these two subgroups. What is particularly striking is how few of the control subjects were found to have significant suicidal ideation (10%), compared to the study groups where the incidence approached 50%.

Although a content analysis of the suicidal ideation has not been completed, some general comments can be made about the ways in which subjects scored as *significant* differed from those scored *not significant* from this point of view.

SUBJECTS WITH SIGNIFICANT SUICIDAL IDEATION

These subjects often reported ideas of suicide that were relatively more elaborate, more persistent, and of longer duration than those scored *not significant*. Their ideas of suicide often presented in an intense way as strong urges or impulses which were sometimes frightening and difficult to control. Some subjects, in fact, were so strongly moved by their impulses that they sought external help to protect themselves. The themes expressed in their suicidal ideas were often those of profound isolation, hopelessness, and self-hatred, and the theme of death as peace, freedom, or release was sometimes reported. Serious conscious consideration of suicide was a regular occurrence in this group and this was often corroborated by partially or completely formulated suicide plans, near attempts, or actual suicidal attempts. Some subjects maintained collections of pills or other poisonous substances for "consolation," and some had set a deadline for change to occur in their lives after which time they felt they could no longer tolerate hope. In some cases the suicidal ideas were associated with strong homicidal impulses and in many of these subjects there was a history of impulsive behavior, aggressiveness, and accident proneness. These subjects were seldom casual in discussing the topic of suicide, were sometimes disturbed by it, and occasionally excited by it. They often referred to suicide as "making sense" and many saw it as a real possibility for them in the future; even as an inevitability.

A few examples of the suicidal ideation abstracted from the interviews will illustrate the sort of data referred to.*

Example I (Significant Suicidal Ideation) This subject was a 19-year-old science student who came to the Health Service because of persistent depressive feelings interfering with her ability to function academically and socially following the breakup of a recent love affair. She reported frequent ideas of suicide which she had experienced over several months.

I began to associate dying with peace and with freedom, and I just didn't think that I wanted to live very much any more. Because it was just so miserable, and there didn't seem to be anything good about it. And I didn't feel afraid of dying at all. I mean, I know I must have been, but I didn't really feel it consciously, afraid of dying. And—perhaps I didn't really want to die, maybe I just wanted some sort of attention. I never told anybody. . . .I haven't done anything worthwhile, and I cause a lot of people unhappiness, and I had caused myself a lot of unhappiness too. And that maybe everything that they told us about suicide wasn't true and God would really be forgiving or something like that. I always wanted, if I were going to die, I wanted to die in a beautiful place. Not in the country but maybe on a mountain or something. At a beautiful time. Because I didn't really think that dying was anything unnatural. Just another part of living. And it would be nice to die among beautiful things.

The subject reported an occasion recently when she felt these thoughts particularly intensely during an afternoon when she had been lonely and had been unsuccessful in contacting any of her friends. She formulated a plan for getting sleeping pills and was on her way to get them when a chance encounter with a friendly

---

*Examples have been disguised to prevent identification of the subject, although material quoted directly is exact.

professor changed her mind. She felt she could understand others' wish to suicide and felt that there was a real possibility of suicide for her in the future unless her circumstances changed. She saw this as a way of controlling her destiny.

> I guess I'd just like to choose the time and the place, and the age, and everything.

Background information revealed that her father had died following a chronic illness when she was six years old following which she had been raised first by her maternal grandmother and then by her mother who worked to support the family. She had great difficulty recalling any of the events surrounding her father's actual death and the immediate period following, although she had vivid recollections of him during the period prior to his final hospitalization when he was home most of the time. She was visibly disturbed when talking of her father and was markedly defensive when discussing the general topic of death. During the interview she was apathetic, melancholic, and spoke with a kind of persistent sadness.

Example II (Significant Suicidal Ideation) The subject was a 20-year-old girl who came for help because of feelings of panic and depression one week after moving out of home following an argument with her mother. Her parents separated when she was ten and divorced two years later following a chronically unstable marriage in which the father was apparently unfaithful. Following the separation she lived with her mother who went through a period of great instability during which she was indiscreet about her sexual behavior, made a suicide attempt, and had a brief hospitalization for a "nervous breakdown." During this time the subject and her sister maintained contact with the father with whom she had a somewhat sexualized relationship and took most of their meals with the maternal grandparents who lived nearby. Both parents remarried within three years and the situation stabilized considerably, although she and the mother have continued to have a good deal of conflict.

She recalls being depressed since she left home at 17 for a year of travel, and since that time she has had frequent periods of moderately severe depression during which she has felt great pessimism toward the future, self-hatred, and frequent thoughts of suicide.

> I saw nothing but great unhappiness in the future, and if that's the case, then

there's no point in living through it. I even have pictures that . . . would sort of amount to living the same as your parents with unhappy marriage, unhappy children, unfulfilled life, very bleak home. Everything looks shades of—no color, no happiness anywhere. It isn't sort of suicide in actively killing yourself. It's sort of "I do not want to live." If you do not want to live, you've got to kill yourself. The things that are ahead are terrible. I do not want to live through them.

Although she emphasized repeatedly that "not wanting to live" was not the same as "suicide" she also returned again and again to the theme of feeling helpless about controlling the course of her life.

Unless I can get to all this stuff below the surface, I will never be happy.

The passionate love I have and the enthusiasm I have for things that are living, and natural things, I really wish I could transfer to the rest of my life, but it's just nonexistent. It's just something I find myself being drawn into.

SUBJECTS WITH NOT-SIGNIFICANT SUICIDAL IDEATION

In contrast to the subjects with "significant suicidal ideation," these subjects usually reported simple, brief, and frequently intellectualized ideas where the thought of suicide had occurred in the face of some pressing reality situation. The theme of escape was common and was expressed in terms such as: "things were a waste of time," or "I thought it would be simpler if I were dead," as was the theme "they'd be sorry when I'm gone." These subjects usually denied any serious consideration of suicide and rarely thought of it as a possibility for the future. They seldom had ever formulated a suicide plan and often spoke disparagingly of persons whom they knew who had made suicide attempts or who had suicided referring to them as "not adjusting," or "spineless," or "sick." Thoughts of suicide seemed to be something that had occurred in moments of despair but without conviction and without a sense of hopelessness. In the words of one subject, "I've felt that things were a complete waste of time, but I've never felt that there's no use going on."

Example III (Suicidal Ideation Not Significant)

When things get rough I'd like to escape, not commit suicide. I'd like to get away, I'd like to—go back and live the way I feel without having to be a part of the rat race. Suicide?—it's sort of a coward's way out, for one thing. There's too much in my life to worry about to compete with other people to get a place in society.

This subject came from an intact family with both parents living and had come to the clinic for a single consultation hoping for the health service to intervene in what he thought was an unfair administrative decision regarding his course load for the coming year.

Example IV (Suicidal Ideation not Significant) This subject was a 21-year-old law student who sought help because of severe symptoms of anxiety and recurrent attacks of depersonalization which had interfered with his functioning over a period of several months. Although presenting quite severe symptoms, he responded well to a brief psychotherapeutic intervention and was felt to have been having a delayed identity crisis focused mainly over the area of career choice. His ego was considered to be fundamentally healthy.

In responding to a question about thoughts of suicide he replied:

> To personally kill myself—no. I've thought of suicide. I've read in psychology why people do it, but just because I don't feel well I'm not going to go out and kill myself. Things can't be that bad.—I can't understand that the state of depression could be so low that a person could have—I don't know, maybe I consider it the easy way out. If you don't like something—well, my father always makes a joke, like the European joke, "If you don't like the world, you can take the gas pipe," you know what I mean? Just as a joke, that's the way I laugh at it. You know, if you don't like what's happening you just, you know, people kill themselves. Some people say it takes a tremendous amount of guts to kill yourself or something like that. I just can't see it.

This subject's mother died of cancer when he was seven years old following an illness of two years' duration during which time his maternal grandmother who was living with the family took over the primary maternal role. After the death of his mother, his grandmother continued to raise him "like a mother," living as before with the father even after his remarriage seven years later. The subject remembers feeling sad after learning of his mother's death but quickly got over this as life continued in the home much as before. He occasionally still thinks of his mother in an idealized way and has sometimes felt guilty about not feeling worse about her being gone. The father's remarriage has proved successful and he has a good relationship with his stepmother and stepsiblings.

SUICIDAL ATTEMPTS

During the course of the interviews, twelve subjects were discovered to have made actual suicidal attempts of which three had made multiple attempts. Where such behavior was reported a detailed inquiry was made of the circumstances surrounding it and an estimate of the severity of the attempt was made according to multiple criteria including the apparent motivation, the medical risk involved, the method chosen, and provisions made for rescue.

Although the number involved is too small for statistical analysis, it is striking to note than ten of the subjects fell in the parental loss groups, six in the parental-death group, and four in the divorce-separated group (see Table 3).

Table 3 Suicidal Attempt ($n = 114$, $x^2 = 2.88$, $.05 < p < .10$, N.S.)

	Yes	No	
Group I Control	2	48	50
Groups II and III Parental death or divorce/ separation	10	54	64
	12	102	114

Seven of the 12 subjects, all belonging to the early parental loss groups, were felt to have made serious attempts and were judged to be of high risk for future suicidal activity. All of the attempts, with one exception, occurred after the age of 12, with half of them taking place in the early adolescent years from 12 to 15. In 10 of the 12 subjects it was apparent that the actual or threatened loss of an important person was the chief precipitating factor in the attempt. In four of the cases where a serious attempt had been made there was also evidence of dangerous symptomatic behavior such as extreme recklessness or participation in highly hazardous sports.

Example V This subject was a 21-year-old undergraduate who came to the clinic with multiple complaints of anxiety, depression, amenorhea, and constipation of long standing. She gave a history of a chaotic family life with parental separation at the age of seven being followed by frequent dislocations during which she was shifted from one parent to the other, often being left for periods of time in the care of disinterested surrogate figures. She reported frequent, intense preoccupation with suicide from early adolescence and had made two suicidal attempts.

The first of these occurred at the age of 15 shortly following her father's remarriage during a period when she felt him to be remote and unapproachable. She recalled feeling angry at him and decided to "retaliate" by shutting herself in her room and refusing to eat. When this brought no response after two days, she bought some sleeping pills from a drug store, ingested them, and retired again to her room informing no one of her action. The pills proved to be a mild preparation as she awakened after a few hours. It was only two weeks later when taken to visit the family doctor that she revealed she had swallowed pills.

The second attempt was made two years later following her breakup with a boyfriend of long standing which in turn was followed by a period of depression and compulsive overeating. The day prior to this attempt she and her mother had argued bitterly about this boyfriend and she felt tormented by feelings of guilt and unworthiness. The next morning she remained home from school while her mother went to work, and took to her bed following swallowing a handful of aspirin compounds. She remained in bed until her sister returned home from school, discovered her nauseous and took her to hospital where she had a stomach lavage. She revealed during the research interview that in the two weeks prior to this attempt she had "experimented" with various other suicide methods including "toying around with knives," and turning on the gas jets but had stopped each time because of fear of "going to hell."

Both of these attempts were judged to have been serious inasmuch as she was convinced in her own mind, albeit incorrectly, that the method chosen was lethal, she planned her actions in advance, and she made no realistic provisions for her rescue.

The relationship of suicidal ideation to actual suicidal behavior and ultimately suicide cannot be proven from this data although our findings thus far regarding the higher incidence of suicidal attempts in the study groups compared to the control group are highly suggestive. In evaluating these findings, it is important to remember that suicidal attempts and suicide increase in frequency with age and that the average age of the group studied (20.5 years) is not an age at which suicidal activity is high compared to the general population although university students may be at higher risk within this age range than others [19]. It seems likely that the number of suicide attempts among this group will increase as they grow older (simply in terms of the natural history of suicidal behavior), but whether the increase will continue to show itself more in the study groups than in the control group can only be shown by a follow-up study. Certainly, from a clinical point of view it seems highly probable that many of our subjects classified as significant suicidal ideation will act out their fantasies at some time in the future.

OTHER FINDINGS

A number of other variables related to the loss experience of our subjects are being examined but as yet the subgroup samples are too small for definitive statements to be made about these. Some of the findings, though inconclusive, are sufficiently important to bear mentioning at this time.

The first of these is that the age of the subject at the time of permanent parental loss seems to have no bearing on the development of suicidal ideas inasmuch as subjects who sustained losses at all ages were found to have significant suicidal ideation. There was a tendency towards a clustering of losses at a later age in the bereaved group and a reciprocal clustering of earlier losses in the divorced-separated group, but this finding may be coincidental reflecting a tendency for families to break up earlier from marital incompatability than from the death of one of the partners. Previous evidence which has suggested that either very early losses or losses in the adolescent period are the most important are not, however, corroborated.

A finding which supports that of previous workers is a trend noted in the significant ideation group towards same sexed parental loss in the male subjects. Loss of the father by death or by divorce is commoner than loss of the mother in this age group, however, and this combined with a slightly higher ratio of male to female subjects in our sample makes this finding difficult to interpret.

DISCUSSION

The findings thus far in this study strongly support the hypothesis that parental loss in childhood is an important factor in the development of suicidal tendencies later in life and there is some evidence that these tendencies are related to disturbances in current object relationships.

It is of particular interest that there seems to be no essential difference in terms of the development of significant suicidal ideation between subjects sustaining parental loss because of death of a parent from those suffering loss because of parental separation. This would seem to throw into question Zilboorg's hypothesis that it is identification with a dead parent that is crucial in producing suicidal tendencies and would tend to support the belief that separation from key parental figures, regardless of the cause, is pathogenic. Dorpat's hypothesis that the severity of the loss is related to the intensity of the suicidal tendencies is not supported either by our data as no qualitative or quantitative differences were readily discernible between our two parental loss groups. Whether the parental death group will ultimately prove to be more actively suicidal than the divorce separation group remains to be seen.

Comparative scanning of the data at this stage suggests that the breakup of a family through parental death may differ in important ways from the breakup of a family because of parental separation. For one thing, bereaved families are more likely to have been stable families prior to the loss; furthermore, they are more likely to have survived longer as a family than are divorced families. An early analysis of the data from our first 70 subjects indicated that whereas there was a tendency among the bereaved families to become more unstable after the loss, the opposite trend was observed in the separated families.

Interestingly enough, the ratio of favorable to unfavorable outcomes was about the same for both types of families although the problems faced in the two types of crisis were often quite different. The presence of a consistent, stable nurturant figure of some sort seemed to be of great importance in protecting against the development of significant suicidal ideation as did the capacity of the family to find substitute objects. In general it was easier to evaluate the reasons for a positive outcome following a loss experience than it was a negative one as in the latter there were often such chaotic circumstances evident that the relative weight of any one potentially pathogenic factor was difficult to sort out. A great many questions are raised by these preliminary observations as to whether the most pathogenic factors are related to disruption of key relationships, their discontinuity, or to other variables such as the presence of conflict in the ongoing relationships following the experience of loss. One of the more important tasks of our project will be to examine these issues in detail and in particular to compare the subjects with significant suicidal ideation to those without significant suicidal ideation from the point of view of the pre-loss home, the post-loss home, the presence or absence of consistent nurturant figures, and the presence or absence of ongoing conflict with these figures.

Another important task will concern the content analysis of the suicidal ideas, the relationship of the themes contained therein to object relationships past and present, and to the processes of mourning. Practically none of our subjects were felt to have had typical responses to mourning, judged by adult standards, and very few were felt to have resolved psychologically the fact of parental separation. The tasks of mourning a dead parent seem to have important differences from those of mourning the loss of one who is alive although the differences and similarities between these processes have not been mapped out.

It would appear that many factors come into play in the genesis of suicidal ideation and that further research will be necessary before some of the questions raised by the present findings can be answered. Studies of suicidal ideation in normal samples at different age levels would be desirable for comparison and validation of the present data, and more specifically focused studies of the ideation of subjects exhibiting suicidal behavior later in life might help plot out the natural history of such ideas and their relationships to object disruptions. Developmental studies of early ideas of suicide and their relationship to the concept of death in childhood would be of great importance as it is in this cognitive context that the experience of loss must be integrated by the child; yet these are notably lacking in the literature.

Such studies might lead to a concept of suicidal behavior that would be more unitary and consistent than many current concepts and in being both developmental and adaptive might bring the riddle of suicide into the realm of more familiar concepts of psychopathology generally.

Acknowledgments

I wish to thank Dr. J. Lohrenz, Director of the McGill University Health Service, for his valuable collaboration and support of the project described in this paper. I am especially grateful to Dr. John Bowlby of the Tavistock Clinic for his inspiration, advice, and encouragement, and would like to thank as well the members of his research seminar who discussed the research project in its early stages. My wife Gale and Dr. Roy Muir gave generously and patiently of their assistance during the preparation of the final draft.

Bibliography

1. Adam, K. S., Suicide: a critical review of the literature, *Canad. Psychiat. Ass. J.*, 12 (1967).
2. Barter, J. T., Swaback, D. O., and Todd, D., Adolescent suicide attempts, *Archives Gen. Psychiat.*, 19 (1968), 523–527.
3. Batchelor, L. R. C., and Napier, M. B., Broken homes and attempted suicide, *British Journal of Delinquency*, 4 (1953), 99–108.
4. Bruhn, J. G., Broken homes among attempted suicides and psychiatric outpatients: a comparative study, *J. Ment. Sci.*, 108 (1902), 772–9.
5. Bowlby, J., Childhood mourning and its implications for psychiatry, *Am. J. Psychiat.*, December, 118, No. 6 (1961).
6. Bowlby, J., Separation Anxiety, *Int. J. Psychoanalysis*, 41 (1960), 89–113.
7. Bowlby, J., Grief and mourning in infancy and early childhood, *Psychoanalytic Study of the Child*, 15 (1960).
8. Bowlby, J., *Attachment*, Vol. I of *Attachment and Loss*, International Psycho-Analytical Library, Hogarth Press and The Institute of Psycho-Analysis, London, 1969.
9. Dorpat, T. L., Jackson, J. K., and Ripley, H. S., Broken homes and attempted and completed suicide, *Arch. Gen. Psychiat.*, 12 (1965), 213–216.
10. Freud, S., *Mourning and Melancholia*, (1915) The Complete Psychological Works of Sigmund Freud, Standard Ed., Vol. XIX, The Hogarth Press, 1957.
11. Freud, A., and Burlingham, D., *Infants without Families*, International Universities Press, New York, 1942.
12. Friedlander, Kate, On the longing to die, *International J. of Psychoanalysis*, 21 (1940), 416–425.
13. Gay, M. J. and Tonge, W. L., The late effects of loss of parents in childhood, *Brit. J. Psychiat.*, 113 (1967), 753–759.
14. Greer, S., The relationship between parental loss and attempted suicide: a control study, *Brit. J. Psychiat.*, 110 (1964), 698–705.

15. Greer, S., Parental loss and attempted suicide: a further report, *Brit. J. Psychiat.*, 112 (1966), 465–470.
16. Greer, S. and Gunn, J. C., Attempted suicides from intact and broken parental homes, *Brit. Med. Jour.*, 2 (1966), 1355–1357.
17. Greer, S., Gunn, J. C., and Koller, K. M., Aetiological factors in attempted suicide, *Brit. Med. Jour.*, 2 (1966), 1352–1355.
18. Gregory, I., Retrospective data concerning childhood loss of a parent, *Arch. Gen. Psychiat.*, 15 (1966), 354–361.
19. Hill, O. S., The association of childhood bereavement with suicidal attempt in depressive illness, *Brit. J. Psychiat.*, 115 (1969), 301–304.
20. Hendin, H., *Suicide and Scandinavia*, Grune and Stratton, New York, 1964.
21. Hendricks, I., Suicide as wish-fulfillment, *Psychiat. Quart.*, 14 (1940), 30–42.
22. Kearney, T. R., Aetiology of attempted suicide, *Proceedings of the Fifth International Conference on Suicide Prevention*, London, England, 1969, 190–194.
23. Keeler, W. R., Children's reaction to death of a parent, in Hoch, P. and Zubin, J., *Depression*, Grune and Stratton, New York, 1954.
24. Klein, M., A Contribution to the Psychogenesis of Manic Depressive States (1934), in *Contributions to Psycho-Analysis, 1921 to 1945*, The Hogarth Press Ltd. and The Institute of Psycho-analysis, London, 1948.
25. Koller, K. M. and Castanos, J. N., The influence of parental deprivation in attempted suicide, *The Medical Journal of Australia*, 1 (1968), 396–399.
26. Levi, L. D., Foles, C., Stein, and M., Sharp, V.H., Separation and attempted suicide, *Arch. Gen. Psychiat.*, 15 (1966), 158–164.
27. Markhusen, E. and Fulton, R., Childhood bereavement and behavior disorders: a critical review, *Omega*, 2 (1971), 107–117.
28. Mattson, A., Seese, L. R., and Hawkins, J. W., Suicidal behavior as a child psychiatric emergency, *Arch. Gen. Psych.*, 20 (1969), 100–109.
29. Moss, L. M. and Hamilton, D. M., Psychotherapy of suicidal patients, *Amer. J. Psychiatry*, 112 (1956), 814–820.
30. Munro, A. and Griffiths, A. B., Some psychiatric non sequelae of childhood bereavement, *Brit. J. Psychiat.*, 115 (1969), 305–11.
31. Paffenbarger, R. S. and Asnes, D. P., Chronic disease in former college students. III. Precursors of suicide in early and middle life, *American Journal of Public Health*, 56 (1966), 1026–1036.
32. Ross, M., Suicide among college students, *American Journal of Psychiatry*, 126:2 (1969), 220–225.
33. Stengel, E., *Suicide and Attempted Suicide*, Penguin Books, New York, 1964.
34. Wald, C., "Syndromes of Suicidal People" reported in Research and training in prevention of suicide in adolescents and youths, *Bulletin of Suicidology*, No. 6 (1970).
35. Walton, H. J., Suicidal behaviour in depressive illness; a study of etiological factors in suicide, *J. Ment. Sci.*, 104 (1958), 884.
36. Zilboorg, G., Differential diagnostic types of suicide, *Arch. of Neurol. and Psychiat.*, 35 (1936), 270–291.
37. Zilboorg, G., Considerations on suicide with particular reference to that of the young, *Am. J. Orthopsychiatry*, 7 (1937).

The Impact of a Father's Suicide on His Latency Son

Eliezer Ilan, M.A. (Israel)

Introduction

Current clinical practice in the case of families that have suffered the loss of a parent is to make sure that the children receive the necessary factual information, that they are given ample opportunity to talk about the loss, and that the feelings of the family members are not concealed from them. The rationale for this advice is based on the alleged need of children to undergo a period of mourning with the hope that in so doing they will be spared the later development of psychopathology. More recently, however, doubts have arisen as to whether children, in fact, are able to mourn like the adult whose grief normally terminates in a nonpathological resolution of the relationship.

Research and conclusive observations are sparse. Barnes [1] has given an instructive and detailed description of the reaction of two young girls to the death of their mother where wise educational handling and good emotional contact may have averted pathological developments. Nevertheless, the author cautioned about possible difficulties that the girls might have in their future development. Wolfenstein [4] advanced an opinion that only with adolescence does the ordinary process of mourning become possible since, according to her, there cannot be an acceptance and working through of loss before the developmental crisis of puberty with its prototype of separation from primary objects. Bowlby and Parkes [2] have said that "Although today a causal linkage between psychological disturbance and a separation or loss that occurred at some time during childhood or adolescence, or later, is well attested, both statistically and clinically, there remain very many problems in understanding both the processes at work and also the exact conditions that determine whether outcome is good or bad." Bearing in mind this state of our present knowledge, any evidence that can be added, even from single case studies, may have a cumulative usefulness in clarifying the connections between loss and subsequent psychopathology.

This clinical paper describes the short-term therapy (25 sessions) of a 16-year-old boy and documents the later repercussions at the age of ten, resulting from the traumatic loss of the father at which time no morbid reactions were in evidence. At the age of 15 (five years later), there was a pathological upsurge of feeling connected with the father's death and this was then worked through in treatment. The child had not been given the opportunity to work through the traumatic experience when it happened, but it is an open question whether better psychological management of the situation at the time could have prevented the adolescent upheaval and spared him the necessity for treatment.

Case History

PRIOR TO THE DEATH OF THE FATHER

Dov had been the wanted and well-developed child of a middle-class family. The marriage—it was the second marriage of the mother—was described as happy during the early years by the mother. Both parents were devoted to their son. When Dov was five, the marriage began to deteriorate. The father started to seek the company of families with a much higher standard of living than he could afford for his family. He got into grave debts. This brought severe tension into the family and the parents quarreled often. The father was impatient with Dov. He spent much of his time outside the house and his mood steadily deteriorated. The mother too spent a lot of time away from home and her relationship with Dov likewise became strained since she was constantly nervous and tense.

THE DEATH OF THE FATHER

At the age of 10, Dov came back from a football game and found his father sprawling, unconscious, and covered with blood in the backyard of his home. The boy started to shout and raised the alarm. He stayed with neighbors for some days and was interrogated by the police. His mother told him that his father had been taken to the hospital and had perhaps met with an accident while fixing the radio antenna on the roof. After some days he was told that his father had died and that the funeral had already taken place. There was little talk about what had happened and little in the way of mourning. Following the father's death, the mother had to work hard to pay the heavy debts her husband had left her. In spite of her reserve and introversion, a very close relationship developed between her and her son. The latter showed no noticeable reactions to the dreadful situation to which he had been exposed. Two years later the mother met and attached herself to a divorced man but for some family considerations on his side, they decided to postpone marriage. The boy continued to behave well and although very attached to his mother, he had friends of his own. He was also doing well in school. At the age of 14, he had a girl friend, played the flute, had some theatrical interests, and was a member of an amateur theater. He was very devoted to his girl friend's mother and even when his friendship with the girl came to an end, he sent her mother flowers on her birthday. It was at the age of 15 that the mother learned from the school authorities that her son was showing signs of disturbance that worried the school. His scholastic achievements dropped markedly, he quarreled with his peers, and occasionally had impulsive outbursts against his teachers. His mood was described as depressively sullen. The school psychologist suggested psychotherapeutic help and the boy willingly accepted this.

Treatment

PHASE 1. DEPRESSION, GUILT AND ACCUSATIONS TOWARD THE MOTHER

He was 16 years of age when he started once-weekly psychotherapy. From the very beginning, Dov complained that he had been bothered during the previous months by thoughts about the untimely death of his father. He felt himself tense and every mention of the father—accidentally and harmlessly—by friends or teachers provoked him to outbursts of rage and abuse. He brooded about the cause of death, whether suicide or accident. He showed me a picture of his father together with a cut-out notice from a newspaper about the tragic incident where the possibility of either suicide or accident was mentioned. He carried these always with him in his pocket.

During the course of treatment, several distinct phases in the way that he dealt with his father's death could be perceived. At the beginning, he described the relationship with his father as having been very good and expressed anger and dissatisfaction with his mother for not having told him of the death at once and for not having let him attend the funeral. He had never expressed this grudge towards his mother directly as he found it difficult to speak to her about his father. He then told me that his mother had recently decided to remarry. He said that he was on good terms with the man and felt he was a decent fellow. Nevertheless, he found it highly in-appropriate for his mother to remarry so soon (six years!) after his father's death.

Having vented his anger against his mother on this surface level, he entered a second and deeper phase of self-accusation. He men-tioned that on Pesach Eve, a year before the death, he had toasted his father "to Death" instead of "to Life" and recalled this as one of his childish jokes. In spite of "not being superstitious," he won-dered uneasily whether this bad wish might not have influenced the later event. As treatment progressed, he began to understand that he might have had bad wishes against his father but his guilty feel-ings only drove him to further accusations against his mother. May-be he had wished his father evil but from evil wishes a man does not die. It was minor compared to the frequent quarrels between his mother and father. He was now quite sure that his father had committed suicide and he raised the suspicion that his mother had been unfaithful to him. "After all, it was her second marriage and now she has married again a third time and she is a good-looking woman." In his fantasy, mother had driven father to committing suicide as she had had a relationship with another man. There was no memory to prove his accusation and he knew that the mother had made the acquaintance of her third husband two years after his father's death. Even with the knowledge that there was not much substance to his accusations, he was unable to relinquish them. When the therapist suggested that he might be furious with his mother for having married again and for having disrupted her close relationship with him and for having betrayed him as she had betrayed his father, he at once denied it all. Following this, however, he began to consider the possibility that it might be good for his mother to have a husband now. She had grown so dependent on him that it would be lonely for her when he left home to marry. He felt that his stepfather was quite a nice man.

PHASE 2. ANGER AND HATE TOWARD THE FATHER

After having worked through this "oedipal" portion of his fantasies about his father's death, he returned to consider his relationship with his father. After much hesitation, he confessed that the picture he had given to the therapist of his good relationship with his father was entirely false. He proceeded to flood the sessions with memories of his father's extreme cruelty toward him. He had been beaten with a strap for every small transgression without a listening to his explanations. He recalled his father's rage at every harmless pleasure in which he had indulged. All these bitter recriminations culminated in a statement that if anybody had driven his father to suicide, he would go to that person and shake hands with him. During this phase of the treatment, there were periods of heavy resistance when he sat silent, tense, and uncomfortable in his chair with the feeling that the therapist was a police investigator. Time and again, the interpretation of the transference meaning of this eased the situation and brought fresh memories of events and emotions concerning him and his father. A typical reaction to this kind of transference interpretation was: "I think it is right that I feel you to be dangerous because you remind me of father but you are a thousand times better than he," and then there would come a further release of memories depicting the strictness and cruelty of the father. A part of this deep fear was also transferred to the headmaster of the school and at one point, he begged the intervention of his good therapist-father against the bad headmaster-father (who, in reality, showed very little understanding for this problem adolescent and was only too willing to be guided by the therapist). After much resistance and hesitation, he expressed the wish to smoke during the sessions and this together with material relating to a confrontation with a teacher who tried to confiscate a whistle in his possession and with which he had played during lessons brought up the topic of masturbation and his fears of being punished (mutilated) by his father for doing it. In spite of the therapist's permission to smoke, he waited a long time before he finally dared to do so.

PHASE 3. SEPARATION AND SELF-ASSERTION OF THE ADOLESCENT

In the final phase of the treatment, material came up indicating a more positive relationship he had had with his father in the earlier years with memories of pleasant walks with him and moods of quiet serenity. At the same time, he began to mention his involvement with girls and the fights he was having over them with boys. He seemed very uneasy about telling the therapist about his girl friend and peer group and became increasingly reluctant to talk. He started to miss sessions and gave signs of wanting to finish treatment. He used the opportunity of a bout of influenza not to return to treatment in spite of a special plea from the therapist. It looked as if he were closing the door on an aspect of his life that he felt was private and personal but he also seemed to sense some danger to his masculine independence from continuing treatment.

In a follow-up interview some years later, he spoke of the great relief that he had obtained from treatment and pointed to his good adjustment with comrades and authorities in the Army. He had felt especially guilty at not coming to a final session when the therapist had invited him to do so. He had felt then that treatment was a burden and that if he had accepted the invitation, he would have been induced to continue. He was very relieved to be able to discuss this "unfinished business" in the follow-up session.

Discussion

This case confronts us with the problem of a traumatic loss of the father by suicide with no attempt made to work through the experience according to the rules of good mental hygiene. The boy was denied attendance at the funeral and given little opportunity to talk about his loss and the distressing circumstances surrounding it. At the other extreme, he began to enjoy many of the advantages brought about by his father's death: cessation of tension in the home; a mother who was more relaxed; and, above all, an undisturbed close relationship with the mother. The prospect of the mother's remarriage had unleashed his depression and guilt feelings and his behavior had become disordered (the Hamlet complex). It is interesting to note how a partial realization of oedipal fantasies by his close contact with his mother for some years had held in check the pathological reactions to the death of the father. This phenomenon was also present in the case reported by Barnes [1] where the death of the mother did not interfere with the four-year-old girl's enjoyment of the oedipal relationship with the father. The father had tried to forestall the development of guilt feelings by some attempt at explanation.

The strong attachment to a love object after bereavement seems to be decisive in mitigating the reactions to loss. The fact that the death of the parent of the same sex is the fulfillment of an oedipal wish does not appear to rouse strong guilt reactions as long as the child can enjoy an undisturbed close relationship with the parent of the opposite sex. However, when Dov, at the age of 15, was forced by outer and inner events to give up his mother attachment, to separate from her, and to find his own identity, the traumatic loss of the father and the deep guilt feelings associated with it came up with great force.

One can speculate as to what results good preventive measures after the death of the father might have achieved in this case. The boy later complained that the mother had excluded him from the funeral and had not given him the true information about his father's death but these were only the superficial grudges he held against his mother. At a deeper level, he also accused her of betraying his father and driving him to his death. This represented a projection of his own guilt feelings, a reflection of his own hate that could scarcely have been touched even by the most sensible handling or even psychotherapeutic management of the acute crisis situation. The development of adolescence together with the change in marital status of the mother brought about a critical situation that mobilized these feelings and allowed the boy in a relatively short period to work through a major part of his relationship to his father. In therapy there was an opportunity to reactivate past fantasies and feelings but the main curative factor in this case was in relation to what Strachey [3] termed a "mutative transference interpretation."

For a decisive period in the treatment, he strongly reexperienced the therapist as a dangerous father figure. Interpretation of this fact helped him to differentiate the actual therapist from this transference image. It enabled him to internalize a new father image that was neither punishing nor accusing and helped him to recall good memories of his father and thus to make peace with the father of his childhood. From the good father-therapist, the boy was then able to separate himself in the characteristic adolescent manner.

One would therefore conclude that preventive measures in the case of latency loss can have only limited possibilities as long as the inner feelings are covered up by a strong relationship to the remaining parent. During the developmental phase of adolescence, however, when the problems of separation and identification are again accented, even a relatively brief period of psychotherapy may be effective in redirecting the child along a healthier channel.

Bibliography

1. Barnes, M. J., Reactions to the Death of a Mother, in *Psychoanal. Study of Child, 19,* International Universities Press, New York, 1964.
2. Bowlby, J. and Parkes, C. M., Separation and Loss within the Family, in *The Child in His Family* (Int. Yearbook for Child Psychiatry and Allied Disciplines, Vol. 1) E. J. Anthony and C. Koupernik, Eds., John Wiley, New York, 1970.
3. Strachey, J., The nature of the therapeutic action of psychoanalysis, *Int. J. Psycho-Anal.,* 15 (1934), 127–159; 50 (1969), 275–292.
4. Wolfenstein, M., How is Mourning Possible? in *Psychoanal. Study of Child, 21,* International Universities Press, New York, 1966.

Children Who Torture and Kill*

S. Lebovici, M.D. (France)

Introduction

The crimes committed by children provoke, at the same time, horror
and astonishment. It is hard to understand, indeed, how young individuals are able to torture and to kill other young ones without
concluding that such deviant activities must be the product of the
miasmas engendered by social life. The crimes of adolescents are
more often in the news, and it is easier to attribute them to the
faults of society and to educational disadvantages than is the case
with younger children whose criminal behavior seems even more
mystifying.

I will be concerned with this last situation. The studies to date
devoted to the rare observations of crimes committed by children
have not furnished any account of their genesis and execution. The
medico-legal appraisals have limited their objectives to questions of
responsibility in the psychiatric sense and implicate constitutional
factors in a generally oversimplified way.

My approach here will be based on clinical experience and on observations that have come to my knowledge relating to cruelties practiced by children. I will then follow this up by descriptions of actual
crimes committed by them.

*Translated by E. James Anthony, M. D.

Some Clinical Facts

THE CRUEL CHILD AND THE CHILD WHO TORTURES

In many of their games, children permit torture. The cowboy and Indian theme envisages the stake to which the prisoner is attached, the scalping, the killing, etc., but generally these games do not go beyond the customary conventions. I will return later to the meaning of these games and to the fantasies that sustain them.

Certain children will choose to act cruelly with playmates who are generally younger and thus unable to defend themselves. One can observe in this situation an alliance between the tormentor and his victim, the alliance being played by the rules of the game.

Many years ago much importance was attached to the acts of certain children often labeled perverse as signifying an amoral proclivity that directed them toward delinquency and crime.

Such subjects, it was claimed, manifested a cruel streak from very early on, pulling the wings off flies, killing small animals, and even strangling cats and dogs. They appeared to observe the slaughter of domestic creatures for food with a peculiar sort of pleasure. Such anamnestic reconstructions always pose a problem since both parents and psychiatrists sense that this early behavior is used first to justify the diagnosis of perversity and then to account for the subsequent criminal act of cruelty. The earlier conduct, of itself, rarely obtains psychiatric consultation but is generally recalled when some major episode of sadism later gets the child to the psychiatrist. One can then question if any specific significance can be attributed to this antecedent behavior outside those cases where it is integrated into a characteristic psychopathological structure.

This may concern manifestly psychotic children where the cruelties are part of the bizarre behavior making the diagnosis fairly evident. More often one has to deal with a composite and complex pathology organized around primary behavior problems which, if followed up, gradually evolve into psychopathy or serious character disorder.

In such cases, the killing of animals at an early age, especially when accompanied by needless acts of cruelty, is likely to impress the clinician but, there again, the limits are by no means distinct apart from the very blatant cases. How does one differentiate a child who kills birds with a slingshot from another who, with better coordination, becomes precociously a little hunter like his father or like many other adults that he has heard about.

ILLUSTRATIONS

A mother leaves her oldest son, a very retarded child and so far relatively placid, for a few minutes in a room where a few-months-old baby lies in his crib. When she returns, she finds the baby dead with his older brother still beating him. It seems that the boy threw the baby on the ground after pulling him around the room and then smashed his skull with a blunt instrument. This simpleminded individual displays a primitive and apparently obvious jealousy that motivates his act or, at least, this is the kind of explanation that adults would tend to give.

The family of a seven-year-old boy who had disappeared from his home received a ransom demand from his kidnappers with proof that he was really in their hands. The parents pleaded to have their child back and were ready to pay the required sum. The police were able to effect an arrest quite rapidly to find that the kidnapper (and murderer) was a 14-year-old boy who lived in the neighborhood. In fact, at the time that the ransom was still being negotiated, the little victim had been dead and buried for some time. The boy confessed without difficulty and explained that having suffered from the separation of his parents, he had decided to commit a murder and earn the death penalty in order to make his father aware of *his* crime in deserting the mother and their three children, the kidnapper being the middle child. Following the father's desertion (for the purpose of remarrying), the relationship between father and son had deteriorated badly and the boy had refused to have his father visit him in the prison where he had been taken after the crime. Up to this time, he had lived with his mother, his grandparents, and an aunt in an old family house. Within this unstimulating environment, he had felt himself isolated and devalued. In school he had been a sad and mediocre student. A few years before the crime, he had undergone a psychiatric evaluation and was recommended for psychodrama. This was not pursued but the intensity of his sadistic anxiety appeared obvious. The crime was certainly premeditated. He had been impressed by the happiness prevailing in the family of his intended victim. He had kidnapped him one evening, carried him off in a handcart, make-believing that it was a game, to his own house where he had killed him quite rapidly and then buried him in a forest close by.

He later on gave another version of the facts. The victim, he claimed, was murdered by someone else whose accomplice he was. Both wanted the ransom in order to leave France and get far away. The killing had not been premeditated but had occurred when the victim had attempted to escape. The second version was not confirmed but agreed in many points with the psychological findings in the case. The boy identified himself with his victim and also imagined that his little sister of the same age was taking the victim's place. His fantasy life, which was still relatively rich at the time he was arrested and put in prison, was organized around homosexual wishes directed toward his father whom he detested because he had left him for the young woman. If one wants, therefore, to understand the unconscious motives of the crime, both versions put forward by the young murderer have to be discussed: he wanted to take revenge on his father at the risk of the death penalty, and he had wanted to kill the innocent victim because he was well cared for in the way he wanted to be cared for by his own father. It must be admitted that these motives cannot of themselves explain the carrying out of the criminal act. During his stay in prison, he made pretense of continuing his studies with the help of his mother and older sister. He struck those observing him with his loneliness and coldness, and his references to what he called "The affair" were made with increasing indifference. During the last period in prison before the trial, he tried to mutilate himself sexually with a knife after his mother had reproached him with his criminal act. When asked, during an interview, what associations the mutilation evoked for him, he suddenly recalled, without feeling, striking his victim with an iron bar to finish him off. Distancing himself from the criminal act did not prevent the guilty feelings from being stirred up and directed to the symbolic act of auto-mutilation. This enables me to discuss the psychopathological core of the case and its predictable outcome. On the other hand, the prison conditions and particularly the loneliness imposed on him could have led to the actual psychoticization; this assumption has been made by certain criminologists.

The example, however, makes clear that the descriptive psychiatric nosology is insufficient to explain the specific features characterizing the transition to a criminal act.

The psychological motivation underlying a crime and the carrying out of a symbolic act may make a criminal child even more of "a stranger" in the eyes of society than a chronic mental patient who inspires pity or contempt. Thus "the stranger," as Camus showed so well in his novel of that name, calls for condemnation and punishment which, in such cases, is little more than a pretext.

The Genesis of Sadistic and Murderous Behavior

CHILDHOOD CRIME AND UNCONSCIOUS GUILT

By reason of his prolonged biological dependence, the human infant experiences a series of emotional dependences in relation to parental figures as a result of which his drives become gradually organized in parallel with his development. One such organization is the oedipal one in which incest and aggression are brought together dynamically and dramatically in the form of an inevitable and ubiquitous complex occurring between the third and fifth year of life in its classical form. The dark legend of ancient Greece is used to account for the emergence of conscience. The complex provides the nodal organization for unconscious guilt feelings that determine, in a vicious cycle, the transitions from aggressive to guilty feelings. Within the oedipal framework, the superego represents a condensation of internalized prohibitions that under certain circumstances could eventually lead to masochistic and self-punitive behavior. It is possible, as suggested by Klein [9], that excessive strictness of the superego may also conduce to criminal activity.

The biblical legends are equally rich sources for the exploration of unconscious guilt. In one story God asked Abraham to sacrifice Isaac and the father was prepared to comply. In the light of this, one can understand the circumcision by the Jewish father of his son as part of the covenant between God and his chosen children whereby they symbolically sacrificed the son's masculinity. The rites of circumcision are the rites of transition to adulthood. In his recent work, *Symbolic Wounds,* Bettelheim [1] views circumcision as more than a symbolic castration inflicted by the father. He considers it in terms of the inverse form of the oedipal complex, the negative phase, in which the son submits to the father out of guilt. He behaves as if he wished to identify himself with his mother and have a child by his father. Castration would then represent the symbol of the bloody delivery the boy must endure in order to become a man. Although this thesis may seem debatable, it is, nevertheless, metaphorically speaking, an illustration of the way in which the disappointments of the inverse oedipal position may conduce to criminal acting out of perverse fantasies related to sexual inversion.

The murderous games of childhood are activated by fantasies generated by the positive and negative phases of the Oedipus complex. Sometimes we can observe the aggressions in free play and sometimes in organized games. For example, a five year old was referred to the clinic because he would often be found standing in front of his father's picture with a pistol pretending to shoot him. The family was worried and interpreted the game as an antecedent to an adult killer. This is only one example among many others where one can observe children, boys as well as girls, enacting stories of violent death long before they have even developed an authentic concept of death.

The war games of children can be looked at, psychoanalytically, in two ways. According to Anna Freud [5], boys, in our culture at least, are extremely prone to assume military roles which she interprets as an identification with the aggressor for the purpose of counteracting castration anxiety.

These warlike games can also be understood, according to Klein [9], as manifestations of archaic fantasies expressing a sadistic relationship to the object. The drive organization presupposes an object to which the desires are directed as evident in the cannibalistic fantasies that seek to devour and thus incorporate the mother (or originally the breast representing the mother). The good mother-breast, however, thus incorporated is then transformed through the workings of the *Les Talonis* into the bad mother-breast. These reciprocal mechanisms, therefore, render the mother into both a desirable and threatening object. Such fantasies are regarded as the source of the early organization of the superego and their persistence has been put forward as an etiological factor in the subsequent sadistic behavior of the child. Although it is true that psychoanalytic observation can uncover these primitive sadistic fantasies in the play of children, it does not explain the transformation of symbolic games into sadistic and murderous reality. The process of transformation can be seen during psychoanalytic treatment when there is an inadequate working through of the transference relationship.

One might conclude from this, according to Freud's concept of working through [6], that the carrying out of the act is nothing more than a repetition in action of a fantasy and indicates an inadequate working through in thought.

Later Freud evoked the operation of what he referred to in his two instinct theory as the death instinct. Deeply embedded in our mental functioning, the death instinct shows a tendency to externalize itself and attack the object adding another source of understanding to the emergence of sadistic and hyperaggressive behavior.

One knows that at this same time, Freud [7] had begun to regard anxiety as a danger signal that was activated when deflected aggression toward our love objects exposed us to the possibility of loss. The possible loss of the love object to some extent holds in check any over-intensification of the libidinal drives that constantly threaten the individual.

A long while before, he had demonstrated that the desire for the object, which was always deeply ambivalent, invariably entailed a certain amount of frustration that helped to inhibit the drives. Similarly, gratifications from the object also exercised its effect and, as a consequence, there was a mixing of this with the aggressive forces that develop within us. But it must be emphasized that the aggressive drive that is always associated with libidinal drives does not imply increased aggressiveness. The assumptions of Freudian metapsychology on displaced aggressiveness do not explain the carrying out of the act, the practice of cruelty or the acting out of fantasy. We need more elaborate hypotheses regarding the psychopathology of such cases and must study them specifically within this field.

The Psychopathology of Crime in Childhood

Psychiatrists, specializing in this area, when examining criminal subjects and adolescents in particular, have the opportunity to investigate their developing sense of responsibility. To some extent they have to make a diagnosis. Quite frequently they find themselves dealing with borderline psychosis, and it is an accepted fact that crime may be the first manifestation of the pseudopsychopathic type of schizophrenia. But often, one cannot go further in defining the underlying criminal structure than to label it "psychopathy" which is sufficiently vague and nebulous nosologically to suggest a number of nuances that bear little relationship to the field of psychiatry.

In the case of younger criminals, the pathology is even more uncertain since immature and developing structures are concerned that are hard to evaluate so that one can only talk of prestructures except for those cases where the crime is integrated into the structure of a profound personality defect or a beginning childhood psychosis.

This raises the question of whether one can speak of prepsychopathic structures in the child. French authors who describe precociousness and "constitutional" perversions are no doubt recalling cases where the child has apparently been unable to acquire a moral sense and is therefore ready to commit the strangest and most atrocious acts without any detectable guilt feeling. This conclusion, however, must be carefully examined in depth and not accepted without first looking for a better understanding of the genesis of such terrible behavior. Already in their studies of the so-called "affectionless character," Friedlander [8] and Bowlby [2] have emphasized the importance of the very early difficulties in relationships that these children have. It is not only a matter of early frustrations but also of incoherence on the level of both gratifications and frustrations, particularly when the superego is being established as well as the relations of the anal phase which is therefore likely to be deficient. The carrying out of an act by these subjects takes place without delay and without restraint as if they were unable to retain or to control their fantasies.

A careful observational study made over a long period in a day hospital [3] has allowed my co-workers and myself to reconstruct the fate of primary narcissism as one of the major psychopathological characteristics of the prepsychopathic child. There was no doubt that in these subjects the oedipal level of development was reached and, therefore, there seemed to be no need to examine the causal significance of the pregenital organization. The identification seemed, at first glance, differentiated in the style of those found in the evolving oedipal situation but a study of the conflicts involved did not fit with the structural definition of the psychopathology of these cases. Further reflection led us to envisage the problem in terms of the vicissitudes in the operation of the most primitive identifications that Freud referred to as primary identification that functioned even before the recognition of the object itself. They are formed under the influence of the primary narcissistic imprint. It is known that it is the projection of primary narcissism in the form of a feeling of self-esteem that leads to the formation of the ego ideal and to the organization of the narcissistic foundation of the superego, the final constitution of which is tied to the final resolution of the Oedipus complex.

The development of these cases and the rapid appearance of psychopathic behavior indicate that as long as a child can project his narcissism, either on one of the parents whom he puts on a pedestal or on a teacher whose authority and strength seem to him utterly respectable, the carrying out of the act is impeded.

This is why the progressive educational systems in specialized institutions can pose so many problems for the management and treatment of these cases. The actual physical presence of the teacher or parent personifying the ego ideal is constantly required to contain, in a concrete sort of way, the carrying out of the act where the drives manifest themselves directly without recourse to symbolization and sublimation. Everything carries on as if the mode of functioning of the superego were not possible under normal conditions and as if guilt feelings did not exist.

The thesis advanced in this work [3] was that the deficiency in the constitution of the superego makes it impossible to establish a validly functioning ego ideal and that this reflects the narcissistic basis of the personality precisely because the projection of the ego ideal, due to the unsuccessful experiences of introjection at this level, has constantly to be made in a megalomanic mode.

When one reflects on these observations, it is difficult to understand how one can explain, genetically and historically, the notion of an early deficit in the organization of the primary identifications of narcissism and of the ego ideal. It is not possible to retrace all the detailed considerations that would provide an historical foundation to these hypotheses. They go back to pessimistic conceptions of nineteenth century French medicine subsumed under the rubric of degeneracy that resort to constitutional hypotheses similar to ones accepted by certain contemporary psychoanalysts when they talk of dysmaturation and disharmony leading one to conclude that it is at the earliest and most basic level of organization that these narcissistic disburbances arise. From varied and prolonged observations, I have become convinced that there is always a profound family pathology. This can be best demonstrated by a case illustration.

ILLUSTRATION

Fabian, under diagnostic observation at day hospital, behaves, all things being equal, like a child psychopath. His fits of temper are completely out of control. It is interesting to note, in the context of what we have been discussing, that his mother so as to be able to work placed him in a day nursery soon after his birth. He underwent experiences of early deprivation but of greater interest to us, his mother displayed a strange piece of behavior when taking him home at night. She said that she felt compelled to bring him a present each day and he had developed the habit of asking for it. It seemed to her the only way that she could make up for her absence as if her presence and maternal care were not sufficient to meet his needs.

This example, in my opinion, illustrates very well what is understood by a deficiency of narcissistic supplies in the mother-child unity.

It is understandable that psychopathy, in its precise sense, is more diagnosable in the adult and the adolescent since the psychopathic behavior brings out the relationship with others whereas the child can only be psychopathic in relation to an adult representing his ego ideal. As in the case of those called "perverse" by the classical French authors, the guilt feelings are missing. In some observations that I have been personally able to make, the conflicts were sufficiently complex and the guilt feelings sufficient to deceive the observer and even make him hopeful with regard to psychotherapy. The guilt feelings are missing, however, in relation to the act or crime. Once the act or crime has been committed, the unconscious guilt, undetectable in the act itself, gradually begins to produce its effect resulting, in part at least, in psychopathic behavior of the self-punitive and moral masochistic type, not as a primary but as a secondary class of symptoms.

As we have come to see it, psychopathy appears finally as a clinical category that, on the level of psychopathology and prognosis, seems to have a closer relationship to psychosis than to perversion and neurosis. It can be specified on the clinical, prognostic and metapsychological level even if certain perplexing developments give one cause to wonder. Certainly, when a child meets the definition of psychopath, there are reasons to believe the diagnosis has little chance of being revised even though certain psychotic (and not exceptional) developments raise the question of psychoticization of the case (as a result, for example, of prison experiences) or the question of pseudopsychopathy in an incipient psychosis.

So, the diagnosis of psychopathy, if made early, especially, should not represent a label inculcating therapeutic skepticism or be taken to mean a final diagnosis (although this would not be unjustifiable in the light of subsequent development in these criminal children).

THE CHILD CRIMINAL AND HIS ENVIRONMENT

Penal history shows that the imprisonment of a child criminal is rarely avoided. There is an almost general consensus that measures of segregation and the protection of society must be taken with regard to such subjects who often seem incorrigible. We should not hide the fact that jail conditions, in themselves, generate further developments in these cases. In one study [10] it is clearly shown that imprisonment and the milieu of the prison may cause psychoticization in addition to whatever other causes that have been cited as activating this process. Anyhow, the fact of bringing together psychopathic criminals can only lead to an increase in prison sentences and offers nothing except, at best, a protection for society. In the conditions that they were treated and are still being treated, it is quite understandable that criminal children become criminal adolescents and criminal adults unable to develop into anything better than psychotics evolving in a more or less characteristic manner.

But it must be equally emphasized that the relation between the criminal and his victim can also be considered from the viewpoint of perverse sadism. In every case, through the transgression represented by the criminal act, the psychopathic child provokes social reactions analogous to the counterreactions observed with respect to sadistic acts of sexual perverts.

One should also note that the sexual pervert finds an accomplice in his victim. One can say [4] that the masochist proposes a real contract to the one he claims as his victim. Is this not also true, at least to some extent, of the victim of the criminal child? In the case described, it was striking and indeed very strange that the seven-year-old little victim agreed to be carried away, in the pretense of playing, in a cart covered with a blanket and was transported through most of the city where he lived.

More generally, one cannot exclude the influence of the cultural milieu in which we live nor the influence of the mass media that finds technical excuses for the criminal act inducing certain children to try it out. Not so long ago in San Francisco, two brothers, seven and ten years old, killed their 20-month-old little brother, beating him to death with a brick. The seven year old declared that he was playing with his oldest brother when the brick he was holding in his hands hit his baby brother. The baby fell down and the two brothers then struck him unmercifully until he died.

Conclusion

This example, which has no obvious explanation, will be an opening for my concluding remarks. One cannot exclude the fact that the psychopathological hypothesis that has been offered in an attempt to explain the carrying out of a crime must be completed by a reference to cases when the game becomes a crime because it is very natural to kill.

It seems to me then that the psychopathological understanding of crime and of cruelty in childhood compels me to refer to the genesis of fantasies, to the understanding of insufficient control over the act and, finally, to a certain apology for violence and destruction which has perhaps its biological roots but which also includes some specific aspects of our culture.

Bibliography

1. Bettelheim, B., *Symbolic Wounds*, Free Press, New York, 1954.
2. Bowlby, J., *Forty-four Juvenile Thieves*, Baillère and Cox, London, 1947.
3. Braunschweig, D., Lebovici, S., and Van Thiel-Godfrind, La Psychopathie chez l'enfant, *Psychiatrie de l'Enfant*, XII (1969), 5–106.
4. Deleuze, G., *Contribution à l'Etude du Masochisme*, Edition de Minuit, Paris, 1967.
5. Freud, A., *The Ego and the Mechanisms of Defense, Revised Edition*, I. U. P., New York, 1966.
6. Freud, S., Remembering, Repeating and Working-Through (Further Recommendations on the Technique of Psycho-Analysis II) (1914), *Standard Edition, XII*, Hogarth Press, 1958.
7. Freud, S., Inhibitions, Symptoms and Anxiety (1926 (1925)), *Standard Edition, XX*, Hogarth Press, 1959.
8. Friedlander, K., Formation of the Antisocial Character, in *The Psychoanalytic Study of the Child*, I, International Universities Press, New York, 1945.
9. Klein, M., *Contributions to Psycho-Analysis*, Hogarth Press, London, 1948.
10. Roumajon, Y., Considérations sur certaines formes de délinquance juvénile, *Evolution Psychiatrique*, 31 (1967), 51–90.

Children Who Kill Their Mothers

John E. Mack, M.D. (U.S.A.), Donald J.
Scherl, M.D. (U.S.A.), and Lee B. Macht,
M.D. (U.S.A.)

Introduction

Matricide is the primal crime. It represents the ultimate discharge
of aggression against the parent figure who has thwarted the child
and inspired its hostility. It is an act which seems to be aimed at
the original offender without displacement or modification.

Concluding his study of 15 intra- and extra-familial juvenile
murders, which included three matricides, Russell stated that "the
basic murder is seen to be that of the mother" [1]. By this he
meant that all of the murders he studied were rooted in frustrations
and deprivations related to the mother although the mother herself
was killed only when the primitive hostility toward her could find
no outlet against another person. A specific understanding of cases
of matricide thus requires an elucidation not only of the evolution
of the criminal event as it derives from the mother-child relationship but also of why no alternative outlet for the murderous impulses was possible.

Literature

MYTHOLOGICAL AND ANCIENT LITERATURE

Of the matricides of ancient mythology the retributive murder of Clytaemnestra by Orestes in collaboration with his sister, Electra, is the best known. The central elements of the myth are familiar. Clytaemnestra has taken a lover, Aegisthus, while her husband, Agamemnon, is fighting in the Trojan wars. She sends her only son, Orestes, away before her husband's return. When Agamemnon returns Clytaemnestra and Aegisthus murder him in his bath. Orestes, perhaps ten at the time, remains away for eight years. He consults the Delphic oracle and Apollo, authorized by Zeus, counsels him that unless he avenges his father's murder he will become an outcast from society, debarred from entering any shrine or temple, and afflicted with leprosy [2]. In spite of this authorization, following the murder of his mother and her lover by his sword, Orestes is mercilessly pursued by the Erinnyes (Eumenides), the Greek goddesses who embodied the vengeance of conscience. They torment him with such anguish he can not eat or sleep until finally he loses his wits. In some accounts he bites off a finger in his frenzy [3]. The Erinnyes are pacified and peace of mind is restored to Orestes only following a trial for murder in Athens during which Apollo speaks on his behalf and Athene casts the deciding vote in his favor.

What deserves to be stressed about this myth is the sexual license of the mother before the child, and the fact that even for the ancient Greeks, among whom expressions of incestuous sexuality and murder seem to have been commonplace, matricide could be committed only when there was the utmost provocation by the mother and justification for the murder supported by the insistence of the highest authority. Even then, the perpetrator suffered terrible tortures of conscience to the point of madness until the guilt could be relieved by still another resource to a higher judicial authority. The issues of justification and the establishment of standards of justice are central themes in the Orestes legends.

In the other well-known Greek legend of matricide, Alcmaeon similarly can only murder his faithless mother with the bidding of the Delphic oracle and the insistence of his father that he avenge the betrayal. He too is pursued by the Erinnyes to the point of madness until half purified of his guilt by one of the Arcadian kings who later has him murdered.

Recorded history contains few matricides. Perhaps it requires an impulse-ridden figure such as Nero to perpetrate a crime so tabooed. The provocation of his mistress, Poppaea, who aroused his jealousy and fear, led Nero to have his mother, Agrippina, killed. Nero, like Orestes and Alcmaeon, was troubled by conscience and sought justification in the official argument that his mother had treacherous designs against the empire and himself. His cruelties eventually brought such hatred upon him that he committed suicide to avoid execution at the hands of his enemies.

PSYCHIATRIC LITERATURE

Ernest Jones in a chapter devoted to "The Theme of Matricide" in his *Hamlet and Oedipus* stresses that the parent who is killed may not be the one more hated [4]. Rather, it is the parent who generates the more intolerable conflict. If the mother is unfaithful to the father, or too openly sexually provocative for the boy to tolerate, he may, according to Jones, commit matricide to remove the incestuous temptation and end his torment. Jones discusses Hamlet's incestuous conflicts and matricidal impulses but does not offer an explanation as to why he chose the course of killing his uncle-stepfather rather than his mother. Wertham, dealing also with the question of why Hamlet's matricidal wishes are not given overt expression in action, suggests that Hamlet's ability to use words against his mother and to get away from Elsinore for awhile diverted and diluted, and thus defused, the murderous intensity of his feelings [5].

Much of the psychiatric and criminological literature on matricide is anecdotal with authors providing brief summaries or sensational highlights of the murder cases. More detailed case material is provided by Wertham, Scherl and Mack, and Russell [5, 6, 1].

Frederick Wertham, in his book *Dark Legend,* has provided the most complete clinical account of a case of matricide in the psychiatric literature [5]. The book tells the story of Gino, a 16½-year-old Italian-American boy who stabbed his mother to death in her bedroom after harboring a resolve to murder her for five years. Gino had idealized the images of both his father and mother. His father died when Gino was 11½. After this, according to the boy's account, the mother withdrew her love from him and began a series of sexual affairs, two of which were with his uncles, that were carried out openly before him. The breakdown of the incestuous taboos and the destruction of the idealized image of the mother created unbearable tension for Gino which he could relieve only through destroying the mother herself who had become the object of his conflict and pain. As in the Greek myths, Gino's father appeared in his fantasies and dreams sanctioning and even demanding the mother's punishment. Although later he felt remorse over the deed, Gino justified and even glorified the murder at the time asserting that his mother deserved this punishment and that he was upholding the family honor.

Wertham stresses the significance of the theme of matricide in the history of civilization, noting the importance of the Orestes legend in the establishment of a patriarchal civilization in ancient Greece, the prominence of the theme in the greatest tragedy in the literature of Western Civilization (Hamlet), and the increasing repression of matricidal themes in Western society as the patriarchal system has become more firmly established. Perhaps the current challenges to this system will see a revival of interest in the matricide theme.

Some of the brief accounts, particularly if studied in conjunction with more detailed reports, furnish valuable insights into the psychology of the person who has committed this crime. Mittleman describes the case of a 16-year-old Caucasian boy who stabbed his mother to death with a scissors, then choked her and batted her head with a hammer when, according to him, she had refused him permission to marry a Negro girl [7]. Cuthbert tells of a 16-year-old boy who killed his stepmother with a hammer after first killing his pet rabbits with the same implement [8]. The mother was described as a demanding person whose last order to her stepson—a punishment for his staying out all one night—was to dispose of his pet rabbits. The rabbits were the only living objects upon which the boy was allowed "to lavish any sort of affection." Szondi, in a letter to Theodore Reik, describes a rather celebrated case of matricide in Central Europe in which a 14½-year-old boy killed his mother with an axe [9]. There were many murders and suicides in his family genealogy. His mother was a severe cleptomaniac, a prostitute who lived a sordid life openly exposing herself in front of the boy. This behavior, together with her quarrels with her husband

and son, led to a divorce. The father remarried, the mother lost custody of the boy, and he lived for a time with his stepmother and father. However, his father expelled him from the home, accusing him of being a "traitor" in "secret league" with his mother. He was committed to an institution, escaped, and returned to his mother. She continued to berate him, and during an unusually vituperative attack he seized a hatchet and killed her with several strokes.

In many of the cases that are only briefly described a pattern of enforced exclusive intimacy between the mother and son can be discerned which allows for no alternative outlets and makes the matricidal outcome seem almost inevitable.

The grossest and most lurid example of matricide related to such enforced and restricted intimacy to come to our attention occurred in the case of a 19-year-old boy who claimed to have been forced by his mother to have frequent sexual relations with her during his adolescence [10]. As in the Mittleman case, during his sophomore year at college he found a girl friend. When he told his mother about the girl and that he wished to see more of her, she became enraged. She "fought" with him and "forced" him to have sexual relations with her the night he told her. The next night when he brought the girl friend home for dinner, the mother insulted her and she left. The young man and his mother fought again, though not seriously. Later that night while his mother slept he stabbed her to death with a knife. After killing her he ripped out, with his own hands, her eyes and uterus. When arrested, and later when interviewed by a psychologist, he justified his action with the observation that "she was evil."

Incidence

The incidence of matricide is difficult to establish as no national or even state records specific to this crime are maintained as such. A large percentage of the recorded offenders are adolescents, reflecting perhaps the special intensity of the conflicts that may influence the mother-child relationship during this period. Dr. David Lelos of the Harvard Laboratory of Community Psychiatry, in collaboration with Dr. Louis McGarry, Director of the Massachusetts Division of Legal Medicine, found 7 matricides among 101 murders committed by psychotic (adjudicated not guilty by reason of

insanity) individuals in Massachusetts between 1890 and 1971, four
by males and three by females [10]. The psychotic murders represented approximately 3-4% of all homicides in the state during this
period. The figures for matricide among the nonpsychotic murders
were not obtained.

Surveys of large groups of murders generally show a high percentage of intra-familial killings. For example, of 14,590 murders reported by the F. B. I. in 1969, approximately one-fourth occurred
within the family. No specific statistics for matricide are provided
[11]. Morris and Blom-Cooper reported 20 matricides among 245
family murders, 19 of the mothers being killed by sons and one by
a daughter [12]. There were only ten patricides reported of which
nine were committed by sons and one by a daughter. McKnight
et al have reported twelve matricide cases (11 successful and one
attempted) hospitalized at the Oak Ridge Division of the Ontario
Hospital in Penetanguishene, all but one admitted between 1942
and 1964 [13]. The average age of the group was 24.5 years, with
seven in the 15-22-year age group. This was 11½ years younger
than the average age for other homicide cases in their patient population. Only one patient was married (a 16-year-old boy) in contrast
to 48% of the total homicide group. In 1963 O'Connell reported
13 men, admitted to the Broadmoor Hospital, who had killed their
mothers within a five-year period, presumably 1957-1962 or there-
abouts [14]. Only 14 cases had been previously observed at this
hospital since 1936. We are not told from what population this
sample was drawn. "About half" the men were said to have "showed
close interest in their mother's sexual conduct." Gillies found four
matricides among 70 killings committed by 66 murderers he examined in the west of Scotland between 1953 and 1964 [15]. There
were no matricides among 54 juvenile murders committed in Ohio
between 1921 and 1947 [16].

Russell found three matricides and three patricides among 15
juvenile murderers committed to the Youth Service Board in
Massachusetts in the early 1960's [1]. Not all adolescent murderers
(and no adults) are committed to this agency so that this figure does
not necessarily reflect the total incidence of this crime in a given
population. Reviewing the records of this same agency, Kearney and
White found two matricide cases among 15 juvenile murders committed between 1964 and 1967 [17]. The authors are personally

familiar with, i. e., evaluated and/or treated, four adolescents, three boys and one girl, who killed their mothers in Massachusetts between 1961 and 1965. In addition, one boy who killed his grandmother was evaluated and treated. Although we searched intensively for other cases in newspaper articles and through contacts with various state agencies and professionals, no other Massachusetts cases came to our attention. The crime can reliably be said to be rare.

Clinical Material

No attempt will be made to provide detailed case reports in this short article. Rather, clinical material will be presented that illustrates the salient points which, in our opinion, deserve particular emphasis in these unusual cases.

The best studied of our cases of matricide remains the boy, Richard, who shot his mother to death when he was 14 years and 11 months [6]. In addition we have evaluated and treated, or supervised the treatment of, two other adolescent boys and one girl who killed their mothers.

We maintained contact with Richard for five years, during the last three of which he was in a continuing therapeutic relationship with one of us (first D. S. and then J. M.). A pattern emerged of a life-long highly erotized sadomasochistic relationship between the mother and son with relentless provocation on the part of both. The murder was the culmination of a seemingly relentless sequence of events which included battles over the possession of the gun itself, a hunting rifle belonging to the father. The mother-child relationship was characterized not so much by deprivation as by hostile, sexual and brutal intimacy dating from age three and perhaps earlier. Exposure of her body before him and sexual provocation of the boy, together with open marital infidelity on the mother's part, inflamed Richard's hatred, outrage, and frustration. This was combined with intense restriction of Richard's freedom of movement outside the house, curtailment of any other human relationships and treatment of his efforts to seek outside help as a betrayal of the parents which should be further punished.

The father was seen as a mere adjunct to the mother's brutality, in Richard's words, "the point of the spear," administering beatings after the boy became too big for her to be able to punish him effectively. The murder itself occurred in her bedroom and, as in other cases described, after a seemingly trivial incident, an argument over the sale of a radio that was not unlike many similar arguments they had over equally unimportant matters. In the course of the killing, which was planned, deliberate, and propelled by intense hatred, an exciting struggle between Richard and his mother for the gun ensued, culminating in his grabbing it from her to complete the shooting. Richard killed his mother to relieve himself of the unbearable anguish which his hatred and incestuous impulses, for which no extra-familial outlet was permitted, brought about in him. He felt that unless he were rid of his mother he could find no independent existence and would be utterly swamped.

In no case that we have studied were justification mechanisms so highly developed or extensively employed both for permitting the commission of the crime and for accounting for it afterwards. Throughout his treatment Richard remained adamant in the justification of his hatred and allowed no consideration of the possibility that he had had any positive feelings toward his mother. "I felt she was one of the world's vices that should be gotten rid of," he insisted, "and that I was doing the world a service to kill her." Whereas there had been some evidence of remorse if not guilt in the months immediately following the crime, Richard became increasingly adamant in his sense of justification and devaluation of her as the years passed.

In neither of the other two adolescent boys we studied was the motivation for the murder as clear, perhaps in part because we did not have the opportunity to study them as intensively.

Michael was 16 years and 5 months when he killed his mother, also in her bedroom, by striking her repeatedly with the blunt edge of an axe blade. Again the precipitating incident was manifestly trivial—she had ordered him to do some work around the house and chop down a tree in the backyard. Michael's mother was a severely hypochondriacal woman who remained bedridden much of the time. She kept Michael confined to the house and perpetually close to her demanding his continuous attention and nagging him incessantly. Michael, in turn, felt used and mistreated and deeply resented her restrictions of his life and demands for intimacy and constant attention. He was unable to find any outlets outside of the home for the expression of his aggressive or sexual impulses or for his need for human relationships. Like Richard, he would run away from home only to be forced to return to his mother. The father was described as distant, cold, and punitive, and argued continuously with his wife, the couple living a socially isolated life. The father was unable to help the boy to find any outlets or "way out" of his cloistered situation. Michael's hatred and tension mounted within him throughout the years of puberty. The murder was for him, as for Richard, a solution to an intolerable dilemma.

Luiz was 16 when he stabbed his mother to death. His father had deserted the family when Luiz was born, returning briefly when he was four and to stay permanently 15 months prior to the crime. Luiz had lived in a close, intimate relationship with his mother who lived only for him. They had much fun together and she called him her big man and used to brag about how strong he was when he would carry her downstairs over his shoulder. Although he felt great hatred toward his father, Luiz was largely unaware of aggressive impulses toward his mother. The only argument he recalled was a chronic one they had had for years over his left ear which he wanted to have operated upon as it looked different than the right. She would not listen to him and this infuriated him. Around the time of the father's return the boy began sniffing glue which activity he continued increasingly up to the murder. Under the influence of the glue he would indulge in regressive grandiose fantasies in which the limitations of his increasingly frustrating life would be overcome. Tension and hatred mounted between Luiz and his father who was interfering with the boy's intimacy with the mother. He stole $1000 from his father and confessed it to the mother who kept his secret.

One month prior to the murder, a girl with whom Luiz had been going steadily broke up with him because of his delinquent activities and companions. The day prior to the murder he argued with his father and resolved, while sniffing glue, to kill him. Luiz got a knife, but when he went upstairs toward the father's room to attack him his mother saw him, stopped him, and wrestled the knife away. As they wrestled he was stabbed in the leg. She tried to flee but he caught her and knocked her to the floor where she lay dazed and moaning. He said that he could not stand to see her suffer so he throttled her with a broom handle and then stabbed her three times with a stilletto and once with a butcher knife.

Luiz's case was particularly pathetic as he had been unaware of his primitive hostility toward his mother and had consciously intended to kill his father. Luiz could in no way justify to himself the matricide in subsequent years, and in fact suffered hideously over the crime, missing his relationship with his mother intensively. The role of the glue in loosening his controls or distorting his perceptions prior to the crime remained unclear.

Nell, the only girl in our series, was 16½ when she shot her mother to death. She told a police officer she had intended to kill her father too. She was the third child and only daughter of an upwardly mobile perfectionistic black family which placed considerable emphasis on social respectability and guarded itself against revealing inner conflict to the outside world. Nell was described by all who knew her as a sullen, quiet, and uncommunicative child who was said by her father to be much closer to her three-years-younger brother than to her two older brothers or her parents.

In contrast to the boys who killed their mothers, Nell told her psychiatrists that she had never had a close relationship with her mother and had felt unloved by both her parents since early childhood. She recalled many beatings by the mother with a belt from age seven to twelve and thought about revenge at that time. At age nine she asked her parents for a dog and ran away when it was denied her. The suitcase she took with her was stolen and she was beaten for this.

As in the case of the boys, the mother was highly restrictive and critical and, according to Nell, kept her locked up at home during adolescence. The summer before the murder Nell went to camp where she enjoyed the free and informal atmosphere and could go around in shorts and slacks. In contrast, at home she was forced by her mother to wear dresses and skirts whereas she wished to continue her tomboyish ways.

The immediate events leading up to the killings and the factors which determined Nell's final resolve remain unclear. Nell told her therapist that she killed her mother because she felt neither the mother nor father nor anyone had ever loved her and she had to kill someone. "I wanted her dead. I hated her so, but I didn't feel it," she told him. Another time she told him, "sometimes I think that if I didn't kill my mother no one would know something was wrong with me."

Several months after the murder Nell developed a paranoid psychotic state with delusions and hallucinations in which she feared and expected she would herself be murdered by the dead mother returned to earth to take revenge or by some other agent of vengeance. Although at first she had insisted her mother deserved to be killed, she could not maintain this attitude and 18 months after the crime wrote a letter to God: "Dear God, I am sorry for killing the mother you gave me. I had no right to do anything like that. If you would only forgive me, I wouldn't have to kill anymore. I only know that I feel very much like dying, and if you don't forgive me I must surely have to die or kill more people till you forgive me for my many sins. Respectfully yours, Nell T." Unlike the three boys who made a form of clinical recovery within months of the crime, upon follow-up three years later Nell remained hospitalized in a deluded, paranoid, and child-like state, plagued with continuing homicidal and suicidal preoccupations.

Discussion

The crime of matricide is too complex in its determination, too rare, and too insufficiently studied to permit confident generalizations about the characteristics of the murderers or the causation of the act. There is evidence that those who commit matricide are younger than other murderers or at least than murderers of non-parents. The crime seems to be committed most frequently by adolescents rather than by younger children (no cases under 14 have been reported), perhaps requiring the intensity of the instinctual drives of puberty to provide sufficient motivation for completing the act. In addition, in reviewing our cases and those in the literature we were impressed with the power of conflicts over independence between these children and their mothers who seemed to allow them no autonomy whatsoever. Possibly its greater rarity among adults can be explained on the basis that once the adolescent period is past the immediate intensity of the mother-child relationship is reduced and other avenues of instinctual and emotional expression become available. Stated slightly differently, it might be expected that if the mother survives her child's adolescence she is unlikely to become its victim thereafter. The crime seems to be more common among boys than girls, but biases in sampling and reporting may be operating here.

As in most crimes of passion, conventional diagnostic categorizations are not especially useful. Generalizations such as Gillies' that matricide is "the schizophrenic crime" are not corroborated by other work and fail to take into account such factors as whether the sample under consideration is taken from the records of a mental hospital or the time relationship between the examination of the murderer and the commission of the crime. A number of murderers suffer transient psychotic-like periods of disorganization with varying disruptions of reality testing, confusion and perceptual distortion during the weeks and even months following the murder as they attempted to integrate the devastating impact of the crime, the loss of the mother and their personal responsibility for it.

Duncan and Duncan in a study of adolescents who murdered or attempted to murder family members have tried to assess the factors which may indicate the potential for homicide [18]. These include the intensity of hostility by verbal expression or behavior, evidence of poor impulse control in response to stress, unavailability of nonviolent alternatives, a sense of hopelessness (see also [19] in this regard), provocativeness and/or helplessness of the victim, availability of weapons, and a history of specific threats.

Both in our cases of matricide and in the literature some more specific patterns may be discerned, keeping in mind the small size of the population being considered. Wertham observed the excessive attachment of his young patient, Gino, to his mother with an idealization of her image, an attitude which changed to intense hatred when she betrayed him by turning to other men after the father's death. No alternatives were available to Gino, no escape from the excessive intensity of the ambivalent mother-child relationship. Russell stressed the deep, primitive hostility toward the mother, controlled in a symbiotic relationship up to midadolescence when, with the "implicit fostering" by both parents of the boy's incestuous drives, the inadequate defenses break down.

Our review permits some further tentative generalizations which apply principally to males as the single case we have reported appears to be the only matricide by a girl described in the published literature. An intense, exclusive deeply sadomasochistic attachment between the mother and son has existed since early childhood if not infancy. The father, if not physically absent, is unable to, or declines to, intervene or otherwise interrupt this hostile intimacy with its destructive outcome which he may covertly promote if not actually demand as in the Greek myths. More likely the father is seen by the child (if not actually serving) as the mother's agent or servant carrying out her punishments or otherwise enforcing her efforts to maintain the exclusiveness of the attachment. The advent of puberty, rather than forcing steps to be taken to afford greater distance between mother and child, serves only to intensify the attachment. The mother responds to her son's adolescence by further restrictions and demands for exclusiveness. Efforts on the part of the child to gain distance and independence or to form other attachments, especially with girls, are met by the mother with hostility and with renewed restrictions, prohibitions, provocations, and demands. An increasingly intense sadomasochistic and sometimes brutal struggle may ensue between mother and son with mounting hatred on the boy's part as he finds himself unable to escape his conflicts. Abortive efforts to seek alternative "ways out" such as running away or desperate turning to others outside the family may be met with further admonition or punishment on the part of the mother. To murder the mother becomes for the boy the only *solution* to his incestuous conflict, the only way to relieve his tension and anguish. If he can devalue her sufficiently and find justification for the murder in convincing himself of the mother's perfidious nature, declaring to himself that she *deserves* to be killed, then the superego prohibitions and ego controls against murder may be overcome. These justification mechanisms serve also in the post-murder period in helping the boy to deal with the crime. We have seen a number of cases of near matricide where many elements in this constellation were present but where the act itself was not committed, or was aborted, because some element in the cycle was interrupted or an intervention, perhaps psychotherapeutic, occurred.

In the case of the one girl studied, different mechanisms seemed to be operating. Rather than an intense sadomasochistic attachment developing between mother and daughter, profound maternal deprivation in early childhood was followed by intense restrictiveness in adolescence. The hatred and aggression toward the mother was more starkly overwhelming for this girl and justification played a lesser role. She was the most disturbed of our cases and remained chronically psychotic following the crime.

Matricide, the ultimate solution to problems of intimacy and conflicts over dependency is, fortunately, a rare crime. For most of the world's adolescents other solutions in the intrapsychic, intra-familial, and extra-familial spheres are available. The rarity of such cases, male or female, may, hopefully, not provide too many ready opportunities to see whether these generalizations will stand.

Bibliography

1. Russell, D. H., A study of juvenile murderers, *J. of Offender Therapy*, 9 (1965), 55–86.
2. Graves, Robert, *The Greek Myths*, George Braziller, New York, 1959.
3. Seyffert, Oskar, *Dictionary of Classical Antiquities*, Meridian Books, New York, 1962.
4. Jones, Ernest, *Hamlet and Oedipus*, Victor Gollanez, Ltd., London, 1949.
5. Wertham, Frederick, *Dark Legend*, Duell, Sloan and Pearce, New York, 1941.
6. Scherl, D. J. and Mack, J. E., A study of adolescent matricide, *J. of the American Academy of Child Psychiatry*, 5 (1966), 569–593.
7. Mittleman, E. and Murphy, F. J., A matricide—a community affair, *J. of Offender Therapy*, 5 (1961), 15–16.
8. Cuthbert, T. M., A portfolio of murders, *Brit. J. of Psychiatry*, 116 (1970), 1–10.
9. Szondi, L., A letter to Theodore Reik, *American Imago*, 25 (1968), 21–26.
10. Lelos, David, Personal Communication to Leila Josephs, July, 1971.
11. F. B. I., *Uniform Crime Report* (1969).
12. Morris, T. and Blom-Cooper, L. J., Murder in microcosm, *The Observer*, London, reported in McKnight et al., see Reference No. 13, 1961.
13. McKnight, C. K., Mohr, J. W., Quinsey, R. E. and Erochko, J., Matricide and mental illness, *Canadian Psychiatric Association Journal*, 11 (1966), 99–106.
14. O'Connell, B. A., Matricide, *Lancet*, 7290 (1963), 1083–1084.
15. Gillies, H., Murder in the west of Scotland, *Brit. J. of Psychiatry*, 111 (1965), 1087–1094.
16. Growden, C. H., *A Group Study of Juvenile Murder*, Ohio Bureau of Juvenile Research, Columbus, Ohio, October, 1949.
17. Kearney, M. and White, S. L., Juvenile Murderers, Unpublished Essay, Newton College of the Sacred Heart, Newton, Massachusetts, 1968.
18. Duncan, J. W. and Duncan, G. M., Murder in the family: a study of some homicidal adolescents, *American J. of Psychiatry*, 127 (1971) 1498–1052.
19. Malmquist, C. P., Premonitory signs of homicidal aggression in juveniles, *American J. of Psychiatry*, 128 (1971), 461–465.

Adolescent Girls Who Kill or Try to Kill Their Fathers

**E. James Anthony, M.D. (U.S.A.) and
A. Rizzo, M.D. (U.S.A.)**

Introduction

In one set of statistics, furnished by the Federal Bureau of Investigation in the United States, the murder of one family member by another constituted about a third of all homicides. Fifty-three percent involved the killing of one spouse by another, 17% the killing of children by parents, 23% the killing of other relatives, and 6% *the killing of parents by children.* Although the last category has a relative infrequency, the theoretical implications are considerable and have prompted a number of literary and psychological studies. Many of these have been focused on the male patricide and the classical theories have attempted to clarify his motivations. The female patricide is not only comparatively rare but has received scant attention from investigators. The fact that girls are far less prone to homicidal aggression than boys is also consistent with the fact that girls are far less likely to kill their fathers than boys. What kind of girls, therefore, commit the "primal crime," as Freud termed it, and why? Before addressing ourselves to these questions, we would like to discuss, as a prelude to subsequent theory-making, the homicidal tendency of juveniles in general and its relation to parricide.

The Homicidal Adolescent

Malmquist (1971) investigated 20 adolescents charged with murder with ages ranging from 13 to 18 years. There were three females in the group. With the exception of one girl, all functioned intellectually within the normal range. Three were diagnosed as schizophrenic, ten as depressive, and seven as suffering from personality disorders. The investigator focused his attention on the prodromal period stretching between the onset of a recognizable psychological shift in functioning and the homicidal act. Characteristics of prodromal behavior were brooding, pessimism, and self-hate; often unperceived and muted "cries for help"; a change in the relationship with the victim involving the loss, or possible loss, of narcissistic supplies; an increase in the use of drugs, perhaps in an effort to contain impulses and affects; the loss of a significant relationship and attempts to deal with it by means of unhelpful, "wild," quasi-therapeutic relationships; an exacerbation of headaches and other chronic physical symptoms; homosexual or incestuous experiences or threats leading to panic; homicidal and suicidal preoccupations; feelings of helplessness, hopelessness, and self-damage; and, most typically, an "emotional crescendo" of agitation, motor restlessness, disturbed eating and sleeping habits, loss of emotional control, and gradual depersonalization.

Sargent (1962) put forward the hypothesis that the child who killed a parent was acting as the unwitting lethal agent of the spouse who unconsciously prompted the act for his own reasons. On investigating a series of such cases, he concluded that there was strong suggestive evidence to support the hypothesis. The children were often stunned by the fact that the murderous act had culminated in murder as if this had been far from their intention and displayed a curious protectiveness not only toward the parent who (in the opinion of the investigator) had indirectly engineered the killing but also toward the victim. The surviving spouses could all recall some occasion when they had wanted their partners "out of the way." They reacted guiltily to the murder as if it were somehow their responsibility but at the same time, there was undeniable relief that it had happened. They also expressed guilt that the child killer had become involved in their marital conflict.

Sargent made three further inferences from his data: First, that the child had his own unconscious motive for aggression toward the parental victim based on his oedipal rivalry and distinct from that of the instigating parent who was however able to exploit it—dreams and fantasies after the killing invariably showed evidence of the earlier oedipal death wish; second, that the child's susceptibility to the covert wishes of the parent was proportional to his immaturity and to the degree of his attachment to the instigating parent; and third, that the child's guilt and depression after the act suggested not the absence of conscience but the presence of a strict and punitive one whose effect had been temporarily suspended. This meant that the deficit lay in the ego and not in the superego. The entire complex of persons, events, and feelings supported the scapegoat theory that children who kill their parents were *simultaneous victims of an unconscious family conspiracy.*

Easson (1961) studied seven boys who had made murderous assaults and one who had actually committed murder. The children all came from apparently "normal" homes, but an investigation disclosed a marked degree of family psychopathology involving hatred associated with brutal violence, sadism, barely concealed incestuousness with seductiveness and infantilization, and a family expectation of murderous attack by the children. Associated factors included the presence of physical illness or deformity, convulsive disorder (temporal lobe type), a confusion of sex roles, and intense sibling rivalry. A striking feature indicating collusion was the way in which the parents permitted and even encouraged the children to collect lethal weapons and sometimes even to retain them after the murderous act. This lent further support to the overall conclusion that *the parents of these children fostered, condoned, and vicariously enjoyed a destructive expression of aggression.*

Bender (1934), in her study of child and adolescent killers, also pointed to this quality of permissiveness with regard to violence on the part of the parents and a similar association with sibling rivalry, organic inferiority, and learning difficulties (see, also, Gardner, 1971).

The child killers so far considered have been, for the most part, male in keeping with the traditional view that delinquent females resort to sexual acting out rather than to physical violence or murder. Judging from more recent surveys, however, the number of aggressive acts committed by females seems to be on the increase although this does not seem to be the case for female patricides. The latter is not only sparsely represented in the current psychiatric literature but far less explicable in terms of available theory. We will now consider predisposing and triggering factors in the expression of undue aggressiveness as well as factors concerned in patricide in general and female patricide in particular.

1.   *Predisposing factors* include, first of all, gross family psychopathology as evident by a climate of brutality and violence, a low threshold for aggressive reactions, a subculture of permissiveness with regard to physical attack, a tendency to find aggressive "solutions" to interpersonal problems, a need to act out rather than verbalize anger, a lack of positive feeling to "neutralize" negative feelings, and a deficiency in overall control; second, the scapegoat use of children to enact unconscious parental homicidal wishes, family conspiracies against a member, or family expectations with regard to impulsive behavior; and third, the presence of some physical handicap (organ inferiority, epilepsy, cortical immaturity, mental subnormality, or mental disorder such as psychopathy or psychosis).

Raybin (1971) found that a particular family mythology could predispose to aggressive behavior when, for example, aggression became equated with being bad, with being masculine, with being loving, or with being free and therefore necessary for the demonstration of these attributes.

2.   *Triggering factors.* Malmquist (1971) postulated a sudden rise in the "homicidal index" during the emotional crescendo of the prodromal phase prior to the murderous attack.

Wertham (1941) described five stages in the transformation of the wish, feeling or impulse into the homicidal act which he referred to as the "catathymic crisis," a concept not too dissimilar from Malmquist's "emotional crescendo." (The stages are summarized in Table 1.) The catathymic crisis can be regarded as an action abreaction in which the urge to act takes precedence over the need to verbalize or express feeling. However, like any cathartic event, it is followed by an effort to regain equilibrium. In the first part of the post-cathartic period, the subject appears bland, emotionally indifferent and unrealistic in his appraisal of what has occurred. In its final phase, in the event that equilibrium is restored, there is a recapturing of some of the original feelings involved and at least partial insight into the meaning of the act. During this phase, "amnesias"

Table 1 The Five Stages of Catathymic Crisis

Stage I	Stage II	Stage III	Stage IV	Stage V
Initial Thinking Disorder	Crystallization of a Plan	Extreme Tension Culminations in the violent Crisis	Superficial Normality	Insight & Recovery
Uneasiness	Intense inner struggle	Overwhelming emotional tension	Immediate lifting of tension	Reestablishment of inner equilibrium
Holding outer situation responsible for inner tension			Superficially normal period	Gain of Insight
Thinking becomes self-centered			Continuing lack of insight	Recovery

Precipitating injurious experiences

Crystallization point in the idea that violent act is the only way out

Preoccupation with the violent act becomes acute and all-absorbing

Execution of violent act

Realization that outer situation does not sufficiently account for the violent act committed

337

are lifted, twilight states are clarified, and causal connections are made permitting a new level of adjustment to ensue. An irresistible impulse during a period of diminished consciousness describes but does not explain the triggering mechanism; however, no explanations are presently available to do this satisfactorily. Wertham recalls a comment made by Freud on a book analyzing a case of murder: "Now we know everything," he said, "except why the murder was committed." In murder, as in other circumstances, it is easier to be wise after the event in recognizing a propensity but not wise enough to postdict the actual event with conviction.

According to Berkowitz (1963), the triggering factor might well reside in the victim so that a target with appropriate stimulus qualities could be envisaged as "pulling" agressive responses from a person who is angry or ready to become angry. The disliked or frustrating subject is seen as a "conveniently chosen outlet" who "invites the discharge" of aggressive energy (Hartmann, Kris and Loewenstein, 1949). This concept of Berkowitz is somewhat similar to the ethological concept of "releaser" meaning a cue or sign stimulus in the external environment that provokes reaction from an organism ready to make such a response. In his search for explanations, therefore, the clinician might do well to focus his attention on the proverbial "red rag" or "inviting" element in the victim.

3. *Psychodynamic factors involved in patricide.* The possibility of patricide was never very far from Freud's mind and he returned to it over and over again throughout his life. It first appeared in his speculation on the "primal horde" concerning a primitive period in which sons banded together, murdered, and devoured their father (1955). It reappeared in his elaboration of the Oedipus complex and it was more than a coincidence that his choice of the three greatest literary masterpieces of all times included the *Oedipus Rex* of Sophocles, Shakespeare's *Hamlet,* and Dostoyevsky's *The Brothers Karamazov,* all having to do with patricide. He assumed that Dostoyevsky was a latent father killer because of his "instinctual character," his entense emotional life, his strong destructive propensity, his marked sexual aggressiveness, his well-developed sado-masochism and his repressed homosexuality embedded in a bisexual tendency. Additional background factors included the development of epilepsy following the murder of his father when he was eighteen and his lifelong guilt because his earlier death wishes had anticipated

the actual killing. The theory of patricide, outlined by Dostoyevsky (1879) in his book, contained the following postulates:

In every man there is a wish amounting to a need to kill his father; this he shares with other members of the family so that when patricide occurs, each member shares the responsibility for it; the actual agent for the killing is generally one whose resistance to the act (because of immaturity or epilepsy, etc.) is less than that of the others; sexual rivalry on an incestuous basis is overtly present; and lastly, there is often little doubt that the father represents an "inviting" target who more or less "asks" to be killed.

Moreover, his behavior is often so obnoxious that he no longer deserved the name of "father." This explained Dostoyevsky's famous paradox of patricide without the killing of the "father." The triggering mechanism, as in the *Oedipus Rex*, was an act of authoritarianism on the father's part.

4. *Psychodynamic factors involved in female patricide.* When Ivan Karamazov asks at the trial: 'Who does not want to kill their father?" He himself answers: "Everybody," meaning not only sons but daughters as well. Female patricide is not an integral part of the Oedipus complex nor of the primal horde theory. When it occurs, therefore, is it because of a concatenation of accidental factors or some, as yet undescribed, variant of a deep-seated complex? Classical theory can be bent to fit the problem by inverting the Oedipus complex and making the father the hated rival for the homosexual possession of the oedipal and pre-Oedipal mother. Alternatively, the intensity of the girl's oedipal love for the father may bring about a transformation of love into murderous hate as an outcome of rejection. As Jones (1910) has pointed out, one can never be certain in the triangular complex who is to be killed—the loved one or the lover. An intense feeling of guilt often follows the patricide but Freud has also called attention to criminal actions stemming from guilt.

That the admixture of incest and patricide is not a Freudian invention or simply a "dark legend" but a living fact of psychopathology is demonstrated from the following two cases.

Case Illustrations

CASE 1. FATHER-KILLING BY AN ADOLESCENT GIRL AGED FIFTEEN

Early Development. The patient's birth and physical developments were uneventful but from a very early age, she was regarded as far more nervous and aggressive than her siblings. In this poor socioeconomic culture, this was attributed to her "tonsils." Her nervousness expressed itself in nightmares, rocking, pulling out her hair and extreme fearfulness, especially of accidents, blood, death, knives, and guns. She became panic-stricken if left on her own. Temperamentally, she was moody, excitable, tense, and given to excessive worrying. Her attendance at school was poor and she performed well below her intellectual capacity (IQ 106). Her feelings of rejection together with oversensitivity made her quarrelsome, boastful, and difficult to get along with. The teachers described her as a "fiery redhead" defiant toward all authority and constantly in fights. However, she was as constantly seeking out help for herself and spent a lot of time talking over her problems with counselors. In short, she appeared to have a lifelong problem in controlling her feelings and aggression.

The Aggressive Climate of the Family. The most startling feature of family life was the juxtaposition of primitive religious beliefs, violence, and bizarre sexual practices. The father was the central figure in the household and his aggressive and erotic activities were the main determinants of family transactions. His behavior oscillated with his drinking habits. When he was "on the bottle," he became unpredictably aggressive or seductive but even when sober, he could be irritable, erratic, and unrealistic so that the family still suffered, although differently. He gave up drinking a few months before his death because of persistent "visions" in which he would see himself murdering his whole family. He also developed suspicions that they were out to kill him and when a can of hair spray exploded in the house, he immediately concluded that there had been an attempt on his life. He became extremely upset when they started to laugh at him over this and threatened to kill them then and there. His relationship with his wife was equally violent. He had beaten her regularly until about six years prior to his death when he stopped dramatically after a drunken incident. She was pregnant at the time and he had slapped her on the stomach whereupon she had drawn a gun on him and threatened to kill him. He had not touched her since, aggressively or sexually, but had turned his attention, in both respects, to his children.

The Sexual Climate of the Family. The father had had sexual relations with three of his four daughters as well as his son "from behind." His regular practice had been to start sexual intercourse with each daughter as she reached puberty and to discard them in turn as he started with a new victim. Two of them, one being the patient, had been made pregnant; one he had aborted with a television antenna, and a full-term baby had been delivered by father and mother and later drowned by the father in the kitchen sink two hours after birth. The mother had helped to bury the baby in a field not far from the home. In spite of all this, he was extremely strict about any extra-familial sexuality. He repeatedly warned his daughters that if they had dates he would kill them. When any adult male, even a relative, so much as laid a friendly hand on one of the girls, he would make a violent attack on him. According to the mother, her husband had always taught his children "to guard their sexuality." Even as babies, while their diapers were being changed, he insisted on having their genitalia covered. She said that he had also taught his son not to look up the skirts of little girls. He was very proud of the fact that his daughters had no boyfriends. He had told them that their virginity, lost through incest, would return to them if they refrained from all sexual contact outside the family. For many years, he had not bothered his wife at all for sex although when he had first married her, he had wanted it three or four times every night and had, in addition, been going around with other women. The wife felt that this was "just fine" since she was usually very tired and, in fact, disgusted by sex.

The Murderous Attack. On the night of the murder, the subject mentioned that she walked barefooted across a ditch with a lot of broken glass in it without cutting her feet. She had also known, from the way that her father looked, that he had some premonition that he was going to die on the day that he was killed. On this particular night, he had forbidden them to go to a drive-in theater but they had disobeyed him. He found them there and accused them loudly of having sexual relations with the men around them. He took them home and when they started to argue with him, he seized one of the girls and started to strangle her. The patient later stated that as soon as she entered the house that evening, she had felt that something violent was going to happen so she went in and hid the guns so that nobody would find them. She had always done this in the past whenever her father had shown signs of becoming violent. When she saw him attacking her sister, she went and fetched one of the guns and threatened to shoot him unless he stopped. Since he continued and the girl was becoming cold and blue, she shot him.

The Aftermath—The Girl's Reaction. Following the killing, the patient became extremely depressed and cried a lot. She said that she had not wanted to kill her father but just to threaten him in order to save her sister. She had always felt very close to this particular girl and did not want her to die. She was surprised that the rest of the family now felt so hostile toward her when, at the time, they all seemed to be in full agreement with her action. She felt that because she was nervous and impulsive the family had always used her when they wanted some "dirty business" done. She reiterated that she wished that her father were still alive even though he was a very sick man because she still loved him. She talked almost continuously about his brutality and the sexual relation with her. She still insisted that he was "a wonderful father." She was very angry that he showed interest in other females. She said that she still considered herself "a virgin except for what Dad had done." She felt that no one could ever understand how she had come to murder her father. A recurrent dream during this period was that her father had not died due to the "accident" but had come out of the mental hospital and was, apparently, well. He had then attempted to seduce numerous women and found that he was incapable of completing the sexual act because "his body was inactivated by the *accident* when he wanted to take one of us but not me." She could not understand "why he did it to us and left one of us undone," meaning the daughter who had been spared. She resented being in the hospital and threatened that if she were kept in she would kill herself because staying in hospital was "like my father's revenge on me—because I took his life and he wanted to live, otherwise he would have taken his own life a long time ago."

The Aftermath—The Mother's Reaction. The mother's reaction was not unlike that of the girl's. She wept and said repeatedly that she loved her husband and that you could not stop loving someone. She felt very lonely now that he was lying in the grave. When asked about the incest, she replied, "My daughters are perfect other than what he did to them." She said that he had always been affectionate and that "all six of us could crawl on top of him at times." He had always been a "flirting man," as a boy with his mother and later when he was courting her. She showed a picture of herself and her husband having sexual intercourse, the picture having been taken by one of the daughters. She also showed another in which her husband was dressed up in her underwear. She said that he frequently liked to dress up in her clothes. She resented the killing very much and added: "I would rather that all the kids were dead rather than him." When asked why she had not reported the incest, she said: "I loved him"; "I was very afraid of him"; "I was afraid he would kill me if I told about it." Before her husband's death, she herself had been accused of voyeurism with regard to neighborhood children.

The girl was not regarded as psychotic in any way but was thought to have a borderline personality characterized by immaturity, egocentricity, poor control, confused thinking, a shaky sense of reality, and a poor self-concept. Diagnostically, she was not unlike the father that she killed.

CASE 2. AN ATTEMPT AT FATHER-KILLING BY AN ADOLESCENT GIRL, AGE FIFTEEN

Early Development. The patient was the fifth and last child born to her parents. Pregnancy, birth, and physical development were all within the normal range. At an early stage she was very sensitive to the idea of death and became extremely distressed when anyone that she knew, even remotely, died. From early childhood she had maintained a very close relationship with her father and was always referred to as "Daddy's little tomboy." He treated her very much like a favored son. He took her everywhere with him, played "rough" with her, taught her to fish, to shoot and to play baseball, and generally "spoilt" her. He babied her, petted her, and gave her everything that she asked. Not only did she have difficulty in accepting herself as a girl, but the family always thought of her as a boy. The onset of menstruation at thirteen was a profound shock to her. She threatened to jump from the second-floor window or throw herself in front of a car. It was not only dirty and repulsive in itself but more importantly, it caused her father to reject her suddenly and completely. He had no time for her anymore and did not want her around him. His authoritarianism, always shown toward the rest of the family, was now no longer tempered by her seductive wiles. Although he seemed to want no contact with her, he strictly forbade her to have any boyfriends or to go on dates. The relationship between them was almost continuously abrasive and she began to "act out" her seething resentment. It seemed that as a result of turning boy into a girl, her father had turned completely away from her. Her behavior became markedly disordered. She lied constantly, showed off "obnoxiously," kept away from the family, disobeyed every order, and exhibited marked jealousy of her sisters.

The Aggressive Climate of the Family. The family atmosphere was extremely authoritarian and the father ruled his group with an iron hand. Everything within the family was encapsulated and insulated which was one reason why it gave the impression of normality to outsiders. The father became increasingly hostile to his daughters as they reached puberty so that all of them experienced a transformation of the relationship. He appeared to have no understanding at all of teenage girls and would criticize every aspect of their adolescent behavior, especially where this touched on their femininity. After the daughter's attack on him, he said: "If I'd only beaten her and shown her who was boss when she was younger, I would be able to see now." The father's hostility toward the patient was paralleled by an angry relationship with her mother. However, it was much easier for her to be openly aggressive with her mother than with her father. Her hostility toward him could only be shown covertly and indirectly.

The Sexual Climate of the Family. The extrafamilial attitudes were extremely puritanical but, prior to puberty, the father was inclined to be very "free and easy" with his daughters. The oldest girl said that he had spoken to her many years previously about the mother and the maternal grandfather having incestuous relationships with each other, and she herself suspected that not only was the mother sometimes unfaithful to her husband but that some "sort of homosexuality" was going on between the mother and the patient. She also hinted darkly at unwanted pregnancies, abortions, and the

the use of dope. She diagnosed her father as being extremely suspicious and her mother, extremely nervous. The mother's brother was chronically psychotic.

The Murderous Attack. In her first version of the shooting, the patient felt that either her mother or her boyfriend was responsible for the act. She simply remembered her father watching TV that night while she was ironing and her mother was taking a bath. She asked her father if he wanted a soda and he had not responded. She had not reacted to this because he often ignored her in this way. She then recalled returning to her room and packing her things for a trip the next day. The next thing was her father shouting and her mother screaming. She ran into the kitchen where she saw him bleeding and got an ice pack for him, at the same time calling her uncle for help. At this point she had become hysterical. In a subsequent version, when the amnesia had gradually lifted, partly with the help of amytal, she recalled further trivial provocations. The father had made a derogatory remark about her boyfriend following this up with a critical comment on her marksmanship. He seemed unable to interchange with her except in a very negative way. She felt the small provocations piling up in her mind and when he paid no attention to her offer of a soda, she felt suddenly so enraged and beside herself that she went and got the rifle, loaded it and shot him at short distance. Miraculously, the bullet severed both optic nerves without killing him. She later admitted that she always knew, somewhat vaguely, that she was responsible for the shooting and yet, somehow, she could not accept it as real. It seemed that her boyfriend had been present in the back of the house on the day of the shooting and had actually watched her undress in preparation for going out with him but he was not there at the time of the shooting.

The Aftermath—The Girl's Reaction. She felt very confused about the family. "I tried to be what they wanted me to be but then I got confused and goofed it all up!" She could not understand their combined hostility toward her when she had only tried to "please" them. She also felt that she had anticipated it all before it happened because of her ESP that she had inherited from her grandfather. She was always able to foresee in dreams when a family member was going to die and she twice saw her father in a

coffin in the weeks before the "accident" took place. She sometimes saw "visions" in the form of designs like abstract painting
and occasionally heard her dead grandmother talking to her. She
also believed that her grandfather had come back to earth as the
family dog who was there to help her as he had once done. When
she shot her father, the dog disappeared from the home. The
effect about the shooting was at first shallow to the point of indifference. Later on, she reported a great deal of frustration and
aggression and said that she was always on the point of "blowing
up." She also displayed a great deal of suspiciousness and behaved
at interviews with marked paranoid alertness. Her self-absorption
was such that she never expressed sympathy or affection for
others. She made use of the defenses of denial and isolation to the
point of depersonalization. Her surface conformity covered a
primitive explosiveness only very poorly controlled. She described
herself as "rotten" inside. In spite of having tried to kill him, she
still felt that her father was a wonderful person but she did admit
that she felt quite confused in her feelings toward him. She said
that she had tried to kill her father to stop him from criticizing
her; she felt that if she killed him, he would be able to love her
from Heaven. She had a recurrent dream following the shooting
that seemed to her to be very absurd. In the dream, she is sleeping
in her own home and yet able to hear what is going on about her.
She has several children and two husbands, a tall one and a short
one, both faceless. She knows that both of them are many years
older than she is. She has requested a gift of a toy duck from one
of them but, instead, receives a live duck with something vaguely
human about it. Next, she finds that there is a large tank in the
back porch filled with water and her children are floating on the
surface while the duck is sinking in distress to the bottom. She
feels she has to rescue the duck from drowning. The scene rapidly
changes to the bathroom where she is giving the duck a bath. However, it drowns in the bathtub and she feels that although this is an
accident, she may have helped it along. She looks up to see her
short husband saying: "That was my duck." The scene changes
again and she has now placed the duck on a railroad track feeling
quite resentful toward it and wanting to rid herself of it. The duck
is killed for a second time and once again the scene shifts. She has
now tied the duck to a tree and is trying to kill it by running into

it with a car and this is where the dream ends. She wakes up feeling annoyed at herself for having dreamed it. She was concerned about leaving hospital because she was afraid that she might try again to kill her father.

The Aftermath—The Parental Reaction. The father was understandably bitter about his blindness and refused to participate in any rehabilitation program. When he came to see his daughter, his hostility toward her was often extreme. He constantly reminded her of the great Commandment that one should love one's father and mother and felt that she must have been out of her mind or "possessed with the Devil" to have made the attempt. He also felt that it was part of her general plan to kill her mother as well in order to run away with her boyfriend. He offered to send her to a religious home for people "who had lost God in their lives," and if she chose not to do this, he wanted her committed to a mental hospital "where the boys are kept on the one side and the girls on the other so that they cannot get to each other." Her resentment against her mother at this point was extreme and her hostility was mainly directed towards her. The mother, in turn, insisted that her daughter was a liar and treated her with great mistrustfulness.

Conclusions

The relationship of father-killing to mother-killing has obtained some discussion in the psychodynamic literature. With regard to matricide, recent studies have tended to implicate pre-oedipal as well as oedipal factors so much so that Rubinstein (1969) feels that there has been a tendency to underrate the significance of the "nuclear" complex in this particular situation. Whereas he is inclined to regard matricide as a regressive and thinly disguised substitute for incest, Kanzer (1948) saw it as a defense against patricide. Arguing along these same lines, it is conceivable that female patricide could be a defense against matricide. Whichever way it works, it would give support to Rubinstein's comment that "the love that kills is incestuous love."

The two cases are like and unlike in a number of ways. In both, the coming together of incestuous and homicidal forces for the act of patricide appears to have been an essential ingredient. In case 1, the incest is overt and in case 2, covert, and this distinction holds true for almost every other aspect of the two cases. The girl in the first case was openly aggressive throughout her history and she lived in a family where open aggressiveness was the rule. The girl in the second case displayed a surface conformity that helped to conceal the increasing rage that possessed her The rejection by the father also took a somewhat different form; the first girl was used as a sexual object and then discarded for the next sister; the second girl sacrificed her femininity and identified herself as a male in order to establish a close relationship with her father only to be rejected out of hand at puberty. The conflict of ambivalence was intense in both; during the prodromal phase, the hate became predominant but following the act, the equilibrium was restored and love and admiration reentered the picture. The mother is spared each time because the hostility towards her is less ambivalent and much more easily expressed. The hate towards the father can only be expressed in action under conditions of a catathymic crisis.

The Karamazov formulation is more evident in the first case: The father deserves to be killed; he has strong premonitions that he will be killed; the girl has strong premonitions that he will be killed; every member of the family appears to have some reasons to kill him; and the one who eventually does is "chosen" because her life-long aggressivity and impulsivity make her, in the eyes of the others, the most suitable agent of destruction.

In the second case, both father and mother are hated but for different reasons. The father is probably right when he accuses the girl of wanting to kill them both. After the rejection at puberty, the girl is caught up in conflicting male and female identifications. The murder attempt is, therefore, an act of liberation from the father's dominance. She feels that she can only become a woman after she has destroyed the father although it becomes evident later that she cannot destroy the father inside her. She, therefore, tries to revenge herself for her father's rejection and, at the same time, attempts to take him away from her maternal rival.

The premonitory dreams of the father's death in both cases seem to indicate the gradual surfacing of the latent death wish and the intensification of the destructive impulse. The dreams after the shooting suggest the resumption of ambivalence. In the first case, the dream is characteristically out in the open whereas in the second case the dream is symbolized. In case 1, it seems that the father has not really been killed but only "inactivated" (or castrated) as a punishment for his turning to other women and other daughters. In case 2, the tall and short husbands would seem to represent the father and phallic mother. She gets children from both of them (one part of the oedipal wish), but what she really wants is the gift of a toy duck (or penis, the other part of the oedipal wish). She receives instead a live duck and not the make-believe one that she had wanted (as if she wished to be a tomboy and not a real boy and thus enjoy the best of both worlds). The rest of the dream has to do with the consequences of the unexpected wish fulfillments. The children are apparently drowned and the duck is in danger of being drowned. (The duck here would seem to represent the father's penis.) She manages to rescue it but then in giving it a bath, she manages to drown it feeling that although this was an "accident" (which is how she always referred to the shooting), she "may have helped it along." She then looks up to see her short husband (that is, her mother) standing there and saying: "That was my duck." The result is that she now becomes extremely resentful towards the duck and kills it, for the second time, by placing it on the railroad track. (One of her concerns in hospital was that she might get out and have a second try at killing her father.) She next ties the duck to a tree (because it seems that it will not allow itself to be permanently killed) and attempts to run into it with a car. At this point she gives up and gets up. It would seem that the duck, or the idea of the duck, is indestructible. It is repeatedly killed but it will not die. There is, apparently, more than one triggering factor in the dream; the father (or tall husband) does not give her what she wants and the mother (or short husband) emphatically asserts her rights. She, therefore, ends up by punishing the father and depriving the mother, killing two birds (or two ducks) with one stone or bullet.

The two cases illuminate the dynamics of patricide at different levels. In the first case, it is a pre-oedipal murder since the father's incestuous relationship with the girl provided her with the only emotional satisfaction that she had ever experienced. The motivation in the second case is more oedipal than pre-oedipal. The fact that one father was killed outright and the other permanently blinded is a commentary on the marksmanship and not on the dynamics of the two cases.

Bibliography

1. Bender, L., Psychiatric mechanisms in child murderers, *J. Nerv. & Ment. Dis.*, 80 (1934), 32–47.
2. Berkowitz, L., Aggressive Stimuli, Aggressive Responses and Hostility Catharsis, in *Violence and War with Clinical Studies*, J. H. Masserman, Ed., Grune & Stratton, New York, 1963.
3. Dostoyevsky, F., *The Brothers Karamazov*, 1879–80.
4. Easson, W., et al., Murderous aggression by children and adolescents, *Arch. Gen. Psychiat.*, 4 (1961), 27–35.
5. Freud, S., Dostoyevsky and Parricide, in *The Standard Edition of the Complete Psychological Works of Sigmund Freud, Volume XXI*, Hogarth Press, London, 1961.
6. Freud, S., Totem and Taboo, in *The Standard Edition of the Complete Psychological Works of Sigmund Freud, Volume XIII*, Hogarth Press, London, 1955.
7. Gardner, G., Aggression and violence—the enemies of precision learning in children, *Amer. J. Psychiat.* 128 (1971), 445–450.
8. Hartmann, H., Kris, E., and Loewenstein, R. M., Notes on the Theory of Aggression, in *The Psychoanalytic Study of the Child, Volume III-IV*, International Universities Press, New York, 1949.
9. Jones, E., The Oedipus complex as an explanation of Hamlet's mystery, *Amer. J. Psychol.*, 21 (1910), 72–113
10. Kanzer, M., Dostoyevsky's matricidal impulses, *Psychoanal. Rev.*, 35 (1948), 115–125.
11. Malmquist, C., Premonitory signs of homicidal aggression in juveniles, *Amer. J. Psychiat.*, 128 (1971), 461–465.
12. National Center for Health Statistics, U. S. P. H. S. Bulletin, 1971.
13. Raybin, J., Aggression, mythology, and the college student, *Amer. J. Psychiat.*, 128 (1971), 466–472.
14. Rubinstein, L. H., The theme of Electra and Orestes: a contribution to the psychopathology of matricide, *Br. J. Med. Psychol.*, 42 (1969), 99–108.
15. Sargent, D., Children who kill—a family conspiracy?, *J. Social Work*, 7 (1962), 35–42.
16. Wertham, F., *Dark Legend*, Duell, Sloan & Pearce, New York, 1941.

SURVIVAL

Editorial Comment

By a curious reversal of psychological perspective, victims and survivors are in the process of reaping a psychopathology of their own. If the victims have been battered and murdered, to what extent have they provoked it? If they have been seduced or raped, to what extent have they "asked for it"? If they have survived disaster, how much do they need to suffer? To survive is to be presumptuous, to cheat the gods, to defy fate; to survive is to do so at the expense of someone else and to feel triumph, joy, relief, but also guilt and shame; to survive is to feel loss and abandonment; to survive is to be angry, indignant, resentful, and embittered; and to survive is to be fixated forever on the moment of survival. Everything thereafter leads back to it. Survival has been referred to as a disease, a psychiatric syndrome in which the sufferers constantly atone for the unfairness of their escape. They are perpetually obligated toward the dead, bound up with them through indestructible ties, seeking scapegoat formulations, purging the death guilt, and always needing to justify existence. The death wish is never far away in the mind of the survivor.

The various chapters in this section focus on different aspects of the survivor's predicament following the concentration camp experience, and the formulations are mostly couched in psychodynamic terms. Lifton, in his investigation of the Hiroshima survivors, has made use of the psychohistorical approach in which the sequence from disintegration to reintegration is followed mainly through the recollections of survivors, and the protocols are then searched for universal tendencies, cultural factors, and historical forces.

In dealing with the child's response, one has to remember both his greater vulnerability as well as his surprising resilience to disaster, his response to the trauma as a savage and overwhelming force, and subsequently as bereavement and abandonment, his age at the time of the occurrence, the surrogation available to him, and the extent of his identification with the dead. Lifton has described the survivor syndrome as a "lifelong psychic numbing."

What happened at Hiroshima was so much more impersonal than in the concentration camp where brutality was a daily experience. Hiroshima was quite different.

A blinding flash—a burning heat—a dead silence—a huge boom—a violent rush of air—a series of shattering noises—and then, a monstrous mushroom with the shape, color, light continuously shifting and changing. . . .

In the wake of this came a total immersion in death, "a sudden and absolute shift from normal existence to an overwhelming encounter with death"; "a sudden loss of a sense of invulnerability"; "a sense of world collapse"; a feeling of being "without self, without a center"; a state of dreamlike somnambulistic, ghostly automatism, a ghastly silence, and then a process of "psychic closing off."

How would the children remember this "ultimate horror?" The images would be superimposed one on top of the other—the explosion itself, the scene of desolation that followed, the decomposing dead, the suffering of the mutilated, the invisible contamination by radiation, and the development of A-bomb disease. This was the total *hibakusha* experience with its combined physical and mental sequelae. It was not surprising that there was a rise in the suicide rate of the survivors. In contrast, there was also the development of a strange kind of group cohesiveness.

For many observers, the most striking feature of the cataclysm was the ensuing silence: no weeping, no screaming, no explaining; not even the children died noisily. Here are some of the memories that children carried away from the experience from Dr. Osada's collection in 1951, six years afterwards.

A girl who was five years old at the time had this to say: "My mother was changed to white bones before the family altar. When I think that for all these years I haven't been able to talk to Mother, I can hardly bear it."

A girl, four years at the time, said: "When we came to the river, there was a man who was really suffering; he was black all over, and he kept saying, 'Give me water.' I felt so sorry for him I could hardly bear it. Many of the little children were crying, 'I'm hungry!' because they hadn't had their breakfast before the bomb fell. At the end of August a baby was born, but only the baby's head was born, and then the baby and mother died together. I was terribly sad."

And another five-year-old girl was resistant to remembering: "I really hate to think about war, and I hate to remember the day when the atom bomb fell. Even when I read books, I skip the part about war. And I skip the newsreels when scenes of war appear."

A boy, 11 years old at the time, recalled only a vignette: "My three-year-old brother with his arms and legs all wrapped in bandages used to run outside every time an airplane passed and shout, 'Give me back my sister.' He was afraid even to look up at the sky."

And another 10-year-old boy had traumatic recollections: "At the side of the river, burned people were moaning, 'Hot! Hot!' and jumping into the river. The river became not a stream of flowing water but of drifting, dead bodies. I wondered why human beings had to kill each other like this."

With many, there seemed to be a permanent sensitivity.

The tragedy of Aberfan in Wales, which occurred on October 21, 1966, was an unusual disaster in that apart from five teachers the victims were all children, 114 of them. A huge complex roared down the mountainside engulfing farms, houses, and much of the school. Unlike Hiroshima, the area was familiar with tragedy. In addition to big disasters, minor accidents occurred, and small numbers of men were killed and disabled. In addition, many of the men suffered from pneumoconiosis and were old before their time, spending their last years in a weakened condition, struggling for breath.

Rescue operations began immediately after the landslide and the bodies of children were recovered for several days afterwards. This constituted one of the enormous strains for the parents, and the business of identifying their dead children was harrowing. The local people were hostile to news reporters, cameramen, the education authorities, and a variety of other scapegoats.

Cases were referred to the child guidance clinic, and five years later a total of 56 children had been seen who were referred for difficulties which the parents thought were directly connected with the disaster. Of these 56 children, only 19 had actually lost siblings in the disaster. The symptoms were varied and included sleeping difficulties, nervousness, lack of friends, unwillingness to go out to play, instability, and enuresis. Those children who were most severely affected were those who had other anxiety-creating forces in their background. The degree of disturbance was not related at all to the degree of physical injury. What seemed most important was the reaction of the parents. The more grief the family had had to endure in the past, the more upset were they by the disaster. Many had a great need to go to the cemetery very frequently and were reluctant to leave the district although offered jobs elsewhere. Many children would speak of their experience when questioned but did not volunteer information. Bad weather—wind, rain, snow— was very frightening to some. Loss of friends was very important, and many of the children had lost all their friends. They found it especially difficult to begin going out to play. Educationally, many seemed to stand still for some time but made progress later on. Three children played "burying" but later gave it up to go on to other play situations.

In Aberfan the full community felt bereaved so that they were unable to give support to one another, and the grief became something that each family had to try to deal with alone. The manner of death was particularly horrifying, for the fact that mostly children were killed made it unlike other tragedies. There was a great need to work out aggressions and to find scapegoats.

As further disasters strike the world, whether natural or man-made, the survivor problem will grow. As was hinted in the Aberfan tragedy, not all survivors show the characteristic syndrome; not all become symtomatic; not all develop into clinical cases. Those survivors who find it difficult to adjust to their own survival often have a prior history of maladjustment to other exacting situations in life. The premorbid history should then suggest who are the survivors at risk. We need more work in this particular area.

E. James Anthony

Bibliography

1. Lacey, G., *Aberfan,* Paper given at the meeting of the Association for Child Psychology and Psychiatry in London, 1971.
2. Lifton, R. J., *Death in Life. Survivors of Hiroshima,* Random House, New York, 1967.

Symposium: Children of the Holocaust

Introductory Remarks

Judith S. Kestenberg, M.D. (U.S.A.)

Some years ago I treated a young adolescent who appeared psychotic and yet was "miraculously" cured by psychoanalysis within a relatively short period. Recovery became possible when the analyst was able to overcome the resistance of the parents to reporting what they had experienced in the holocaust and her own resistance to listening to their report. The patient himself enacted the fate of a lost family member and not what the parents had undergone in reality. It was only when I was able to confront him with what had actually happened that it became possible for him to rid himself of the unconscious desire to sacrifice himself in place of the deceased relative whom he never knew.

How far-reaching this chain of events can be was further exemplified in my analysis of an adult who had lost cousins, whom he had also never met, in the concentration camps. Influenced by the guilt of his mother, he had carried an unconscious guilt within himself that caused him to go from country to country in an attempt to escape it. It also provoked him to want to drop out of analysis because he felt that he had "sacrificed enough already."

My inquiries have revealed that while emotional disturbances are

---

*Proceedings of a symposium at the joint meeting of the International Congress of Child Psychiatry and Allied Professions and the American Association for Child Psychoanalysis in Jerusalem, August, 1970.

relatively frequent and severe in the children of survivors, sometimes amounting to a pseudopsychosis, not many of them have had psychoanalysis, the figures being larger for Israel and England (the Hampstead Clinic) than for the United States. Survivor-parents seem to resist the treatment of their children even more so than their own. Legal interviews, conducted by M. Kestenberg with survivors seeking compensation, disclosed a profound wish on the part of the survivor-parents to see their children as messianic redeemers rather than as patients.

A number of important questions suggest themselves for this symposium:

1. Whether the treatment of these children requires a special *trust-inspiring preparation* of the parents.

2. Whether the *analyst's own alienation* from the disturbing problems involved can be sufficiently overcome to allow him to penetrate them in depth.

3. Whether the pathology of parents who have been exposed to Nazi persecution can produce *bizarre sadomasochistic interchanges* between parent and child as a result of "identification with the aggressor" (suggested by Dale Meers).

4. Whether the ego-resilience of survivor-parents has generated *a special type of personality development* in their children.

5. And, finally, whether there are *unique dynamics,* discoverable by psychoanalysis, operating in these children.

Some scanty but suggestive information is already available. For example, in the only published case of an analysis of a survivor's child by H. Z. Winnik (1968), there is evidence that the horror stories communicated by the father to the son did indeed induce nightmares and terrors similar to those reported by Nazi victims. However, communication need not be explicit. Open or latent horror has been found in survivors' children whether they have been told or deliberately not told what happened to their parents.

It is important to add, in order to give balance to this symposium, that although survivor-parents can and do behave pathogenically, they can also manifest a surprising vitality, stability and strength in the upbringing of their children. The difference between one or other response may be a function of variability in experience but this is not, by any means, the whole answer which must also include variations in ego strength stemming from constitutional and environmental factors. Is it possible for psychoanalysis to disclose what constitutes strength or weakness in the dynamics of children of survivors?

Bibliography

Winnik, H. Z., Contribution to psychic traumatization through social catastrophe, *Int. J. Psycho-Anal.*, 49 (1968), 298–301.

The Analysis of a Child of Survivors

Moses Laufer, Ph.D.

The case of Michael was discussed in a previous paper from the viewpoint of the loss of a parent and the mourning processes in adolescence. This presentation has tried to focus on Michael as a person
who grew up in a family of people who had been in concentration
camps. The facts that Michael's father died in a concentration camp
before he was born, and that his mother remarried when he was four
and a half, and that she died during his adolescence were very special features of this case and aggravated the difficulties in isolating
the essential problem connected with being a survivor's child. Superimposed on all this was the biological advent of adolescence and the
new feelings about his body that came to occupy the center of the
analysis. Michael came into treatment at the age of 14.8 and left
treatment at the age of 18.6. He had been reluctant to start, but
his mother had forced him, threatening punishment if he refused.
The first part of treatment was spent in working on card tricks.
His mother worried because her boy was not doing well in school
despite a high I. Q. She expected him to follow in his real father's
footsteps and become, unlike his stepfather, intellectual. She also
constantly worried that she had done something wrong in bringing
him up. She told him stories about the strength and high quality of
his real father; of how she fled with him to Sweden when he was two
years old, keeping him in a basket and admonishing him to be quiet

so that he would not be discovered; of how emaciated she had been when he was born and how he was nursed by another woman who had also had a child. In addition, his mother constantly admonished him to be grateful to England, the country that had taken him in and given him haven. As a mark of appreciation she wanted him to be kind, quiet, and polite. They had come to London when he was seven and being unable to speak the language, he felt shy and conformity to this later became his rationalization for an inhibition of aggression that was ego syntonic.

The analyst's earliest and biggest concern was that Michael was suicidal. He felt that the frequent reiterations of "you don't have to do anything you don't want to," and "there is always a way out if things prove unmanageable," contained a wish for death. These phrases also expressed his identification with and aggression against his real father "who had 'allowed' the Nazis to do to him whatever they wanted."* Then feelings, stemming from his early experiences, had to be analyzed before he could cope with his mother's death which occurred when he was about eight months in analysis.

In an early interview mother described how Michael shed no tears when she visited him in the hospital where he had been confined for three weeks at the age of eight with pneumonia. When his mother died, he also could not cry. No attempt had been made to prepare him for her death although his stepfather and grandmother understood well that she was dangerously ill, and he was bewildered, shocked, and full of guilt because he could not grieve for her. He would not change his clothes and refused to see people or listen to his records for several weeks. Despite all this and despite the guilt he felt on seeing his stepfather and grandmother cry, he assumed the responsibility of running the home, shopping for food, and cooking it.

As one reaction to his mother's death, Michael found himself unable to touch his penis. He became aware in the analysis of his incestuous, oedipal fantasies and his desire to have intercourse with a middle-aged woman. He understood the oedipal meaning and reacted with shame and disgust. This connected up to an earlier idea that

---

*The implication here might be that his father had to do what they wanted him to do, starve and die. It could also imply that his mother had to do what they wanted her to do (the sexual implication of this will be seen later). Last but not least, it could represent Michael's protest against the survivor-mother who taught him to submit(to be quiet and grateful) in order to survive.

his mother was a whore and that he was illegitimate. He wanted the analyst to guess which of the men in a photograph given to him by his mother was his father. At the same time he accused himself of injuring his mother through his birth. He also wondered whether she would have lived longer if she had not been pregnant at the time. He debated within himself whether he, his father or his step-father were to blame.

At this point, his analyst was concerned lest he might look upon his body as a source of destruction and seek to destroy it in a suicide that would also serve to reunite him, in fantasy, with his mother and real father. He decided cautiously against focusing on these connections at the time and concentrated instead on helping Michael to work through his mourning. He showed Michael how much he wanted to keep his mother alive. Although mourning could not be completed until the oedipal feelings were understood, this acquisition of insight was postponed until the suicidal risk lessened.

When Michael was able to concentrate on the positive feelings he had felt towards his mother, he began to feel an urgency to decide about his future. He gave up the idea of following his father into an intellectual career, and with the guidance and help of an admired friend of the family, he entered a catering school. So strong was his desire to become a caterer that a subsequent disappointment in his adult friend did not deter him from pursuing his career.

At this time he talked about his stepfather and his real father and realized that he was identified with both. In transference, he saw the analyst as having great power over him. Perhaps the analyst thought of him as stupid or ugly; perhaps he wanted him to become someone special. He was fearful of his passive wish to give in to the analyst as he had given in to his mother. He assured himself that he could manage without anybody. At the same time he felt forced by the early death of his father and by his mother's subsequent death to experience a feeling of loss for those he loved. He wondered what life might have been if his father had not died in a concentration camp. It took many months of analysis before Michael realized that he had lived with a fantasy that his real father may have died of starvation. He knew that his mother was emaciated during her pregnancy which, he thought, contributed to her premature death. Through caring for his stepfather and grandmother and by means of his catering he was able to keep active the relationship to his real father that he had been able previously to nurture only through his relationship to his mother.

When Michael began attending the catering school, he became preoccupied with gambling and although this had roots in homosexuality, there were more obvious connections to his mourning and masturbatory conflicts. He had need to feel that he was in control of his own destiny. It made him take unusual risks but always with the intensity that he could win. His losses he attributed to lapses in attention. He bragged about his winnings and described the physical excitement that accompanied the gambling. From his need to eat before his analytic sessions and before gambling it was possible to reconstruct some of his earliest guilty sexual activities. He used to vomit at about seven years of age when left in the care of a neighbor. Next door lived a girl whom he bribed with sweets to allow him to touch her anus. Now when he saw this girl on the street, the thought occurred: "I used to be able to get her to do anything by giving her sweets." By continuing to reconstruct his childhood and by revealing more and more of his fantasies about his real father, he was able to work through his mourning for his mother.

Even though his problems were far from being completely resolved, he wanted to see how he could go on without analysis. His analyst considered this to be a normal move for an adolescent and felt that the suicidal risk was sufficiently diminished to allow treatment to be terminated. He has followed up on Michael to his present age of 25 years. He had finished with catering school and had become attached to a girl whom he wanted to marry. He was able to enjoy sex but was not sure whether his attachment to his girl friend was lasting. Therefore, he decided to go to another country both to specialize further in catering as well as to give himself time away from the girl to decide whether he really needed her or could do without her. Although he was functioning well, he still experienced feelings of sadness that caused him to worry at times. He enjoyed his catering work but considered it second-best. Some of his earlier shame could be detected in this.

His pathology could be considered under four headings all relating to his status as the child of a survivor.

1.   The damage to the normal infantile omnipotence that came about because of his father's inability to survive and the

atmosphere of vulnerability and death within which he grew up.

2. His feminine identification with the victim.

3. The enormous inhibition of his aggressivity that increasingly tied him to his mother and made his awakening adolescent sexuality feel very dangerous.

4. The disturbed relationship to his own body as observed in his special attitude to death and dying. The crucial sentence: "You don't have to do anything you don't want to do", was related not only to his masturbatory conflict but also to the idea that he could kill himself if he so wanted. The idea of dying was a way of fulfilling the fantasy of reunion with the dead, idealized father and later with the dead mother as well. He also used it as a defense against his passivity and inability to protect himself that made him dependent on others.

In conclusion, it is clear that there were very special circumstances in this case over and above the survivor problem. Michael never knew his real father, he lived alone with his mother until he was four and a half, and then he lost his mother in adolescence. However, it was still possible to recognize certain areas of vulnerability that seemed characteristic of children of survivors.

Discussion

Miriam Williams, M.D. (U.S.A.)

Dr. Laufer in his sensitive perception and treatment of this patient chooses four areas in which to evaluate Michael's specific problems. Out of the multitude of traumatic events in Michael's life it could not have been easy to crystallize out that part which can be considered specific for the patient's pathology due to being the child of a parent survivor.

To start with point one of Dr. Laufer's discussion: That is, "the damage to the normal infantile omnipotence": The question is whether the stories of Michael's rescue and his father's death had only a detrimental effect on the patient's development, depriving him of the sense of infantile omnipotence. From Michael's subsequent omnipotent behavior during adolescence—the gambling and the card tricks after his mother's death—we see a good deal of evidence of the survival of infantile omnipotence. It is not possible that Michael used those stories of his own miraculous rescue to perceive himself as a very special person? In fact, he believed himself luckier and smarter than anyone else. I believe that the concept of his omnipotence served him well during the mourning period as an important function of helping him through a most difficult time of life.

To Dr. Laufer's second point: "The identification with the victim"—"Michael's readiness to identify with people in authority not in a normal adolescent way in emulating them but in wanting to be protected by the authority." This and certain aspects of sexual behavior are interpreted as being signs of Michael's feminine identification. This is true in some aspects and understandably so. However, when the so-called protector-friend, for instance, turned out to be an unreliable person, Michael did not give up his plans of going to catering school. Had his passivity supervened he could have blamed his friend for being let down and given up his plans. This Michael did not do. Like a typical adolescent who wished to be independent, he left the analyst-parent out of his making decisions and unaided went on with constructive arrangements for a career.

It is in no way that I wish to minimize Michael's neurosis. I saw one way of pursuing the discussion would be to explore further Michael's pathology of which Dr. Laufer gave us such a full picture. However, while thinking on those lines, I was struck by the opposite: the many areas of strength and comparative mental health dormant in the patient that enabled him, with the help of analysis, to grow and develop. My contribution to this paper will focus on these aspects.

The question is: *How was it possible for this boy, who appeared to be a very disturbed young adolescent and whose life had been cruelly disrupted so many times, to emerge as a comparatively well functioning human being?* I believe that it is due to the great potential of Michael's capacity for adaptive functioning.

In following Michael's development, we see the mother's impact on Michael as being probably greater than we ordinarily assume it to be. Similarly, Michael's mother-transference onto the person of the analyst must have been of almost equal quality. When the death of his mother deprived Michael of the only close relationship he had had, we can understand and almost expect Dr. Laufer to develop also a parental concern for his young and bereft patient.

From this point of view there must have been an important interplay between the transference and countertransference that gave the analysis an added and valuable dimension. This mutual responsiveness between analyst and patient gives us a clue to Michael's early relationship to his mother which was decisive in the patient's ability to respond to analysis.

In many ways, Michael must have felt a very loved child. Like in the episode of the biblical Moses, a woman, in our case the strong and aggressive mother, hid Michael in a basket and smuggled him out from a country that did not hold much promise for his future. At the age of four and a half, when to have a father figure is crucial in the life of a child because of the Oedipal situation, Michael's mother happened to remarry. This gave Michael a chance to lessen the intensity of the relationship to his mother.

In her moves and deeds we recognize Michael's mother as a person of great zest for life whose wish for continuity made it possible for her to survive the most grueling conditions. It seems that her authority aroused Michael's envy and hostility making him afraid of retaliation for his aggressive and ambivalent feelings towards her. It is to the credit of the mother that in spite of the difficulties she must have encountered with her son, her concern and insistence that Michael undergo treatment became a reality. For it was due to Michael's analysis that the patient was able to integrate the healthy parts of his mental functioning. From a negative point of view one could look at the mother's influence on Michael in terms of her grief and depression. But this assumption omits the influence of her drive and determination which are outstanding features of courage. It is this quality in her that supplied Michael with the ego strength and the ego ideal of a continuous thrust towards life and achievement. That we have learned about the background of Michael's father, it is not surprising for the mother to have wished to see in her son the fulfillment of his father's and her own ambitions.

Michael, it seems, felt most of the time that he could not live up to the aspirations his mother had for him. But it was also a sign of the hopes his mother expressed for his future and her caring for him.

Michael's mother was unusual from a very specific point of view and that is her positive and almost objective attitude towards having her child analyzed. *In my own experience it is uncommon for parents who are survivors to encourage or to pressure their children to undergo analysis.* Parent survivors might consciously think that they want help for their children but often withdraw them when they show signs of improvement. Unlike these parents, Michael's mother was able to encourage him to establish a relationship outside of herself and the family in order that he be helped. Most of the parent survivors appear to be bound by an unconscious symbiotic-like relationship to a particular child or children and cannot allow them to enter into the close relationship with a therapist. In that way they defend themselves against the intrusion into a part of their own feared and dark past.

A word about Dr. Laufer's two other points: One, about Michael's aggression and two, the possible threat of suicide. Point one: The mother's inhibiting influence on Michael's expression of aggression: For instance, in urging him particularly after the move to England to be a nice and polite boy. Was a nice and polite male the mother's ideal that might have been a representation of her dead husband that she projected onto England? The question is whether we can attribute Michael's shyness and unaggressiveness entirely to the mother's influence or could it not have been that her demands in this area met in Michael fertile ground for his acceptance of her pronounced ideals. The important fact in this connection is that though the mother expressed her preference for the inhibition of aggressive behavior, she herself tackled life in a practical, constructive and assertive, aggressive way. The example of her deeds, not just her words, must have helped Michael later to take his life into his own hands and carve out a future for himself. In this he did not ask for the analyst's immediate help. Though Michael's attitude appeared to be a negative transference to Dr. Laufer, in reality it was a healthy move towards object removal—so decisive in the development of an adolescent. Michael's choice of a career contained determinants that might have been called neurotic; however, under the circumstances they proved to be an excellent adaptation to his background. In his work he got himself an attainable and practical goal and tried to perfect himself to a high degree.

To point two: The patient's possible suicide. This, of course, presents a problem with which the therapist of the adolescent is often faced, in particular when dealing with a very depressed patient. As I followed the material of Michael's analysis, I hesitated to share the analyst's concern. Though in the last resort only the analyst can judge such a dangerous situation. Michael's saying, "You don't have to do anything you don't want to do," is not necessarily to be taken as a suicidal threat only, but amongst other meanings it can also be seen as a frequent adolescent expression of a new found sense of power and discovery of one's separateness and individuality. In Michael it was no doubt also associated to his conflict about masturbation and death. In general, I would not consider the threat of suicide as specific for Michael's pathology. It seems that Michael did not attempt suicide.

To conclude, we would have to know and review many more analyses of children of survivors before arriving at an evaluation of the kind of harm they have suffered. We understand that there must have been damage done to them, but we have to keep on searching and decide each patient individually, particularly as to his ego and adaptive functioning.

Discussion from the Floor

Dr. Albert Solnit (U. S. A.) felt that the paper had raised an extraordinary number of questions. He thought that Dr. Laufer had not suggested that Michael's treatment had really been completed and it certainly seemed likely that the patient might seek further analysis later on. The present analysis had been massively influenced by his mother's death, and a good deal of the treatment material had to be directly related to this event. One question that is relevant to the whole theory of object loss arises: Do we see delayed reactions at a point when new demands are made on the individual who has expressed loss? In Michael's case, the whole situation may well be reactivated later in Michael's life when he tries to enter into and sustain close relationships. Another question that comes up is the role of fantasy in the formation of identifications. In orphaned children, one may often see a subtle or, at times, not so subtle discouragement of this by those looking after them. The children may ask or feel—who am I like? what is making me what I am?—and be left mystified. In this case, the mother's permission for Michael to have a fantasy about his real father seems to have helped him very much. These features among many others provided some reason why there were so many different kinds of children of survivors. A third question had to do with the quality of instinctual development and whether the passivity as described in the clinical material was indeed central, but this might require Michael to elucidate completely. Dr. Laufer had been careful not to give the impression that Michael's analysis had terminated, and it was clear that the boy needed more help.

Dr. Fischer (Canada) wondered how much of the story of Michael having been carried across the border was perpetuated by the mother fostering the idea that the son had nearly caused the mother's death. He felt that Michael had successfully prevented the analysis from giving him anything. What we are able to see is Michael's great struggle with orality and of making it impossible for the analyst to symbolically feed him. He speculated as to what might have happened if Dr. Laufer had actually fed Michael food. Michael's catering could be regarded as an attempt on the boy's part to say that nobody could really give him anything. The catering was not an expression of his ego strength but an expression of his wish to give himself something rather than to give to others. Dr. Fischer was not impressed by the success of the analysis.

Dr. Stahl (U. S. A.) spoke briefly about the question whether Michael thought that his father died an unnatural death because he wanted to die. Could Michael not think that if his father had wanted to live very badly he would have survived?

Mrs. Bielitzki (Poland) adhered herself to the question of what kind of father Michael would become. She spoke of her experience with fatherless fathers and with the children of fatherless fathers during the recent exodus of Polish Jews. These Jewish survivors and their children did not identify with being Jewish but felt a loyalty to Communist Poland. This circumstance made the problem of formation of an identity, continued from an unknown past, an especially difficult one. She emphasized strength of the denial observed in the people. Some of these people had felt that they did not have the right or the opportunity to feel grief. It was as if they felt that they had to smile, however great their grief was. Later in their lives, there was extreme denial by these people of their geneological background, of their Jewish background, and of their identifications. This denial was the most characteristic part of the families of survivors with whom she had contact. She met many more aggressive than shy, withdrawn children, and they seemed unable to understand how people could die without fighting. Many of them had no past, and it appeared crucial for them to try to have a future of some kind. Some of the boys had difficulty in assuming the male role.

In his reply, Dr. Laufer said that although he agreed with Dr. Williams' comment that Michael had got a great deal from his mother, he did not agree with her explanation about the use which Michael had made of the infantile omnipotence. Dr. Laufer felt that Michael was still a very vulnerable person and that the reasons for the underlying depression were not yet clear. Although there were signs of strength, he still considered him to be somebody who would eventually need further help and whose pathology might easily emerge in some future situations of stress. The possibility of suicide was related to Michael's feeling that he had lost the person who created the link between himself and his real father and also that his mother's death was for him a kind of confirmation that his body was no good. Dr. Laufer did not feel ready to think of Michael as somebody who was functioning comparatively well but more as somebody who seemed to be getting on. He agreed with Dr. Solnit that Michael would very likely need further help as an adult and that his present behavior should not be viewed as a sign of good functioning. He felt that Dr. Fischer may also have assumed that Michael's treatment was complete—instead it would be correct to say that it had seemed appropriate for Michael's present life to allow him to leave treatment. The question of actually feeding his patient did not seem to belong to the treatment situation. He felt that Michael did not need a "corrective experience" at this point in his life but more appropriately insight into the nature of his disturbance.

Children of Survivors*

L. Rosenberger, M.D.

The author's experience in the Child Guidance Clinic at Shalvata, Tel-Aviv, coupled with the analyses of two adolescent children of survivors, has strengthened her conviction that children of survivors show no distinctive psychopathology and that any differences there are can be attributed to the particular handling by the parents as a reflection of their own personalities.

Two types of survivor-parents can be postulated:

1. Those who disregard the children's emotional needs and are obsessed instead with the need to provide food and goods in order to prevent hunger and material deprivation such as they had experienced in Europe. This type of parent does not respond well to counseling.
2. Those who identify almost totally with the growing child, reliving their childhood through him or believing in identification with their own deceased parents. They lack emotional maturity and use their children for the fulfillment of their own narcissistic needs.

The Case of A.

A., now nineteen and a half, had been in analysis for two and a

*Summarized by J. S. Kestenberg, M. D.

half years because of problems in school and depression. His father had lived in a ghetto with his parents and younger siblings. He and his younger brothers would steal food for the family. When he was nine, he* and his father were deported to Auschwitz where his father was put to death. Only he and his mother survived; he in Auschwitz, she in the ghetto. After liberation he emigrated to Israel and became a leading member of a kibbutz. He ingratiated himself with adults and shared with the children. His preoccupation with food had been replaced by a thirst for knowledge and a rigid code of morality. He proved a good husband and father but retained the quality of an adolescent.

When A. was nine years old (the age at which his father had to leave his brothers), the family left their first kibbutz because his father was offended at the kibbutz's committee's refusal to support his aged mother. A. missed his peer group and began to associate with street gangs and to skip school. At 13 he left the family and joined the high school of still another kibbutz of which he has remained a member. In his late teens he asked to be referred to a psychologist because of depression. This had begun with an obsessive need to succeed in work over and above what was required from his group. In the kibbutzim, work is highly valued and the esteem of the group depends on good performance. A. began to skip school to work in order to do more than the required work-norm. (In this conflict, it is worth recalling that his father's survival depended on his energy to work. Weak or sick people were sent to the gas chamber.) He became attached to a young girl who had been in treatment for some years. When a new teacher encouraged independence, A. stopped studying and became depressed again. He slept during work hours, withdrew from social activities, and began to "borrow" cars driving without a license. (His father had stolen in order to survive.) He felt all alone, not understood by his parents and wanted to die. [The father had been left alone after many of his family had died and had been attached to a young girl (A.'s mother).] Analysis brought him, step by step, insight and understanding of the turmoil within himself and gradual improvement in the repressed aggressivity. The most important turning point came when he understood that his morality (his superego) was not yet internalized but still represented by his father.

The strong relationship with his father was pre-oedipal in nature.

*That is A's father (Note of the Editor).

He spent his leisure hours with him and away from his mother. His father played with him very permissively but never allowed any transgressions with other people, especially women. In analysis, A. thought at first that he hardly knew his mother until he was 14 years old. Later, he recaptured memories of crying when she left him at bedtime.

After working through his inverted oedipal attachment to his father, he was able to establish a healthier post-oedipal identification in its place. Many modifications in the analytic approach had to be used as the patient progressed from pre-oedipal to oedipal developments because of his inability to function within a purely analytic parent. Only after he listened to and assimilated his father's concentration camp experiences (that he was compulsively repeating in his current behavior) did it become possible for him to report dreams and associate freely.

The crucial question is: What will the father's reaction be to the narcissistic deprivation that would follow the son's liberation from his dependency on his father and his turning to the mother at the end of the analysis? Even at this juncture, although he expresses satisfaction with some changes, he is full of criticism.

The Impact of the Nazi Concentration Camps on the Children of Survivors

Erna Furman (U.S.A.)

Introduction

The phenomenon of the Nazi concentration camps deserves serious study from many points of view. In my professional field I have been able to view it from one aspect only, namely, that of the individual's psychological experience. It is this aspect, above all, which is most highly invested emotionally by everyone and therefore easily distorted. It is also the aspect which least lends itself to generalizations. *Each individual came to camp with a different personality and at a different point in his development, each underwent different specific experiences in camp, and each has lived under different circumstances since then. The more anyone has worked with people exposed to a camp experience, the more he is aware of these enormous individual differences and the resulting difficulty in making meaningful comparisons. Perhaps the only shared factors are those of having experienced a stressful interference of more or less traumatic proportions and the task of coming to terms with having survived it.* All individuals have to grapple with these factors throughout their continuing lives. For each, his manner of integrating them is in turn affected by all that he faces in his on-going life, good and bad alike. This painful, endless process of gradual integration is again a most highly individual one and affects differently the many aspects of personality functioning. Even for the individual, it varies from time to time so that no person can be characterized as using a set form of mechanisms. The specific, direct effects on the child of his parents' camp experiences are therefore not only difficult to isolate but may become meaningless unless seen in the context of the parents' and child's individual personalities and their interactions.

I hope that this brief report will illustrate the above points and help focus on the need for understanding the great complexity of interacting factors in individual cases.

The material comes from the intensive analysis of a child, Danny, who was born in the United States several years after the end of the war, whose parents had both undergone concentration camp experiences. The direct analytic work with the child also included weekly interviews with his mother throughout the course of the treatment. For the purpose of the presentation I am singling out one personality aspect, namely that of mothering and its effect on the child.[1]

The Case of Danny

Danny was brought for help by his parents at the age of three and a half. He was an atypical child, grossly lacking in basic ego-masteries such as independent eating, not to mention such functions as speech, self-differentiation, and reality-testing. He was constantly in dread of being overwhelmed from within and without, a fear which he tried to ward off by manipulating and controlling people and material objects. This mechanism frequently failed exposing him to severe anxiety tantrums. His mother, passive and apathetic with outsiders, maintained an intense primitive relationship with him characterized by tyrannical and violent mutual control in some areas and in others by treating him as a part of herself. She dared not as much as look out the window lest Danny scream for her to look at him only, but *she* would decide when he needed to urinate, would hold his penis, and pour warm water on it to produce the flow of urine. Danny's father, most of the time absorbed in studies

[1] Dr. Kestenberg points out that Israeli psychoanalysts have emphasized the crucial importance of parental handling in the children of survivors.

and work, expected the boy to behave like a much older child. When Danny could not follow the father's rigid and meticulous instructions for operating the electric train set, the father demanded, "Go and read something."

Danny was accepted into the Hanna Perkins Nursery School and I saw the mother weekly for a few months preparatory to individual daily treatment for Danny which was to go on for five years and which, in turn, was followed by intensive after-care till Danny's nineteenth year.

Mrs. Z., an only child, grew up in Eastern Europe where her parents were comfortably off and esteemed members of an isolated close-knit orthodox Jewish community. Her intellectual father traditionally shunned manual work. His not even tying his own shoes was quite acceptable. Similarly, her mother's obsessional housewife neurosis was quite well absorbed into the rituals of kosher housekeeping. Her nagging sadomasochistic relationship with Mrs. Z. was viewed as one of the trials of child-rearing and diluted by the customary participatory care of members of the wider family. Nazi domination broke up this way of life when Mrs. Z. was in her late teens. For a time many managed to hide out. During this period circumstances forced Mrs. Z. to betray her uncle and aunt in an attempt to save her parents but, soon after, Mrs. Z. and her parents were also caught and followed their relatives to a concentration camp. Whereas they miraculously survived the next three years, the rest of the family was killed.

Immediately after the war the family tried unsuccessfully to settle in a bigger modern town. Much to her parents' dismay, Mrs. Z. fell in love with Mr. Z., an atheist. He had grown up in the same country but in an assimilated atmosphere. His mother died when he was about 12. Unable to tolerate his father's flagrant promiscuity and his new stepmother, he had wandered off on his own, supporting himself for a few years till he was sent to a concentration camp. To console Mrs. Z.'s parents, Mr. Z. promised to adhere henceforth to orthodox rituals, a promise he kept without a shred of religious belief but well in keeping with his obsessional character. The young couple married and shortly emigrated to the United States, in large part to escape their early emotional ties and the associated memories of the camp experiences.

In the United States their big hopes were dashed. Mr. Z. had wanted to undo the past losses by becoming a learned professional but had to settle for a "lesser" specialty. This severe narcissistic blow intensified his rigid defenses. Later he displaced his disappointment and self-criticism onto his son whom he expected to be perfect and whose immaturity and later limitations he could never accept. Mrs. Z.'s adolescent rebellious dream centered on having a baby and being a better mother than her own mother had been. Her underlying dependency broke through in her fury and panic when she had to leave a sheltered job because of her pregnancy. The next blow came when, unexpectedly, she gave birth to twins of whom only Danny survived after many anxious weeks of hospitalization. As the father defensively withdrew into himself and his work, she spent some lonely, desperate months of trying to mother her child "opposite from my mother." When Danny was a little over a year old, they visited her parents who had recently come to live in another part of this country. Not only could the grandparents' personalities not adapt to the changed environment but, in an attempt to atone for their survival and current comfortable circumstances, they had become religious fanatics, their lives distorted by obsessional pseudoreligious rituals. They also blamed Mrs. Z. for betraying her uncle and aunt and warned her to increase her atonement rituals. In her guilt and dependency, she handed Danny's care over to her mother, a disastrous experience of drastic change for him. Within a short time, however, Mrs. Z. rebelled again and left them. On her own once more, she determined to educate Danny as, what she considered, as American boy. He alone was spoken to in English and an open-door bathroom and bedroom policy was instituted. At the same time, however, when the Sabbath came, Danny was expected to sit in the synagogue watching the men pray, and at home he was not allowed to play or to do anything, not even to open doors. This regime was periodically interrupted by the grandparents' visits, at which time they ruled the house and Danny. Although their mechanisms varied greatly, parents and grandparents alike shared a feeling that their earlier life and camp experiences set them apart so that they did not associate socially with "outsiders," particularly non-Jews.

Mrs. Z.'s knowledge that I could speak her language, both literally and figuratively, helped more than anything else in slowly developing a working relationship with her. While our interviews were geared to helping her educate Danny and understand some of his difficulties, Mrs. Z. used me increasingly as an alternate model for integrating past and present and, in the process, for initiating a maternal development based on realistic concepts. She gradually detached herself from her mother and, albeit with much support, was later able to overcome her depressive reaction when her mother died. With her second child she proved herself a competent, realistic mother and supported with pleasure the girl's good progressive development. She could somewhat widen her social circle, reduce her religious rituals, and sustain neutral interests which in turn enabled her to provide a more appropriate home environment. With Danny, her handling improved beyond expectation, but she remained extremely dependent on me as the slightest setback revived her pathological guilt and involvement.

Danny himself improved considerably and achieved a degree of ego-mastery which, for several years, enabled him to function in many areas of the wider community with phase-adequate though precarious personality development. As he became capable of absorbing knowledge, he was given age-adequate information on the parents' camp experiences. In most instances during his prepuberty years, this centered around explaining phenomena he had observed and found confusing, e. g., the number branded on his mother's arm, her panic at police dogs, her reaction to certain topics. In that period of his development, such information reassured him more than upset him as it strengthened his reality-testing. During his early adolescence he became deeply interested in the events of World War II but for different reasons. The Nazi atrocities, his family's Jewishness, and their camp experiences were drawn into his fantasy life as he struggled with pregenital and homosexual impulses as well as with attempting to develop an independent identity.

Danny's mother might have fared much better as a mother had she been able to continue her life in the circumscribed community she grew up in. Instead, in her late adolescence, she had to suffer the traumata of her camp experience and later the stress of a sickly newborn and the pathological interference of her own deteriorated mother. Her ability to utilize the therapist's help and to mother effectively a second child showed that she had many latent strengths at her disposal. Danny's early years, however, coincided with his mother's greatest period of stress and he was destined to remain her "weak point." She handled her conscious memories and knowledge of her war experiences appropriately with her child. She did not burden him with accounts of past events yet answered realistically his questions to the extent of his ability to comprehend. This was brought out during the years of treatment when she required relatively little help, in this regard, from the therapist and when the analytic material of the child showed but little use of these events in his fantasies. The follow-up contact suggested that, as far as the boy was concerned, the parents' actual experiences played an important part in his adolescent emotional life although his mother's attitude did not appear to have changed in this area.

I have commented on a few highlights only to stress the need to study individual cases intensively, avoiding tempting generalizations, in order to understand the impact of the Nazi concentration camps on the children of survivors.

Children of Concentration Camp Survivors

Dov R. Aleksandrowicz, M.D. (U.S.A.)

The Problem

The purpose of this study was to observe possible effects of the Nazi persecution on the children of the survivors of ghettos and concentration camps. The question we posed was: "Do the psychic scars carried by people who survived such an ordeal affect the mental health of their children? If so, do those children show typical or specific symptoms that can be related to the traumas inflicted on their parents?"

Our study was *not* concerned with grossly disturbed parents. Many of the concentration camp survivors are very ill, chronically depressed, irritable, sometimes even regressed to dementia-like states. It is only to be expected that the children of such parents be emotionally disturbed, and thus we have deliberately excluded them from our study. Our purpose was to study survivors who were, at least outwardly, "well adjusted." We were looking for more subtle changes in personality which may not prevent them from functioning in the society and yet impair their ability as parents.

It became apparent at an early stage of the study that a statistical analysis of the impact of concentration camp traumatization was both impractical and unreliable. There were too many individual variables, some of them not susceptible to measurement. Some

385

of the parents survived the war under the protection of their own parents, others were separated at an early age or relatively late. Some were protected by benevolent Poles, others were on their own. There is no way to describe experience in quantitative terms, for example, how can one measure the amount of guilt felt when one sees one's mother being dragged to the death chamber? The most traumatic memories of the concentration camp victims vary as much as the ingenuity of their torturers would allow. Also, there was no way to compare quantitatively the amount of pathogenic influence exerted by each parent. In some cases it was clearly a matter of a neurotic interaction within the marriage. In some cases, however, one parent seemed obviously more pathogenic while the other exerted a moderating influence. The "survivor" parent was not always the more disturbed one. In one case, at least, the survivor parent (a mother) was relatively stable while the father, who came to Israel in 1933, was an ambulatory schizophrenic grossly disturbed in his relationship to his children.

Having given up any attempt at statistical analysis, I have to satisfy myself with purely impressionistic conclusions well knowing that they can serve only as preliminary hypotheses.

A. CASE MATERIAL

Children who met the following criteria were selected from all the cases referred to our clinic:

1. One parent, at least, a survivor of Nazi persecution and born in Poland. (For the sake of comparison we included a group in which the parents born in Poland and surviving the war in the USSR);

2. The survivor-parent not a psychiatric patient and not grossly disturbed;

3. The child not retarded.

The sample was limited to Polish-born survivors in order to make the group fairly homogeneous in social and ethnic background. Most of them belong to lower middle class or to a skilled working class. In addition they had all been under Nazi occupation for about the same length of time which was not the case, for example, in regard to the Hungarian Jews.

Parents who lived during the war in the USSR were included for comparison. They belonged to the same social background and had been exposed to considerable stress during the war: separation from families, hunger, and imprisonment. At the same time, the people under Russian occupation were spared the extreme sufferings imposed by the Germans, e. g., deliberate humiliation to the point of loss of any self-image, perpetual danger of death if discovered while hiding or if "guilty" of an imaginary offense, or being subjected to arbitrary and sadistic tortures.

The investigation included one or more interviews with the child, one or more interviews with each of the parents and/or both parents together, and psychological tests of the child. The sample includes 34 families which fall into the following groups:

a. Both parents survivors of Nazi persecution: ten families.
b. One parent survivor of persecution, the other parent in Israel during the war or born after 1945: ten families.
c. One parent survivor of Nazi persecution, the other surviving war in USSR: five families.
d. Both parents surviving was in USSR: nine families.

B. CLINICAL OBSERVATIONS AND DISCUSSION

The children in groups a, b, and c did not appear diagnostically different from other patients of similar background. There was a relatively high number of cases with phobias, with neurotic (or reactive) behavior disorders, or with a combination of both syndromes (21 patients out of 25 as compared with two among the nine families in group-d families). Parental attitudes in these cases were a combination of pampering with inconsistent discipline because of unresolved guilt and/or overcompensated aggression. In some cases there were also excessive expectations, a wish for the child to compensate the parent for his or her lost opportunities. Such attitudes are common among parents of neurotic children and by no means specific to our group. At the same time it was often apparent in the individual case that the parent's neurotic attitude was caused—or at least greatly magnified—by his or her vicissitudes during the war. As an example we may present a seven-year-old boy with separation anxiety, mild behavior disorder and transitory enuresis which appeared during the "Six Days War." His mother had lost her only brother during World War II, a partisan who shot himself rather than surrender to the police. She had some objective reasons to blame herself for the brother's suicide in addition to experiencing guilt associated with her intense envy of her brother. This conflict was never resolved and she transferred much of it onto her only son. She was unable to curb the child's aggression and could not conceal from him her own anxiety over any subject associated with death.

There was one case of psychosis among our patients, one borderline psychotic (and one in the comparison group), one with minimal brain damage (and four such cases in the comparison group). Although the diagnostic categories did not differ much from those of other children with a similar social background, yet there seemed to emerge some constellations rather typical of families of concentration camp survivors.

1. The Family with "Parental Disequilibrium" In an apparently high number of cases (eight out of 25 families), we have seen that the survivor parent was a strong, capable, usually intelligent, and often ambitious person who had married someone below his level: either intellectually or socially disadvantaged, or weak and ineffectual. As a result, parental authority was not inconsistent but out of balance with one parent respected and admired and the other one rejected and despised.[1]

The family of H. may serve as an example of such disequilibrium. Their younger boy, Eyal, was referred because of encopresis and enuresis. He is a mildly obese boy of seven, passive and fearful, with few friends. Mr. H., the father of Eyal, was an only child who had been brought into the ghetto at the age of eight. His parents were soon taken to death camps and he was left with a grandmother who was half-paralyzed and unable to leave her room. By sheer courage and initiative, he was able to stay alive and to provide food for himself and for the grandmother. He later joined an uncle and they were among a small group of families left behind to clean the ghetto after its "liquidation." The boy managed to smuggle his wheel-chair-bound grandmother out of her home and took care of her until she died shortly after the liberation. He came to this country and married a woman of Iranian descent. Her parents are illiterate and she herself is a dull, ignorant woman who reacts to her feelings of frustration by hysterical outbursts and helpless rage thus giving additional support to the husband's contention that she cannot be

---

[1] In four families, the disequilibrium was very pronounced, in four only moderately so. Among the nine families surviving in Russia, there was only one such case.

trusted with responsibilities and that her opinions as to the children's
education carry no weight.

Mr. H. takes good care of his sons and is proud of his paternal
role. He quoted a teacher saying: "I know immediately when you
are called up for reserve duty: your children's homework shows it
right away." Although cooperative in the evaluation, Mr. H. could
not disguise his resentment about my discussing with the boy the
subject of Nazi persecutions without getting "clearance" from him,
a sensitive matter for Mr. H. He interpreted my questioning of the
child as a threat to his absolute control of the family and also as a
threat to his version of the holocaust. He is justly proud of what he
did in the ghetto but is not, as a rule, inclined to talk about the past.
Nevertheless, he becomes excited when people point out the helplessness and the passivity of the Jewish victims of the Nazis. He
points out examples of heroism and argues, with a great deal of justification, that nobody can judge another person's behavior under
such extreme conditions. He also told me how hurt he was when one
of his children, who idolizes him, asked him why he allowed his
parents to be killed without doing anything to protect them.

The family structure in this case reflects Mr. H.'s need to dominate
and to control which seems to be related to his denial of passivity.
We may speculate whether early childhood experiences had anything
to do with it—quite possibly they did. Yet we have indications that
the extreme and humiliating passivity to which he was subjected in
the ghetto and his inability to save the parents (for which he substitutes his saving the grandmother) have a great deal to do with his
present behavior. The whole family is grossly out of balance along
the activity-passivity scale. Both boys are, in fact, passively attached
to their father and lack a clear-cut masculine identification.

We may suspect that in many cases such an energetic and resourceful personality was, in itself, a decisive factor in survival—as a matter
of fact, in some cases that was clearly so (although in a few of these
"out-of-balance" families the survival of the dominant parent was a
matter of chance, for example, being left in the care of benevolent
Poles). Yet Mr. H.'s problem is not his resourceful personality but his
fear of passivity which, in his case, is related to the narcissistic in-
juries inflicted on him and to guilt over the death of his parents.

2. The "Affective Deficiency" Syndrome and Hyper-repression
Many authors have described the feelings of void and the affective
flatness of numerous concentration camp survivors [1, 2]. This
symptom has been ascribed to massive repression of the traumatic
memories [2].

Mrs. C. is one such survivor. At the age of 15, she was placed in
a ghetto and until the age of 17½ she was in Auschwitz. She lost
her entire family. After having immigrated to Israel, she found work
as a telephone operator. She never complained of any psychiatric
symptoms but led a restricted, lonely life. At the age of 34, she
married Mr. C., a widower one year her senior. She took good care
of his only son (then two years old) and later also of her two boys.
Yet both her children have emotional problems. The older one,
aged five and a half, is a bed-wetter, an aggressive, hyperactive, and
frightened youngster. He describes his future in these terms: "I will
go to the high school, then I will be a soldier, then a father, and then
I will die. Why? Because, when one finishes everything, one dies."
The child's mother is totally unable to comprehend and to face his
terrors.

Mrs. C. used to have anxiety dreams but in the last years she dreams
mainly of her lost family. She cannot discuss her memories with anybody, not her husband nor the people from her town whom she
meets during commemorative services. She cannot tolerate anything
reminding her of the Nazi atrocities or of violence in general, e. g.,
she shut off the radio during the Eichmann trial. She could not tell
the children about her past; she can only discuss the children's problems in terms of physical symptoms. This woman seems to have become so sensitized to psychic pain that she can cope only by avoidance and withdrawal. Having learned to rely on hyper-repression
she cannot accept the children's need to develop their own repres-
sions gradually. Her children feel neglected and emotionally starved
but unable to verbalize their anger and their fears because the expression of such emotions is actively discouraged by their mother.
At the same time she fails to control the acting out of aggression.
Instead, she withdraws from the angry child.

3. Other Parental Attitudes Rakoff [3] and Trossman [4] have
described other problems in children of camp survivors, namely,
overprotection by the parents, excessive parental expectations, and

a peculiar type of cultural conflict: The parents want the child to merge with the culture they live in, to be a bridge between them and the Gentiles, and yet they want the child "to remember," to be a continuation of themselves and their lost families.

These constellations did not seem typical of our concentration camp survivors as compared with other families. Overprotection and overcompensation as defense against aggressive feelings toward the child are common among Jewish parents, perhaps because the Jewish culture places great demands on the parents and overt rejection of the child is strongly condemned. Excessive parental expectations are common too, and they are also common among people who immigrate into a new country and find themselves diminished in their social status.

The conflict between the demand that the child should fit into the Gentile culture and yet be a continuation of the parents' tragic lives [3] is certainly specific to the camp survivors and yet we have not encountered it at all in our sample. The explanation is simple: Rakoff's survivors were lonely aliens in a largely indifferent world; ours could easily acculturate themselves in a Jewish state and indeed most of them did. Moreover, there was less need for the parents to ask from the child to be a sort of living memorial to their tragic fate and their lost families. This function has been taken over and institutionalized by the State itself.

C. CONCLUSIONS

The emotional scars left by concentration camp experience may result in emotional problems in children of the survivors but they appear as only one factor in a complex of pathogenic influences. The premorbid personality of the survivor, his relationship to his own parents, the personality of the spouse, and the surrounding social structure—all these play an important role.

As a group, children of camp survivors do not appear to be different from other children of comparable socioeconomic background referred to our clinic. It is possible that emotional problems are more frequent among these children, but we have no data on that. We do find, however, that in many cases the problems of the child relate to the emotional scars seen in the survivor-parent.

It is difficult to speak about specific patterns of illness or specific family constellations, though some patterns may be relatively more frequent than others. Our survivor-parents are a selected group. Because the children referred to us were between five and 16 years old, the parents themselves were relatively young and most of them were in camps as children or adolescents. Thus, very few of them had lost a spouse or child and for many of them the trauma was related to early separation from parents. Because of their relatively young age they tended to identify more with their new country and their self-image was not primarily that of a concentration camp victim. They were less fixated in the traumatic past. On the other hand, because of the early separation from their parents they may have more of a tendency to suffer from emotional impoverishment and may find it more difficult to identify themselves with the parental role.

Many questions remain open. Further studies, comparing different groups of parents, like the ones in Ghetto Fighters' Kibbutz [5], may help to elucidate the complex relationship between disaster, recovery, and the shaping of a new generation.

Bibliography

1. Bychowski, C., Permanent Character Changes as an Aftereffect of Persecution, in *Massive Psychic Trauma*, Krystal, H., Ed., International U. P., New York, 1968.
2. Niederland, W. G., Clinical observations on the "survivor syndrome," *Int. J. Psychoanalysis*, 49 (1968), 313–315.
3. (a) Rakoff, V., Long-term effects of the concentration camp experience, *Viewpoint*, (1966), 17–21. (b) Rakoff, V., Sigal, J. J., and Epstein, N. B., Children and families of concentration camp survivors, *Canada's Mental Health*, XIV (1966), 24–26.
4. Trossman, B., Adolescent children of concentration camp survivors, *Canad. Psychiat. Assoc. J.*, 13 (1968), 121–123.
5. Klein, M., Survivor Families in Kibbutzim, VII Congress of the Intern. Assoc. for Child Psychiatry, August, 1970, Jerusalem.

Children of the Holocaust: Mourning and Bereavement[1]

Hilel Klein, M.D. (Israel)

Introduction

This paper presents an analysis of the adaptation processes of a group of holocaust survivors and their families. Emphasis is on the issues of death, mourning, and grief in the continuity of life experiences with special attention on the transmission from one generation to another of coping mechanisms and attitudes toward loss. How do the children of holocaust survivors relate to their parents' lengthy oppression, close contact with total destruction, and overwhelming actual losses? What kind of family emerges when an individual who has survived Nazi persecution lives in a framework different from his original milieu?

Method

Psychosocial studies of 25 survivor families on the kibbutz were

[1] I would like to thank Shulamith Reinharz, sociologist, for her valuable help in discussing the material and editing the manuscript. My thanks are extended to Tamar Shushan, psychologist, who interviewed the children and administered the tests.

undertaken between 1967 and 1969. Three survivors received psychoanalytically-oriented psychotherapy. Each family was interviewed as a whole in two sessions of two hours each. Three interviews were conducted with each survivor parent during the course of one month; these were augmented by information obtained from questionnaires which were distributed to each survivor relating to his feelings about his own childhood and his relation to his present family. First-born children were interviewed by a psychologist who administered projective and intelligence tests (Rorschach and TAT, Wechsler Intelligence Scale for Children).

The Survivors

No evidence of manifest individual or family psychopathology was discovered in the early childhood experiences of these holocaust survivors. The fact that they reached the period of the holocaust in their adolescence after having experienced the previous developmental phase in a warm, supportive family atmosphere is perhaps one of the determinants of survival in this group.

With the destruction of their families, communities, and their entire familiar world, the survivors lost their self-image and basic feeling of security as well as their sense of continuity with previous experiences. Their response to persecution consisted of several phases: attempts at mastering adversity, cohesive pairing behavior, and finally, passive compliance to the aggressor. At this time, individual and collective ritualized mourning and bereavement were not experienced and grief was not worked through.

Following their liberation, the survivors gave expression to their previously suppressed aggression in fantasies of revenge, complete compensation, and the resurrection of their families. Their need to deny the liquidation of their families led to searching activities characteristic of mourners; they not only tried to trace missing family members in a realistic way but scanned crowds in unfamiliar environments to discover a face of the past. This "urge to search for and to recover the lost figures" [2] stems from a rebirth fantasy connected with regression to magical thinking—scanning the environment for signs of the departed despite certain knowledge of their death. Conscious expression of grief, however, was delayed until after the initial phase of readaptation to Israel (three to five

years). The fantasies of the restoration of murdered families, which
had sustained many survivors during the persecution, were only
gradually abandoned as the evidence of their death became indis-
putable.

With physical recuperation, gradual satisfaction of their powerful
oral needs in the new surroundings, and the growth of a community
with common interests, the survivors began to reestablish libidinal
ties in intense friendships and marriages. These relationships were
motivated by the attempt to escape feelings of loss and grief and to
restore the lost family. The attempts to establish love relationships
frequently resulted in post-marital crises characterized by depression
and guilt feelings. In some cases this crisis served as the catharsis
for grief connected with the holocaust which had not been expressed
previously. The crisis period was an important transition which
served as a "trial period" for the spouses to attempt to relate to each
other without fearful clinging or projection of their lost love objects.

The theme of personal, family and community rebirth is central
to the survivors' lives in Israel and coincides with the theme of reestablishment of the Jewish homeland. The implicit belief that even
after the overwhelming suffering they had undergone it was possible
to begin again was manifested in an openness to acculturation in
their new environment. The rebirth motif also provided the survivors
with a rationale for their escape from extinction as well as a positive
self-image as pioneers and builders of a new society.

Although their everyday activities do not characterize the individuals in this study as a unique group which has survived annihilation, their extraordinary experiences remain with them as traumatic
memories. A residue of chronic apprehensiveness is expressed in
dreams whose themes are "running away from the Nazis" indicating
fears of the returning threat, extermination of the self and the
family. Despite the conscious effort of the survivors to rationalize
their anxiety, they displayed a very low tolerance for dealing with
painful memories during the interviews.

Illustrative Cases[2]

EVA

Eva is the sole survivor of her family. Her parents, Polish bourgeois religious Jews, were killed during the holocaust. During the interviews Eva at first spoke about herself very reluctantly but later expressed herself with a great deal of force and emotion.

In her childhood Eva felt very strong ties to her father, a member of the mystic Chassidic sect, but a very tolerant man. Her mother was strong and obstinate and more orthodox in her religious beliefs than the father. When, during the Nazi deportations, Eva saw her father try to run away and hide leaving the family behind, she was deeply shaken by his failure to live up to her expectations of a good and strong man. She interprets his fear of death as cowardice and is obsessed to this day with questions about her father's fearful attempt to save his own life rather than his family's. Eva's mother subsequently became a more positive figure for her daughter by going courageously to the Gestapo in an attempt to liberate her husband. Eva now identifies less with her father and more with her mother's suppression of emotions and general attitude toward life.

Eva suffered the persecution of the ghetto and concentration camp but finally succeeded in running away from a transport and lived as a Polish girl on Aryan papers. She attributes her survival to her intense hatred of her oppressors. After her liberation she became a communist in her native country. She incorporates this decision into her self-image as a "woman of initiative" and stresses that she was actively involved in communist activities at the age of 12. Her espousal of communism was based on the conviction that it would liberate mankind from slavery and antisemitism rather than a desire to rebel against her parents.

After liberation she married a non-Jewish member of the communist party and although the marriage was satisfying, it lasted only one-and-a-half years. At this time her work for the security police enabled her to express hatred and revenge directly. She began to feel, however, that she was betraying her parents and her Jewish

---

[2]These cases are also cited in Hilel Klein, Families of Concentration Camp Survivors in the Kibbutz: Psychosocial Studies, in *International Psychiatric Clinics,* H. Krystal (Ed.), International Universities Press, New York, in press.

identity. Finally, she decided she could not live as a non-Jew and had to take her place in the Jewish community. She moved to Israel and married a man 15 years her senior. Her second husband had avoided imprisonment in a concentration camp by escaping to Russia. Although he suffered greatly there, he managed to save his family and his identity. Eva saw in this man a father figure symbolizing security and a return to her Jewish identity.

Eva is fascinated by stories of the holocaust and befriends only fellow immigrants. She has strong guilt feelings about her attempts to deny her Jewishness. In the kibbutz she feels her values of social justice are realized. The kibbutz is for her a source of security that would be impossible to find elsewhere. She feels that the influence on her child of the other parental figures on the kibbutz makes her daughter stronger than her. Her fear that something will happen to her child is manifested in her frequent nighttime inspections of the childrens' sleeping house. During therapy, it was revealed that these fears were connected with memories of nightly deportations in the ghetto.

Eva acknowledged occasional negative feelings about the kibbutz but said that they were offset by its advantages: "Sometimes I feel a need to run away from the closeness of the kibbutz, but the community experience here is so strong it gives me strength. I couldn't live in any other surroundings."

Eva's desire to deny her Jewish identity was overdetermined by her unresolved adolescent oedipal conflicts derived from her disappointment in her father's failing to live up to her positive image of him as loving protector. Her expression of aggression and choice of a non-Jewish marriage partner symbolized among other things revenge against this negative representation of her father. Eva internalized her father's response in following the same pattern of running away and deserting the family. Her attempt to escape her Jewish identity was also motivated by the realistic fear that Jewishness meant annihilation. But after the war, when the source of danger was gone, she continued the pattern of "flight" which had originally saved her life.

Eva's intelligent and sensitive 14½-year-old daughter is involved emotionally and intellectually in the holocaust. She empathizes with her parents' losses and says she "can understand her mother's nervousness because she lost everyone in her family." She blames others (outsiders and persecutors) for her mother's depression and not her mother herself. She defends herself against ambivalent feelings towards her mother by rationalizing her mother's behavior in the light of her traumatic experiences. The mother's neurotic anxieties are tolerated by the daughter since she knows that they are grounded in real experience.

During the 1967 war, the daughter and her peers fantasized another holocaust "with Arabs coming to the kibbutz and destroying everything." In her frequent dreams about the war she imagined that she would not fight the Arabs: "I thought only that we would run away and hide." Early in the war, her teacher was killed. She described the morale as very low after his death; many children responded by writing poems. Not having ever seen her parents cry made her afraid to cry, but at the death of this teacher she was able to cry with the other children. According to Eva's daughter the older generation was unable to cry because "they had so many people to mourn." She stresses the importance of death and separation as difficult issues for her and belittles the value of heroism as compared with survival.

Eva's daughter feels that anger is dangerous and emphasizes that she and her friends in the kibbutz cannot be angry with each other. She is aware of differences between herself and some Argentine immigrant children who are able to express anger and indifference. Her defense mechanism of denying aggression toward her parents and her surroundings is conspicuous. She feels insecure in the adults' ability to defend her against external aggression and depends instead on her peer group for defense against anxieties and feelings of helplessness. Although she feels that the kibbutz adults cannot be relied on for protection, she sees in them certain strengths which her parents lack.

AVRAHAM

Avraham, born in 1930, is married and the father of two children, a boy age eight and a girl age five. His adolescent years between the ages of ten and fifteen were spent in a ghetto and concentration camp. Both his parents and a young sister were killed leaving him the sole survivor of his immediate family. His young daughter is named after the sister who died.

At the age of sixteen Avraham came to Israel where he contributed vitally to the establishment and development of his kibbutz by his leadership and specialization in agriculture. He is now considered one of the founding fathers of the kibbutz.

Avraham's wife did not undergo the holocaust persecution. Her extended family has taken in Avraham with love and care; he serves to replace a son they lost just as they provide him with a new family. Both Avraham and his wife's family recognize each other's need and acknowledge their roles as mutual substitutes. Avraham's wife's attitude to her husband is overprotective. She feels that he cannot fully reciprocate her love because his deepest feelings are tied to his lost family.

During therapy this well-adapted man revealed his recent pre-occupation with the traumatic events of his past. With tears in his eyes he told about repetitive thoughts and fantasies which occurred when he took his child in his lap—young children being hurled against the walls to their death by German soldiers. His immediate response to this fantasy was to shout to himself: "I shall not let them! I shall kill them!"

During therapy the suppressed experiences—scenes witnessed during the extermination action in the town—were uncovered with their emotional content, the shame, anger, and guilt Avraham felt for not having tried to stop the aggressors. The atrocities surpassed the limitations of sadistic, aggressive death wishes, and childish fantasies. The horrors of the holocaust were, in fact, more fantastic than fantasy. The above episode is an example of how suppressed past experiences recur as flashbacks which intrude on everyday life.

A recurring theme developed in which Avraham compared his experiences in the holocaust to Abraham's sacrifice of Isaac in the Bible. He felt that he had been betrayed by his parents who were helpless to protect him and that he, in turn, had betrayed his sister in his inability to save her.

The parable of "The Binding of Isaac" expresses the ambiguous and ambivalent feelings of the survivor toward his family. He is not sure whether he is Abraham, the sacrificer or Isaac, the sacrificed.

Avraham related a striking episode which typifies the conflicts rooted in the holocaust experience and his effort to reconcile them with his first encounter with a German since his liberation. Upon being unexpectedly confronted with the German kibbutz-volunteer in the fields, he reacted with bewilderment and rage and fantasized killing this "anonymous German." Instead he gained control of his rage and handled his feelings by giving the very grapes he had culti-vated to the young man. He accompanied the gift with the follow-ing words: "Your father gave my father Cyclon B. I am giving you the fruit of the land of Israel." They both cried and as a result they were able to relate to each other as individuals rather than as anon-ymous symbols.

The tears served as a mutual catharsis which allowed for the dis-solution of the fantasied aggressor-victim bond. In giving the gift of the grapes, the survivor was able to relinquish his overcompliance to the aggressor and deal with his own aggression within the definition of his new positive self-image. In this act he liberated himself from the negative identity the Germans had imposed on their victims.

The case of Avraham demonstrates the extent to which the kib-butz setting supported the adaptation and growth of the traumatized individual. The kibbutz provided the survivor with a system of values, an opportunity to develop tools to master his conflicts and a framework for experiencing feelings of self-sameness and physical continuity. In the kibbutz he was able to adopt the role of host, "man of the soil", and master in his own home and discontinue the role of displaced uprooted wanderer craving revenge. The kibbutz society functioned as a new extended family to take the place of the one he lost. Through his participation in the struggle for national independence, the struggle against the desert, and the struggle to build his own community, he regained a sense of wholeness and be-longing. The opportunity to exercise initiative and express aggres-sion through the leadership of his group helped him overcome feel-ings of guilt derived from passivity during the holocaust.

Avraham has written a great deal about the holocaust and has submitted articles to the periodical "Yalkut Moreshet" (Heritage) which is devoted to holocaust history. His family has learned much about the concentration camp and the ghetto, and on certain holi-days they relive his experiences in a kind of "mourning feast." The family integrates the memory fragments which he tells them into an image of Avraham as "hero in a fairy tale" who passes through danger, is hurt and wounded, and then comes to life again for the sake of the children.

The profusion of fantasy life, which serves as a coping mechanism for both generations, parent and children, frees ego restrictions and suppressed aggressive tendencies with the achievement of a remarkable degree of neutralization of aggressive energy. The displaced neutralized aggression may then be invested in positive goals, such as "pioneering" and working, or expressing intellectual curiosity about the past in an attempt to abstract some meaning from the holocaust experience.

The children's fantasies, based on fragments of the parents' actual experience, provide a sense of security and cathartic relief from their anxieties. In some cases, the children believed that their parents' triumph over extreme danger left them invulnerable to present or future danger.

The "experienced fairy tales" of the children of survivors, with their recurring themes of danger, death, and salvation, as well as their emotional content, have a telling effect on the resolution of oedipal conflicts in the sons. The internalization of the father-image as victim of aggression and as hero who was miraculously saved for the sake of the children results in the diminishing of castration fears derived from the original oedipal constellation. Instead of perceiving the father as a threatening aggressor who metes out punishment for libidinal fantasies, the sons tend to identify with the fathers and project their fears onto fantasized external aggressors. In the adolescent, the revival of oedipal conflicts brings to the surface the identification with the father as hero, with a reaction-formation-like denial of fear and anxiety about the self. The phenomenon is observed particularly during army service.

In some cases, identification with the fantasy image of the parent is at the expense of libidinal investment. Interpersonal relationships within the family are characterized by awe, respect, and an affirmation of solidarity rather than intimacy. The fantasies and heroic tales preserve a sense of historic continuity for the survivors and their children. The retrieval of lost fragments of the parents' past identity contributes to identity formation during the children's adolescence.

The significance of the traumatization for the individuals in the study group was influenced both by their pretraumatic psychological development and by the later course of their life in the kibbutz community with its specific social structure and its institutionalized coping mechanisms for mourning and working through. Ernst Kris alludes to this subject in an article where he stresses that the significance of a traumatic event is not determined at the time of its occurrence but that the further course of life determines which experience gains significance as the traumatic one [5]. In her discussion of the impact of traumatic events in the development of the child, Anna Freud notes that the actual occurrence of the event is often overshadowed in significance by the psychic response to it and that it is difficult to determine which element of a given experience will be selected for cathexis and emotional involvement [3].

In the children's fantasies there was a marked tendency to deny frightening situations by turning them into pleasant ones and inventing happy, positive endings. Denial was prominent when anxiety-provoking situations such as separation or abandonment were represented. The children unconsciously deny conflict with significant adults and avoid overt expression of anger and aggression. The reaction to the danger of war and to open aggression from others is passive—escaping, hiding, crying, sticking together with the other children. They try to terminate fighting among other children by persuasion of asking for help.

In real situations of separation or abandonment which awakened anxiety, the children's basic defense was denial. There was a similar tendency to deny situations connected with the hostility and/or aggression of themselves and their parents. In the unconscious material, however, the parents expressed their hostility at having been abandoned by their own parents. The children's dreams similarly demonstrated that denial of separation was not successful, as evidenced by themes of abandonment by a helpless mother and rescue by a miracle.

The Process of Mourning

The most problematic issue in the post-traumatic lives of the survivors is the experiencing and expression of mourning. Legitimized institutional occasions, such as the national day of commemoration and memorial days for communities that were destroyed, have changed in nature over the years from a collective catharsis of vengeance towards the tormentors to occasions for the expression of grief and mourning for lost families and demonstration of pride in present achievements with special stress on the continuation of the family. The apparent absence of the intrapunitive mode of handling hostility [1, 6, 7, 8, 9, 10, 11] and the lack of experienced psychic disturbances is attributed to this opportunity for group expression of mourning and aggression among the survivors.

The avenues for coping with the holocaust experience are psychologically satisfying and socially approved. The group expression of grief partially compensates for the inability of the individual to mourn at the time of his loss. In the kibbutz, the suffering is reinterpreted in a collective rather than an individualistic manner so that the survivors feel that they suffered and survived in a group and that their experiences form an integral part of Jewish history. In this respect, the kibbutz has provided an institutionalized coping mechanism which has freed libidinal energies to be used for constructive ends.

The survivors have channeled their aggression into political ideology and an intensified in-group feeling. They are also able to legitimately direct it against an external enemy. These activities tend to alleviate the humiliation, degradation, and helplessness felt during the persecution. We hypothesize that these legitimized modes of aggression diminish the need to suppress rage and reduce the frequency of depressed states resulting from the transformation of suppressed aggressive feelings.

The unique history of the survivors creates highly charged conflicts for them and their children in light of the renewed losses in the present wars. Although they deny associating the Arabs with the Nazis, their dreams and fantasies reveal that such associations do exist: "When I fought for the first time with a gun in my hand during the War of Independence (1948), I thought what a pity I did not have a gun then." Arabs and Nazis are interchanged in their dreams whose motif is the continuing fear of extermination.

Survivors as Parents

Survivors' families are characterized by a distinctive pattern of parent-child relations. This pattern is a derivative of the dominant family motif—restoration of the "lost" family and undoing of the destruction.

In some cases this pattern began during pregnancy. In the interviews a number of mothers said that during pregnancy they feared having been changed from "good mothers" to witches who would give birth to monsters. They thus revealed that, to a certain extent, they had internalized the negative image that their persecutors had tried to project on them. These obsessive fears of survivor mothers were based on real experiences in the ghettos and the concentration camp—the loss of young siblings or offspring, which, according to their inner reality, they had "sacrificed" for their own lives. Anxieties concerning their own motherhood were expressed in their fantasies in symbols of self-degradation derived from the holocaust experience such as that of a prostitute or a hungry animal. Some of these women suffered miscarriages, amenorrhea, or remained sterile for many years.

It is important to distinguish between the obsessive fears of survivor mothers and the fantasies of neurotic mothers. In the former group, the sources of the fears are real experiences while in the latter group, fantasies and obsessions concerning the unborn child are rooted in unsolved pre-oedipal or oedipal conflicts.

Several of the mothers felt that their emotional and physical response to their first-born children was inadequate during the first months of life and characterized their behavior as having consisted of inhibited affect and limited emotional nurturing. The mothers' own fears, which stemmed from the previous danger of physical extinction from external forces or from hunger, were expressed in an overprotective attitude toward their children and a need to give them food. Many of the children of these survivors, especially the first-born, either overate or had general feeding problems. The mothers' overprotectiveness was a response as well to their fears of having been seriously damaged by the holocaust and to the feeling that the future held "something terrible" for the child. In every case, this fear expressed their expectation of a return of the persecution, this time involving themselves and their children. This interpretation is substantiated by the parents' repetitive persecutory dreams composed of unmodified memories of Nazi persecution altered only by the fact that in the dreams their children are trapped with them in the concentration camp.

The fearful attitude of the parents is shared by the children and is manifested in the difficulty of both in separating from each other. This problem is prominent during times of illness or war. In such instances these parents engage in compulsive ritualistic behavior such as frequent nighttime inspections of their children. The separation anxiety partly accounts for the fact that survivors spend more time with their children in their homes than do other families in the kibbutz—a fact recognized by all the members of the kibbutz.

Since the first-born child is usually identified with lost members of the parents' families of origin, their feelings toward him are colored by the guilt they feel toward those who perished. The special meaning of the first child extends to all their other children whom the parents see as lost family members or substitutes for them. They speak of their children as "given to them in the place of the lost ones." This phenomenon is vividly expressed by their naming their children after those who perished or giving them names symbolizing survival. As the children develop, their parents tell them stories about the holocaust. The children respond to these stories by emphasizing the victories of Israel (compensation for the traumatic "lost battles" of the persecution) rather than by identifying with the image of the victim in their parents.

Despite the fears and anxieties which pervade the parent-child relationship, the parents see their offspring as sources of security and gratification. They frequently remark that they "have such good children in spite of all the persecution" they suffered. The parents maintain high expectations for their children. Regardless of their own educational attainments, the survivors share the value of intellectual achievements for their children and demand that their offsprings be socially active and receive training in mastering adversity.

Family Systems of Survivors of the Holocaust

Families of survivors exhibit a unique family life style characterized by much display of affection, overprotectiveness and openness among their members. The affect-laden manner is understood as a reemergence of affect suppressed during the holocaust which has been recathected with restituted love objects—an expression of the libidinization of the overcathected objects which replace lost objects and a defense against an emerging anxiety concerning new losses. The overcathexis of these families is distinguished from that of neurotic families in which the affect-laden quality is rooted in a reaction toward death wishes. In these survivor families, expressions of closeness are especially evident at times when parents relate their terrible past and when they confront real external danger. This overprotectiveness and overcathexis is to be understood as a coping mechanism rather than an expression of pathology.[3]

The very notion of "the family" is highly charged for these survivors of massive persecution. Verbally and nonverbally they demonstrate the strong ties with the present family and with the destroyed one. The overcathexis leads to more conversation about relatives within this group than in kibbutz families who did not endure the holocaust. The family's effort to keep the lost members alive creates a sense of continuity in their existence. The parents implicitly communicate to their children their concern that the youngsters have been deprived of grandparents and other relatives, and the children quickly learn the importance of sustaining their parents' memories. One mother related that her eight-year-old daughter said: "I have been in Poland. I remember your house, I know my grandmother."

The unusual child-rearing arrangements of the kibbutz pose certain problems for the holocaust survivor parent and solves others [4]. Although peer group living for the children intensifies separation anxieties, the mothers are helped in overcoming their fears about being damaged and damaging their children by the intervention of the "metapelet" (house mother) who is responsible for child care and education. The presence of multiple mother-figures who mitigate possible "harmful mothering" provides survivor mothers with a sense of security.

A difficult period in the mother-child relationship is the anal phase when the child experiments with autonomy and separation. The child's strivings create anxiety, aggression, and feelings of helplessness in the mother. The first-born's entry into latency matches an increasing sense of security in the mother. During crisis situations such as war, the parents convey to their children their own feelings of security, belonging, and courage.

Another difficult period for the families of survivors is the child's adolescence which corresponds to the phase during which the parents' traumatization occurred. During their adolescence the children of survivors strive for independence and libidinal freedom which were denied their parents. As adolescents in Nazi Europe their preoccupation with survival prohibited expression of emotional and instinctual

[3] For an assessment of pathology, see the work of the Canadian team [12, 13].

impulses. The striving for sexual freedom in the sons reactivates castration fears in the fathers. On the other hand, the parents try to encourage the children to do what the parents were unable to do during their adolescence.

The parents invest so much in their children that they sometimes overestimate the children's abilities. Their concern for the children's future fulfillment is greater than their concern for their own needs and ambitions. To a certain extent these parents experience their lives as sacrifices for their children, and in some cases it is for the sake of the children that the parents stay on the kibbutz.

Concluding Remarks

The survivors of the concentration camp and ghetto were unable to mourn during and immediately after the holocaust. The kibbutz provided them with a secure supportive environment in which they could finally work through their feelings. On the annual day of commemoration the community mourns together in a collective spirit. The burning of six candles to symbolize the six million who perished and the displaying of fruit and flowers to embody the element of hope and rebirth are rituals through which they express together their feelings of grief and affirm the meaning of the past experiences as a positive force for the future.

Collective mourning integrates the generations and the community and provides feedback through which the individual can affirm his own feelings. This affirmation, a vital aspect of sharing, is continuously reexperienced by the holocaust survivor families on the kibbutz.

Although the survivors in the study tended to suppress the affective quality of their experiences, there was no denial of the past as such. The community norm in the kibbutz is to deny the holocaust experience as a negative symbol and regard it as a positive force linked to the rebirth of the Jewish people in the state of Israel. The children's images of their parents as heroes and resistance fighters and the mutual avoidance by parents and children of the more traumatic details of the past experience reinforces the reconceptualization of the holocaust.

The children participate in the mourning for holocaust victims and show a healthy ability to mourn for their own losses. For their parents they replace the generation that perished and symbolize the roots of the generations to come. They thus fulfill the vital function of maintaining the historical continuity and conviction that from the grief and despair of the past comes the hope of the future.

Our observations lead us to suggest that collective rituals of mourning, such as those discussed above, be undertaken on the family, community, national, or international level. The whole world has yet to mourn for the annihilation of millions of people during the holocaust and other man-made disasters. The recognition and affirmation of the deeds and horrors of the past enable a group to experience a sense of historic continuity and to utilize their experiences as a positive force. Collective experiences allow individuals and families to work through feelings of shame, anger and fear and to release dynamic emotional energy that is otherwise misdirected.

Bibliography

1. Blos, Peter, Maladaptive Behavior: A Private Language, Nunberg Lecture, (unpublished manuscript), March, 1969.
2. Bowlby, John and Parkes, Murray C., Separation and Loss Within the Family, in *The Child in His Family*, E. James Anthony and Cyrille Koupernik, Eds., John Wiley and Sons, New York, 1970.
3. Freud, Anna, *The Writings of Anna Freud 5, Research at the Hampstead Child Therapy Clinic and Other Papers*, International Universities Press, New York, (1969), 131–135.
4. Klein, Hilel, The Kibbutz as a Framework for Psychosocial Adaptation of Traumatized Survivors, in *Mental Health and Social Change*, Louis Miller, Ed., Academic Press, Jerusalem (in press).
5. Kris, Ernst, Notes on the Development and on Some Current Problems of Psychoanalytic Child Psychology, in *The Psychoanalytic Study of the Child*, R. Eissler et al., Eds., International Universities Press, New York, 5 (1950), 24–46.
6. Krystal, Henry, Minutes of Discussion Group No. 6: Children and Social Catastrophe: Sequelae in Survivors and the Children of Survivors, American Psychoanalytic Annual Meeting, Boston, (unpublished manuscript). May, 1968.
7. Krystal, Henry, Psychic Sequelae of Massive Psychic Trauma, in *Proceedings of the Fourth World Congress of Psychiatry*, J. J. Lopez Ibor, Ed., Excerpta Medica Foundation, Amsterdam, 2 (1968), 931–936.
8. *Massive Psychic Trauma*, Krystal, Henry, Ed., International Universities Press, New York, 1968.
9. Krystal, Henry and Petty, T. A., Dynamics of adjustment to migration, *Psychiatric Quarterly*, Supp. 37 (1963), 118–133.
10. Niederland, William G., The problem of the survivor, *Journal of Hillside Hospital*, 10 (1961), 233–247.

11. Niederland, William G., The Problem of the Survivor: The Psychiatric Evaluation of Emotional Disorders in Survivors of Nazi Persecution, in *Massive Psychic Trauma*, Henry Krystal, Ed., International Universities Press, New York, (1968), 8–22.
12. Rakoff, V., Sigal, J. J., and Epstein, N. B., Minutes of Discussion Group, No. 6: Children and Social Catastrophe: Sequelae in Survivors and the Children of Survivors, American Psychoanalytic Association Annual Meeting, Boston (unpublished manuscript), May (1968), 12–25.
13. Trossman, B., Adolescent children of concentration camp survivors, *Journal of the Canadian Psychiatric Association*, 13 (1968), 121–123.

Hypotheses and Methodology in the Study of Families of the Holocaust Survivors

John J. Sigal, Ph.D. (Canada)

The search for effects of survivors of the holocaust on the psychological functioning of their children is based on the following general hypotheses [1]: (a) People who experience the same or similar chronic deprivation, or distortions of other kinds in their psychological environment, will subsequently develop distortions in their capacities for human relations similar to others having had the same experience. (b) The distortion in this capacity will produce distortions common to this group in their relationship to their children. (c) The distortions common to the parent-child relationship will produce distortions in behavior common to their children. This section contains the work of eight authors or discussants in search of an hypothesis—the specific form of the above general hypotheses that would apply to the offsprings of survivors of the holocaust. Dr. Kestenberg's summary of Dr. Laufer's paper and the subsequent discussion suggest that the people at the Jerusalem symposium who discussed data based on clinical work were not successful in their search. This was predictable on methodological grounds. The discussion centered on a case in which so many other important variables—the effect on the patient's mother of the loss of her husband while she was pregnant, her remarriage at a critical age for the boy, her death when the boy was a young adolescent—may have so influenced or determined the content of the patient's psychic world and the form of his personality that isolation of the critical sequence of events or outcomes was next to impossible, a fact recognized by Dr. Laufer and most of the discussants. The widely differing interpretations of the material also supports this contention.

Although they met with little success in achieving the main goal, Dr. Kestenberg noted a certain consensus with regard to the type of treatment or management that met with success. She noted from her experience and from Dr. Furman's case material that the success of a survivor's child's treatment may hinge on the therapist's being able to provide an extremely close, positive relationship with the mother and to help her deal with the problem of telling the child of the realities of the camp situation in an appropriate way. Dr. Kestenberg also wondered if the same set of conditions, namely, a warm, supportive environment, are the bases for the relatively high frequency with which these people turn to the Hampstead Clinic and the clinic in Cleveland. (The deterrent effect on an immigrant population of high fees in private practice should not be ignored when discussing the frequency with which these people seek help and the context within which they do so.) I can give further clinical confirmation of the relevance of a strong supportive environment for the mothers to the adequate functioning of the children. In the course of one of our studies, Dr. Rakoff and I interviewed a family in which the three adolescent boys seemed to be managing extraordinarily well despite the fact that the mother had reacted to her wartime experiences in a manner which we had come to recognize as psychopathogenic. The mother was quite explicit in attributing the integration of the family and the high level of the boys' functioning to the truly remarkable reliability, competence, and affective availability of her husband. He was an emotional giant. A similar situation resulted in two boys, seven and nine years old, not appearing for treatment. Because of their disruptive uncontrollable behavior in school, the teacher recommended that they see a psychiatrist. The father, who had survived the holocaust by a series of shrewd responses to the challenges of the labor camp and who is now an extremely success-ful businessman, forcefully told the teacher that he would not have his children sent to a psychiatrist; that it was the school's responsibility to see that his boys' behavior improved. Cowed and spurred on by the father's challenge the school set about dealing with the problem more actively and the boys' behavior did improve. Again, the mother was potentially of the psychopathogenic type. These cases stand in marked contrast to the typical family that we have seen in our clinic in which the father, often having had no contact with the Nazi persecution, eventually withdraws in despair at ever being able to cope with the relationship with a depressed and agitated wife [2].

Dr. Aleksandrowicz and Dr. Klein also refer to the importance of the environment for the groups they studied, specifically groups in Israel or on the kibbutz, and suggest that the idealism and goals of the country or of the group help the parents cope with the mourning process and the sense of anomia, and Dr. Klein suggests, help the children cope with their aggressive fantasies.

Why is it so hard to find the common denominator to what it is that these parents are helped with by the country, the therapist, or the spouse? Why is it so hard to find a common denominator to what the consequences might be in the absence of such help? Why is it that we have found a consistent pattern in the families that we have studied clinically [3] through a systematic coding of hospital records [4] and in direct observation using interviews and questionnaires [1] whereas others can find no such pattern? The real difficulty appears to derive from considering the survivor group as (a) homogeneous and (b) unique.

Dr. Aleksandrowicz and Dr. Rosenberger have begun to deal with the myth of homogeneity; each has defined two subgroups within the group of survivors. Our observations relate most closely to the group of families Dr. Aleksandrowicz describes under the heading of "Affective Deficiency Syndrome and Hyperrepression." We may even be dealing with a subgroup of this group, one in which preoccupation figures prominantly as the reason for the affective deficiency. Rather than suffering from hyperrepression, our families are of the well-known type in which there is a failure of repression leading to continual preoccupation in the parent with their tragic losses and to their being libidinally unavailable to their children or to their spouses. In these families the spouse first attempts to be supportive, then becomes angry at the libidinal unavailability and unresponsiveness of the survivor and finally withdraws into isolation. In the absence of affective support from either parent, the children lack impulse control and begin to attack each other.[1] Some of the discussants of Dr. Laufer's paper and other authors in this section describe cases that resemble the ones that we have studied.

Let us now deal with the uniqueness hypothesis, i. e., that survivors of the holocaust must have a unique quality to their responses. I would suggest that this is highly improbable given the relatively limited range of people's potential affective responses to any situation. Consistent with the general hypotheses outlined at the beginning of my comments, I would suggest that others, surviving experiences with similar psychological consequences, should manifest the same responses. If my suggestion is correct, then one could arrive at the essential elements in any set of hypotheses concerning the effects of survival by testing them out on other groups with similar dynamics derived from totally different situations. This could be done equally well by those who use interviews, tests and questionnaires as by those who conduct clinical investigations.

This procedure has been followed for the preoccupation hypothesis outlined above. The hypothesis has, as a result, proven to be very useful in diagnosis and treatment [2, 5]. First we studied the family functioning of concentration camp survivors that came to our clinic for help and established that when preoccupation figured prominently in them there was the particular series of consequences within the family described previously. We then noticed that these consequences were the same as in families which were in a hiding or in Russian labor camps and in which preoccupation was a significant factor. Finally we were able to establish that they were the same as in families who had no contact with the Nazi persecution but were preoccupied for reasons as varied as chronic illness in one parent, fear that a child might die, alcoholism in one spouse, etc.[2] When

---

[1] These dynamics have been described more fully elsewhere [2].

[2] I am grateful to Miss Anna Freud for the encouragement she gave me to pursue this line of investigation. She stated "What I like about [this approach] is that you explain the lack of communication between the parents and child by the former's total preoccupation . . . rather than by the specificity of the experience. I think this is true also for parental preoccupation with . . . passions of all kinds" [6].

we observe the type of difficulties in children's behavior that we first noticed in the families of survivors, we now explore the possibility that there is a preoccupied parent around, even if the family is not one of survivors.

Bibliography

1. Sigal, J. J., Silver, D., and Ellin, B., Some Second-Generation Effects of Survival of the Nazi Persecution, Paper presented at the Fifth World Congress of Psychiatry, Mexico City, 1971.
2. Sigal, J. J., Familial Consequences of Parental Preoccupation (unpublished manuscript), 1971.
3. Rakoff, V., Sigal, J. J., and Epstein, N. B., The families of concentration camp survivors, *Canada's Mental Health,* 14 (1966), 24–25.
4. Sigal, J. J. and Rakoff, V., Concentration camp survival: a pilot study of the effects on the second generation, *Canadian Psychiatric Assoc. J.,* (in press).
5. Sigal, J. J., Second-Generation Effects of Massive Psychic Trauma, in *Psychic Traumatization,* H. Krystal and W. B. Niederland, Eds., Little, Brown, and Co., New York, 1971; *International Psychiatry Clinics,* 9 (1971), 55–65.
6. Freud, A., personal communication, 1966.

THE TRANSCULTURAL
EXPERIENCE OF DEATH,
DYING, AND DISABILITY

Introduction: Transcultural Approaches to the Experience of Death

Geoffrey Gorer, M.A. (England)

Introduction

The chapters in this section illustrate the approaches of social anthropologists to a universal human situation and stand in some contrast to the approaches of the physicians, psychologists, and sociologists in the preceding sections.

The differences of approach lie less in the techniques of investigation—all four sciences rely in the last resort on interviews, usually supplemented by observations; the differences lie in the framework, in the context within which the information and observations are interpreted; and this framework or context also influences the type of information sought in the interviews and observations.

The physician is primarily concerned with physical health, with the reestablishment of the appropriate physiological well-being of the patient. The psychologist is primarily concerned with some concept of mental health and tries to help his patients achieve this goal: sometimes an ideal goal of optimum personality development which does not correspond to any pattern in the external world, sometimes to a more vaguely apprehended normative concept of "adjustment" which should result in the patient behaving like the more successful and admired people in the appropriate social class of his or her society at the time of treatment.

Typically, the sociologist is concerned with the distribution of traits or attitudes or behavior within his own contemporary society. Although sociological findings may be used as a basis for recommending social changes, these depend on the private and often inarticulate value judgments of the sociologist or of his clients. Typically, the sociologist takes the dominant contemporary values of his society for granted though his researches frequently discover unforeseen distributions of traits and behavior within his society.

For the social anthropologist the major conceptual unit is not the individual nor a section of society but the whole human society with its unique culture. Ideally, the social anthropologist relates the society and culture he is studying to all human societies and cultures that have been described or deduced from material remains (in which script and the graphic arts should be included); ideally, the social anthropologist relates his observations to all the societies that the human species has developed from the emergence of Homo sapiens to the most complex of contemporary societies. Traditionally, the social anthropologist has been predominantly concerned with recording and analyzing the technologically simple and nonliterate societies of the world; but the generalizations which he draws from the studies of these unique societies—often consisting of only a few hundred people—should be, and generally are, applicable to all known human societies.

The papers in this section would appear to suggest two tentative generalizations. The first, and the more relevant to the theme of this Yearbook, is that in societies with high infantile mortality—and it should be remembered that this means the whole of humanity save for a few technologically advanced societies in the last century or so—the deaths of infants and small children are interpreted differently and mourned for (if at all) differently to the deaths of older children or adults. Dr. Palgi tells us that for the Yemenites an infant has no soul for thirty days; Dr. Collomb illustrates in fascinating detail the concept that young Serer children are half in this world, half in the world of ancestors; and Dr. Khare documents the beliefs of the high-caste Hindus of Uttar Pradesh in the incomplete humanity of pre-adolescents.

Technically, it is interesting that both the Serer and the high-caste Hindus interpret the deaths of infants or young children as being due to the faults of the parents and not to supernatural malevolence; in many societies such deaths are ascribed to sorcery or to ghosts, particularly the ghosts of women who have died in childbirth.

Literary evidence suggests that this differential attitude to the death of infants and young children was current in England at least up till the beginning of the 19th century. In *Mansfield Park,* published in 1814, Jane Austen writes of "the cant of its being a very happy thing (if three or four children had died) and a great blessing . . . to have them so well provided for"; and a mother says of her daughter who died after she had learned to speak: "Poor little sweet creature! Well, she was taken away from evil to come."[1] The second more tentative generalization, suggested by Dr. Palgi's paper and my own, is that mourning tends to become deritualized and privatized as urbanization and technological elaboration increase with the possible implication that grief will produce more psychological disturbance in individual members of "advanced" secular societies than occurred, or occur, in societies with unquestioned mourning rituals.

[1] Mansfield Park, Vol. Three, Chapters XIII and VII.

Death, Grief, and Mourning in Britain

Geoffrey Gorer, M.D. (England)

This chapter will discuss briefly the study of bereavement in Britain which I made in 1963 [3] with such additions and modifications as seem appropriate in the light of my subsequent reading and experiences.

I started my study with the knowledge that (to the best of my information) all recorded societies up to the beginning of this century had elaborated rules concerning the disposal of the dead and their possessions and of the appropriate behavior to be manifested by the survivors who, according to the customs of the society, were emotionally most involved with the dead person. I have had to express this rather clumsily since different societies vary in the way they structure emotional intimacy. To take a well-known example, in many matrilineal societies, the bond between a man and his mother's brother is expected to be much closer than the bond with the mother's husband, even though the mother's husband is the physiological father. Whether a man should mourn for his father or for his maternal uncle is determined by his society's structuring of kinship relationships; but appropriate mourning behavior is (to the best of my knowledge) universally enjoined.

There are very few universal traits or practices found in all human societies from the simplest to the most complex. All recorded human societies speak a language, conserve fire, and have some sort of cutting implement; all recorded societies elaborate the biological bonds of bearer, begetter, and offspring into kinship systems; all societies have some division of labor based on age and sex; all societies have incest prohibitions and rules regulating sexual behavior, designating appropriate marriage partners, and legitimizing offspring; and all societies have rules and ritual concerning the disposal of the dead and the appropriate behavior of mourners.

The great majority of societies have a belief in some sort of survival after death. In these societies, before the body is disposed of, ritual is performed either to help the dead in their post-terrestrial life or to prevent them harming the living; frequently, the ritual is designed to deal with both eventualities. All societies have rules concerning the ways in which and the places at which the dead body should be disposed of; and all societies prescribe the appropriate behavior of the survivors deemed closest to the dead person between the time of death and the disposal of the body. In most societies the behavior of the bereaved is prescribed for a period after the disposal of the body, a period most frequently measured by the solar or lunar calendar.

In the greater number of recorded societies, including our own up to about fifty years ago, mourners go through what Van Gennep [8] called a *rite de passage* (he initially developed this term to describe adolescent initiation rites): a formal withdrawal from society, a period during which the mourner abstains from some social activities and is typically distinguished by his appearance or clothes so that all who come into contact with him recognize him as a mourner and treat him in prescribed ways, and a return to society and to full social participation in one or more stages.

This treatment of mourning as a *rite de passage* is not quite universal. A few societies, chiefly nomadic, have been recorded which limit all public signs of mourning to the few days between death and the disposal of the body. There are also a few societies, chiefly the advanced societies of Asia, which treat or treated mourning as interminable; in Hindu India and classical China especially, the mourning of widows was meant to be life-long. If, however, one takes the society as a unit rather than the size of the component populations, I think one can safely state that the treating of mourning as a *rite de passage* is very general.

If a custom, such as this, is widespread throughout human societies in all stages of development, it seems reasonable to assume that the custom is congruent with species-characteristic human psychology and that those societies which lack such customs and rules of behavior are aberrant.

In a short article I have perforce had to simplify very considerably the information on the social treatment of mourners which recorded human societies have developed. I should like, however, to emphasize that I undertook the study of bereavement in contemporary Britain with the knowledge that for most of humanity mourning is, and has been, *ritualized*; that the behavior of mourners is prescribed in considerable detail and also, typically, their appearance and/or costume so that mourners are immediately *recognizable;* the treatment which mourners are accorded by the *other members* of society is also prescribed. In most societies mourners go through a *rite de passage* determined by the calendar and not by their autonomous feelings.

As far as my reading and knowledge go, there is no record from any society before this century of mourners failing to follow the prescribed behavior; nor is there any evidence that following the social imperatives of ritualized mourning produced psychological maladjustment in identifiable individuals. Negative evidence must always be treated with the greatest circumspection; because behavior has not been reported it need not mean that it has not occurred; but with this caveat it can be assumed that for most people in most societies the prescribed behavior enabled them to work through, and come to terms with, the misery of bereavement without psychological disturbance.

As far as the professional classes of southeastern England are concerned, my personal experience illustrates the enormous change which has taken place in the treatment of mourning in my own society in the last half-century. My father was drowned in 1915 and my behavior and costume, and even more those of my widowed mother, were almost entirely dictated by the prevailing social rules. My younger brother died of cancer in 1961; and there were no social rules available to guide the behavior of his widow and children. Within my lifetime, in my social class, mourning had become almost completely deritualized. A major motive for my undertaking research on British bereavement was to discover whether this deritualization was general in all classes and all regions of Britain and, if this was the case, what were the consequences?

I will only describe very summarily the design of the research. An opinion research company asked a carefully selected stratified proportional sample of 1628 people of both sexes, of all ages over 16 and coming from every region and every social class in Britain, whether they had ever attended a funeral or cremation, when, and who it was for? By these means a group of 359 people were identified who had lost a primary relative—father, mother, brother, sister, husband, wife, son, or daughter—in the past five years. The interviewers asked these informants a series of questions suitable to tabulation such as questions about the behavior surrounding the death and the disposal of the body, their religious beliefs and practices, and whether any physiological changes had accompanied their bereavement. They were also asked if they were willing for somebody—me—to come to talk to them at greater length about their bereavement. Two hundred and twelve expressed a willingness to be interviewed at greater length; I selected 112 from these but in the event only succeeded in recording 80 interviews. These were tape-recorded and were conducted in the bereaved person's home with very few exceptions. A few informants preferred to be interviewed at their place of work so as not to distress some other member of the family, usually a surviving parent but in two cases the second wife.

This survey deals with all eight primary relationships; the other surveys with which I am acquainted concentrate on the death of a spouse (typically a husband) or of a parent. The bereaved were discovered through stratified sampling and not because they were psychologically disturbed (though quite a few were) and had asked for help nor through a hospital contact or selection in a small area. The sample was very extensive socially and geographically, ranging from an admiral's widow to a bricklayer's sister and covering every major region in Britain.

I paid a lot of attention to the religious beliefs and practices of my informants for a number of reasons. First, in Britain, death is a religious preserve; in only two cases out of the 359 was a dead body disposed of without benefit of clergy. Second, the only generally available consolations for the grief of bereavement are phrased in religious terms. Third, the only person who is neither kin nor neighbor who may offer help and comfort to the bereaved after the funeral in nearly the whole of Britain is the clergyman or minister in those parishes where they conduct pastoral visits.

Contemporary ritualization of mourning—treating mourning as a *rite de passage*—is almost entirely determined by the bereaved's adherence to a minority[1] creed.

The group whose mourning is most completely ritualized is Orthodox Jewry. Those who follow its prescriptions have a week of very intensive mourning during which the bereaved have to face their loss and voice their distress without privacy from sunrise to sunset. Those mourners who had performed this very intensive ritual stated that they had found it therapeutic and comforting. Members of the Church of Scotland also have a fairly concentrated ritual between death and the disposal of the body with vigils and religious services in the home; in the days after the funeral the ministers and neighbors make prescribed ritual visits. Roman Catholics of Irish origin (even though the migration may have taken place a couple of generations earlier) maintain the rite of the wake and feel that they can assist the person mourned to attain heaven by having masses said for them. Both Roman Catholics of Irish origin and members of the Church of Scotland tend to wear black costumes, ties, etc., for quite a long time after the funeral thus indicating that they are mourners with much more regularity than the rest of the British population.

The bereaved members of these three creeds who I interviewed appeared to have performed their mourning without undue psychological distress and to have returned to physiological and psychological homeostasis within the year. The two exceptions to this generalization were parents who had lost adult children. On the basis of these interviews, the loss of a grown child appears to be the most devastating of all griefs and the hardest from which to recover— a point I will revert to later on in this paper.

A generalization, derived from my interviews, is one that I should be much happier not to make for it goes against all my personal prejudices and preconceptions. Burial of the dead is enjoined for Orthodox Jews and was for Roman Catholics until 1963; members of the Church of Scotland preferred burial to cremation in the

---

[1] I am using the term of "minority" in a strictly statistical sense. About two thirds of the British describe themselves as "Church of England" though they may have no religious beliefs or practices. None of the other creeds are confessed to by 10% of the population; most have an even smaller percentage.

proportion of two to one. The opting for burial, by those whose
creeds or agnosticism allow a choice, implies the acceptance of a
style of mourning of a different nature to that implicit in cremation;
it also implies a willingness to engage in continuous extra expense to
keep green the memory of the dead. All my personal inclinations
are opposed to the cult of the corpse and the cemetery; but, according to my evidence, there is a marked tendency for mourning to be
worked through more satisfactorily when the person mourned for
is buried than when he is cremated. This is not an invariant rule;
many of those who had chosen cremation worked through their
mourning satisfactorily, a few of those who had chosen burial did
not. I think, though, that it is significant and not an artifact of the
small sample that out of the 15 people whom I considered to be in
despair (or suffering from depression or melancholia), all had had
the relative they mourned cremated without any formal or ritual
elaboration.

For the majority in Britain, mourning is almost completely deritualized. Outside the professional classes, most people indicate the
presence of mourners in the house between the death and the disposal of the body by drawn blinds (shades) or other signs. At the
funeral, four-fifths of the men, but barely half the women, indicate
that they are mourners by modifications of their costumes;[2] but
only older mourners chiefly from the unskilled working class continue the wearing of mourning for any considerable time after the
interment.   Only a very small minority (less than a fifth) of the
English said that they abstained from diversions after the funeral or
cremation, and even for this minority the abstention was measured
in days rather than weeks.

Not only is mourning almost completely deritualized for the
majority of the British who call themselves members of the Church
of England or of one of the nonconformist sects or who reject any
sectarian label; social disapproval is manifested against any public
signs of mourning, both verbally, by stigmatizing it as morbid or
unhealthy and also (frequently) in action by withdrawing from social
contact with the bereaved unless or until they act as if nothing of

---

[2]This difference between the behavior of the two sexes can probably be accounted for by
the expense. Women mourners need a black costume and hat, men only a black tie and
possibly a black crepe armband and hat.

consequence had occurred. In most classes and most regions in Britain, mourning is treated as though it were a shameful weakness to be indulged in, if at all, as furtively and secretively as if it were some sort of analogue of masturbation. There is a taboo not only on people weeping or looking doleful anywhere that they can be observed but also in their talking about their feelings of grief or any of their experiences of bereavement. The prevailing ethos demands that mourners "bottle up" all their thoughts and feelings. At the end of my interviews with them, several of my informants thanked me with obvious sincerity for talking to them without embarrassment about their feelings and experiences. A typical phrasing was: "I've got a lot off my chest"; and clearly for many of these people, even those well integrated in their community and with a happy family life, this was a unique opportunity to put into words the miseries and perplexities which had followed their bereavement.

Two areas where the absence of ritual and the denial of mourning pose particular problems are what to tell children about a death in the family and how to handle the first contacts after bereavement between the bereaved and their friends, neighbors, or workmates.

In general, if British children are told anything at all about the death in the family, they are fobbed off with euphemisms. People with no sort of religious belief, who never say prayers or attend a church and say explicitly that they do not believe in an afterlife, tell their children that the dead parent, grandparent, uncle, or aunt has "gone to Heaven," "gone to Jesus," and the like. A sizable proportion of British parents use God and Jesus in communication with their children in almost exactly the same way as they use Santa Claus. Besides the religious euphemisms, there are the customary verbal euphemisms denying the fact of death: "gone to sleep," "gone to rest," and the like. A common phrasing, which seems to me to have particularly unfortunate connotations, is to tell the children that the dead person has gone away on a long visit.

Nearly half my informants who had children under 16 told them nothing at all about the recent death of a near relative. Sometimes there were legitimate reasons for this reticence: the children were too young to understand or old enough to know about death from other sources, but many parents treated the subject as literally unmentionable. This is capable of having very unfortunate effects; a few of my informants' children seem permanently traumatized by their unmentionable experience. I am inclined to draw a close connection between the treating of death and mourning as unmentionable and the furtive excitement engendered by what I have called "the pornography of death" [4], the horror comic, and the like.

The absence of any ritual or generally accepted etiquette renders particularly difficult the first contacts between friends, neighbors, or workmates and the recently bereaved. Should they speak of the dead person or act as if nothing had happened? Will the bereaved involve them in a distasteful upsurge of grief if they do mention their loss? Will they be considered callous if they do not refer to it? Many people avoid this dilemma by looking the other way, by curtailing as much as may be their contacts with the bereaved.

The mourners I interviewed divided almost equally into those who found spoken condolences painful and those who found them comforting. I have not space to elaborate the evidence; but on the basis of these interviews I would consider that the grateful acceptance of spoken condolences is one of the most reliable signs that the bereaved is working through his or her mourning satisfactorily. My impression was that those who welcomed spoken sympathy were well integrated in their community and happy in their work whereas those who (to use the most common phrasing) "found it easier" when their loss was not mentioned tended to be withdrawn characters, somewhat frightened of their own emotions.

A second indication (according to my evidence) that mourners are dealing adequately with their grief can be found in the manifest content of their dreams. Among the most general physiological responses to bereavement are disturbed sleep and loss of weight; in the main sample, two-thirds of the women and two-fifths of the men reported that they slept less well than previously after their bereavement; just on half the women and a quarter of the men reported loss of weight.

This disturbed sleep after bereavement is frequently accompanied by vivid dreams of the dead person mourned for. When the bereaved person is working through his or her grief adequately there is a very strong tendency for the dead person to be young and in good health in the dreams. Adults dreaming of their dead parents see them as tall: in the typical words of the wife of a salesmanager mourning for her father:

He seemed big in these dreams. Actually he wasn't a tall man. He was very good to us children, you know, he took us everywhere.

Similarly husbands or wives dream of their dead spouses as young. The widow of a Scottish baker said:

I do dream, but I canna keep it long enough. . . He looks younger, aye, nice, nice. Last time I was dreaming he had lovely hair—I told Mrs. X. he was younger lookin' than ever.

A widower working in local government whose wife had died prematurely from tuberculosis said:

I wake up suddenly in the night and think that she's there, you know. . .She is generally younger as when we were first married; that's the time when I dream of her mostly. . .I find the dreams quite pleasant.

When mourning is not being adequately worked through, or when there was (as indicated by the rest of the interview) considerable ambivalence in the relationship with the dead person, the dead person is seen either as he or she was just before death or as a corpse. Thus, a 61-year-old widow said that when she dreams of her husband:

That's a strange thing; when I do he's always one step away from me; I never get any contact; he looks just as he died.

The wife of a van driver said of her husband's sister who had died in their home:

Next couple of nights I could see her; every time I closed my eyes I could see her. . .I seen her when she died. Oh, she was terrible. She must have suffered.

Quite a number of these dreams had a very distressing affect, the quality of nightmares.

As Freud wrote in *Mourning and Melancholia* [2] : "We do not even know the economic means by which mourning carries out its task." I am certainly unable to explain the healing or symptomatic function of these dreams of the person mourned.

Nearly all my informants who reported dreams in which the dead person was seen as young and lively stated that they were comforting. Typical working-class phrasings were: "There was a bit of a laugh in it as well"; "We have a laugh and that." The first statement was made by the widow of a small shopkeeper, the second by the wife of a pensioned bricklayer talking about the death of her younger sister. Men and women mourning for their parents, their spouses, or their brothers and sisters all reported these comforting experiences;

but this comfort was denied to the six desolate parents whom I interviewed who had lost a grown child.

This distinction highlights what I consider to be the most important generalization derived from my survey and which has been confirmed by all my reading and experience since the survey was made; the difference in the quality and content of the mourning process when death is untimely or unforeseen compared with the mourning for a death in the fullness of time or prepared for by a terminal illness.[3]

I am inclined to believe that human beings manifest two different forms of mourning depending on whether the death mourned is felt to be "natural" or not. In my interviews, the mourning of a parent for the death of a grown child was of quite a different nature to the mourning of a child for the death of a parent. With one exception, the parents mourning for a dead child seemed quite inconsolable; with two exceptions—men who had been "exceptionally close" to their mother—the adults who had lost their parents worked through their mourning adequately in a few months.

I consider that this distinction needs special emphasis because the existing literature is very heavily biased towards the descriptions of mourning for untimely deaths. In his pioneering paper, *Symptomatology and Management of Acute Grief* [6], Dr. Lindemann drew nearly all his evidence from people bereaved in a disaster, the terrible restaurant fire at Coconut Grove; in *Widows and Their Families* [7], Peter Marris selected his informants from widows whose husbands had been under fifty years old at the time of death. There is a larger literature about the mourning of children for the death of a parent; save in the most exceptional circumstances, the death of the parent of a young child is, almost by definition, untimely.

I believe that there are components in the mourning for an untimely death which are either absent or only minimally present when the death has been foreshadowed by the age or illness of the person mourned for. I would consider that the most important of these components is anger; anger directed against the doctors for negligence or against God or fate or the government for unfairness, for injustice. This anger may also be directed against the self, in the self-reproaches

[3]This distinction was originally made by Dr. R. Lehrman in an article entitled "Reactions to untimely death" [*Psychiatric Quarterly,* 5 (1956)]. I was only made aware of this article after my survey was finished.

which are a prominent feature of melancholia; perhaps this anger directed against the self is more fittingly described as guilt.

I was aware of the theoretical statements that anger and/or guilt are inevitable components of mourning when I conducted my interviews, and I was alert to any expressions or indications of these emotions. The fact that I found no signs of either emotion in the greater number of cases might be due to reticence during a single interview though most of my informants spoke very freely on most other aspects of their mourning (the interviews were unstructured and did not follow a fixed schedule); but I think it also theoretically probable that typically these emotions are elicited only in mourning for an untimely death. Those informants who did display or recall anger or indulged in self-reproaches and self-questioning were all mourning untimely deaths.

So far I have been writing about "working through mourning satisfactorily" as if we all knew what a satisfactory mourning process was; in doing so, incidentally, I am following nearly all other writers who have dealt with this topic, apart from Dr. Bowlby [1]; and I am not in disagreement with the description of satisfactory "normal" mourning as outlined or implied in the work of psychologists in this century or codified by social custom in the majority of human societies including our own up to the last sixty years.

Like the *rites de passage* of ritualized mourning, the pattern of normal mourning falls into three temporal phases: a short period of shock or numbness typically lasting from the occurrence of death to the disposal of the body or a few days after; a period of intense grief frequently marked by bouts of painful weeping, loss of weight, disturbed sleep with vivid dreams, and a withdrawal of interest from the external world—symptoms which also frequently accompany acute illness; and a return to physical homeostasis and a normal social life in one or more stages. In most traditional societies, the second stage—the period of intense grief—is determined by religious or social prescriptions based on the calendar of the society. When, as for the majority of contemporary Britons, the religious or social prescriptions are no longer accorded any validity, this period of intense mourning is determined by the mourner's autonomous feelings. There is naturally a very wide gamut depending on the personality of the mourner and the relationship with the deceased; it is my impression that the median duration of this phase of "normal" mourning is between eight and sixteen weeks.

I called this three-phase pattern of mourning, which echoes the traditional *rite de passage,* "time-limited mourning"; and I think it is noteworthy that out of the 80 mourners whom I interviewed at length, considerably less than half had mourned in this fashion, even interpreting their statements with as much generosity as possible. As I stated earlier, this time-limited "normal" mourning is more easily available for members of the Church of Scotland, the Roman Catholics, and the Orthodox Jews; but it was also evolved spontaneously by mourners belonging to the other Protestant creeds and by agnostics. Men and women coming from all social classes and in equal numbers mourned in this fashion and all relatives may be so mourned but this "time-limited" pattern is most frequent with those who have lost a parent. It would appear that the death of a person of a generation above one's own can be accepted with more resignation and mourned with more spontaneity than the death of a loved person of one's own generation or of the generation below.

The mourning of the majority of my British informants who did not follow this time-limited sequence can be divided into two major groups: those who, for one reason or another, never reach the second stage of intense grief; and those who, for one reason or another, never get out of it.

I divided the people who never reached the second stage of normal mourning into four subgroups. Most of them can be dealt with fairly succinctly. First, there are the members of the modern elective sects, such as Spiritualism, Christian Science, and various adaptations of Asian religions, who deny the "reality" of death and who would be going against their tenets if they mourned; they are sustained in their denial of mourning by their fellow sectarians. Second there are some bereaved people who had no love for the dead person and so feel no grief. Third, people who have nursed the dying through a long and painful terminal illness may have done most or all of their mourning before the death occurs and may feel the eventual death emotionally as well as intellectually as a relief.

There is, however, a sizable group who consciously refuse to mourn, to give way to grief; they "carry on" and "keep busy" as if nothing had happened, consistently in public and usually in private also. From my observations, this is predominantly a feminine response, women denying their grief for their husbands or (in three cases) for their mothers. Only one man among my informants used any such phrases; he was refusing to mourn for his mother and, on a deeply symbolic level, had taken over her role in tending his grief-stricken father.

This refusal to mourn has several components. One is the generous wish not to make others unhappy in one's misery, particularly to protect children from the infection of grief. A second component might be described as psychological hypochondria, a belief that giving way to grief is "morbid" and "unhealthy" and that mental health will best be maintained by being continuously active, by seeking perpetual distraction. This psychological hypochondria is most evident among middleclass women without the need to earn their living; and though I found advocates and practicers of such behavior in all social classes, a disproportionately high number came from the widows of husbands in the professional and managerial classes. With nearly all these women it seemed to me that, by denying expression to their grief, they had reduced their lives to triviality even though their purposeful busyness warded off any overt symptoms of depression. In the British middle classes, widows who behave in this way are frequently described as "wonderful."

I divided those who never get out of the second stage of intense grief into three subgroups; I am, however, not quite certain that the first subgroup to be mentioned is properly so described. These are the people who proclaim in so many words, and almost always in the same phrase, that they, or the bereaved whom they are describing, will "never get over it." The people who made this statement were predominantly members of the traditional British working classes and over 50 years old. I felt that this statement was frequently made with some complacency. I do not question the fact that the dead person was deeply loved and sincerely mourned; but it would seem that within this older semiskilled or unskilled working-class group, the statement that one will never get over one's grief is a demonstration of how loving and dutiful the mourner is.

Fifteen out of the 80 people I interviewed at length I consider to have been in irreversible despair. None of these people in despair were very recently bereaved; at least twelve months had passed since the death of the person they mourned so insistently. Their unhappiness was of a quite different nature to the intense grief which so many of the "time-limited" mourners reported in the first months of their bereavement. Five of these mourners had lost a husband, six a wife, two were middleaged men who had lost their mothers, and two were people who had lost young adult sons. I found three of these mourners in despair sitting alone in the dark.

A symptom of despair which I had not foreseen before I started my interviewing is what I have called "mummification," using the word in a metaphorical fashion. This type of mourner preserves the grief for the lost husband or wife by keeping the house and every object in it precisely as he or she had left it, as though it were a shrine which would be at any moment reanimated.[4] The visual impression is very striking: a woman living alone with a man's personal belongings all over the room; or a worker in heavy industry tending a room full of brightly polished, feminine knickknacks.

The tending of these domestic shrines at least gave these persistent mourners some occupation; the other mourners in despair lived lives of heart-rending emptiness. The despair is almost palpable: the flaccid face muscles, the toneless voice, the halting speeches in short sentences, the insistent preoccupation with their own misery, often the appearance of undernourishment. These people in despair were all solitary as it seemed by choice; for, with two exceptions, those who lived alone had married children or other kinfolk who were willing to receive them into their house.

I should like to repeat again that only four of these 15 people in despair had had their relative buried; and these four were the only ones who had given even minimal formal or ritual elaboration to the disposal of the body or engaged in any formal mourning.

My research left me with the strong conviction that our contemporary society's denial of mourning and the absence of any social ritual or etiquette for dealing with mourners after the disposal of the body is conducive to a great deal of neurotic and maladaptive behavior, to much theoretically unnecessary misery.

The ritual and consolations of religion are available to the pious minorities; but on the minimal criteria of attending a place of worship once a month or saying daily prayers, or the like, only a third of the population of contemporary Britain can be described as believers. Slightly less than half the population of contemporary Britain give

---

[4]The accounts of Queen Victoria in widowhood suggest strongly that she was a mourner who indulged in "mummification" in a royal fashion.

even verbal assent to a belief in an afterlife; the vast majority of these predominantly bland beliefs have no overt religious content nor congruence with any form of Christian eschatology. Since death is still a religious preserve, this means that our society offers neither comfort nor guidance to the majority of the British with residual or nonexistent religious beliefs in the crises of misery and loneliness following bereavement which are probable occurrences in every human life.

I would suggest that this situation calls for social inventions, inventions analogous to civil marriage. Until a century ago, marriage in Britain was also a religious preserve; only the clergy could give a union social recognition and validity which would legitimize the offspring of the union. Civil marriage was invented; the invention was rather drab and lacks the ritual and ceremony which make a "church wedding" so attractive to many nonbelieving British brides and their parents. But at least the invention was made; marriages can now be solemnized without benefit of clergy.

It would seem possible for lay mourning ceremonies to be invented too. These ceremonies and ritual would have to take into account the need of mourners for both companionship and privacy and recognize the facts that it is (almost certainly) desirable for mourners to give vocal expression to their grief without embarrassment or reticence and that, for some weeks after bereavement, a mourner is undergoing much the same physiological changes as occur during and after a severe illness; further, we need in Britain the social invention and general acceptance of an etiquette to regulate the first contacts between a mourner and his friends, neighbors and workmates; and, at least in Britain, we need the invention of meaningful social roles for widows.[5]

Besides the endopsychic, private, psychological components, grief and mourning also have social components; and the attitudes, values, and institutions prevalent in a given society at a given time can make mourning easier or harder to live through, can facilitate a benign or maladaptive outcome. At present, the majority of British (and, I believe, American) society with residual or no religious

---

[5]The Belgians have invented beguinages, community houses, with shared cooking, etc., where the able-bodied widows engage in some sorts of social work. The Russian *babushka* ("grandmother") is treated as an indispensible adjunct to the household of the more educated where both husband and wife are likely to be working.

beliefs receive very little help during the period of intense grief when most mourners are in more need of social support and assistance than at any time since infancy and early childhood. As Dr. Bowlby [1] has pointed out, crying is always a demand for help; the help which contemporary mourners demand has no explicit content at present; social inventions could, I believe, supply at least some of this content.

Bibliography

1. Bowlby, J., *Attachment and Loss,* Basic Books, New York, 1969.
2. Freud, Sigmund, *Mourning and Melancholia,* 1917, Standard Edition, Volume 14.
3. Gorer, Geoffrey, *Death, Grief and Mourning in Comtemporary Britain,* New York, Doubleday, 1965.
4. Gorer, Geoffrey, *The Pornography of Death,* Encounter, New York, 1955.
5. Lehrmann, S. R., Reactions to untimely death, *Psychiatric Quarterly,* XXX (1956).
6. Lindemann, E., Symptomatology and management of acute grief, *American Journal of Psychiatry,* CI (1944).
7. Marris, Peter, *Widows and Their Families,* Routledge & Paul, London, 1958.
8. Van Gennep, Arnold, *Les Rites de Passage,* Paris, 1909. English translation: *The Rites of Passage,* London, Routledge & Paul, 1960.

The Child Who Leaves and Returns or the Death of the Same Child[1]

H. Collomb, M.D. (Senegal)

> *"The children, they die, they die, then*
> *this name is given in order to gain a child."*
> > *Mossi Country, Haute-Volte [6]*
>
> *"He goes the first time, he passes on again.*
> *He goes the second time, he passes on again.*
> *He goes the third time, the fourth, the fifth, the sixth,*
> *When it is the seventh...."*
> > *Yoruba country, Nigeria [8]*

Two observations can be made immediately about the majority of African countries: (1) the infant mortality rate is very high and (2) the mothers seem to be relatively indifferent to the death of the child.

The infant mortality rate, due to numerous factors (environment, low economic level, very reduced medical assistance) is an objective fact: 50% of the children die before the age of five.

The second observation refers to the attitude of the African in general toward death. The case of the mother is, however, special. According to traditional values, the mother is valued only for or exists only through her children. She is consecrated to fertility; not to have any children or to lose them at an early age is the worst condition: It is social annihilation. The problem is not that of death but rather that of life. If the children die, her anguish will be that of a barren woman.

When the children die repeatedly at an early age, the phenomenon

---

[1] The title expresses the meaning of Serer term "tji:d a paxer" better than the literal translation (evil spirit) does.

receives an explanation. It is meaningful and it is perceived as a message from the spirit beyond the living (the "numineux"). In spite of various cultural differences, these successive deaths are often interpreted according to a model found over and over again in many African countries. It concerns the same child who returns and leaves again after a brief stay among the living; he refuses to remain because a sin or an impurity has, probably, been committed against what he is or what he represents, that is, tradition, the law of the ancestors.

In the course of an investigation in the country of the Serers,[2] the object of which was to evaluate, from samples, the overall health of a rural population, much information had been gathered about the "tji:d a paxer." One mother, Fatou N'D. . ., having learned of our interest in this question, came to Dakar to talk to us of her case.

The Problem of Fatou

Fatou, accompanied by an investigator native to her country, arrives with two children: Moktar, 3½ years old, and Babacar, 2½ years old. She is six months' pregnant. Moktar has infected wounds on his legs; Babacar presents a state of severe malnutrition.

THE STORY OF FATOU

"She is coming to talk; she knows that you are interested in the 'tji:d a paxer.' She does not expect anything definite. She has had nine children; five have already died. The time has come for Babacar and Moktar to leave."

The Dead Children "It is Babacar who wants to leave; he resembles too well the others who have already left. He has the same look about him, the same way of crying. If he cries, it is the same. He is to leave with Moktar; they always leave in two's. I am expecting their death. Perhaps he will depart with the one whom I have within my belly. They are the same child—they die the same month or the same day. This week they are going to die; Moktar and Babacar,

---

[2]The Serers constitute a population of about 500,000 people who make up about thirty ethnic subgroups. The majority of them are located in a peanut basin; the capital is Kaolack, 200 kilometers from Dakar, Senegal. It is a profoundly religious group; in spite of the influence of Islam and Christianity, the belief in animism is still very strong.

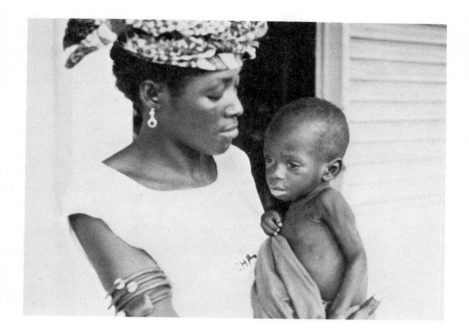

they are the same.

They always die at the same time, at two years of age, at two and a half years of age. The first waits for the second who is within my belly. When the second one comes, they leave. It is the same child. The first child who departed was Seynabou, a daughter; she died at the age of two and a half when I was pregnant. The second and third ones departed together; they were N'Guilane and N'Dèye. They departed the same week; N'Guilane was two years old, and N'Dèye was one. I was six months pregnant. The fourth child, Ibrahima, died at four years of age with his sister, Seynabou, who was two and a half years old. The mother was told, 'It is the same child; they want to leave together.' They told the child, 'We have recognized you.' But he left anyway. And now it is Moktar and Babacar who are due to leave.

Moktar has a sign; you see his legs. He has wounds. Ibrahima, who died at the age of four with his sister Seynabou, had the same wounds. Look at Moktar's head; it is not a true head. Look at the

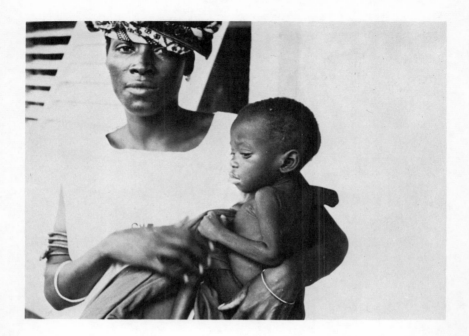

way he looks; he does not use his eyes as the other children do. It is necessary that I do not wash his eyes in the morning because he recognizes everything through his eyes. If I wash his eyes, he sees too much and then both of them are going to leave. Moktar and Babacar, they are the same child. The children have reached the age of dying; they want to depart."

The Rites of Protection "She has tried to keep them from leaving; she has had the *diat* (rite of protection) performed with the baobab (monkey-bread tree) at night. You take a piece of hard wood, well sharpened to a point; you take the child outside and measure the tibia with the wood that you have cut. You must be nude, without clothes, without *gris-gris* (protective amulets). A man of the family performs this ritual, either the father or the uncle. You choose, within the cemetery, a baobab tree which is very solid, a tall tree which resists all things, a very strong tree in order to resist the dead ones who are around it. You say the following formula over the

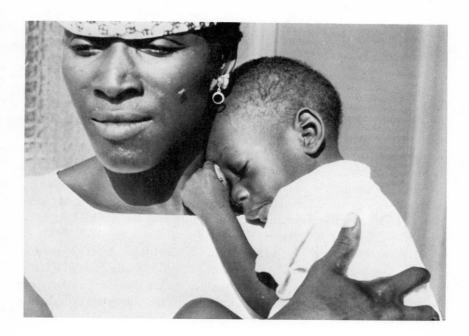

the wood that has measured the tibia; you say, "Baobab, you who are solid, who resists all things, who resists the dead ones who surround you, refuse my child. Do not make him come near you." If the child is a boy, you thrust the stake into the wood four times and then drive it in; if the child is a girl, it is done three times. Afterwards, the man returns to the house. If the baobab falls or if someone carries away the piece of sharpened wood planted within the baobab, the children die.

For the last two children, this ritual was performed; it was of no use. For these two (Moktar and Babacar), even that will not keep them. They do not have any amulets; it is not worth the effort. The amulets cannot do anything against them; they do what they want. The roots can sometimes help: you wash them with the sap of the roots. But for these two, this is not doing any good; they want to depart. . . .The dispensary is useless. The hospital? She does not know anymore; she is discouraged. It would surprise her greatly if

they could do something at the hospital; at the hospital, they do not
know about these things. Everything there is medical, and it is the
tradition which can help the children. She expects the death of the
children; it is the same sickness. They are the same signs."

The Children The story is told without apparent emotion. It
would seem that she is telling a story that does not concern her.
She speaks of what she does with the children who are going to
leave. If the child cries, she puts him on her back. She thinks that
if the child is angry, he is going to leave immediately. If she separates herself from the child, he may die. If something annoys him,
he is going away. She cannot leave them even if she sleeps. She must
never leave them; she must always be with them. It is necessary that
she does not pronounce his name; in order to speak of him, she only
points to him but he must not see it. You must not strike him; if
you do strike him, he dies.

"He knows everything; he understands all things. You say something and he understands. Yesterday, you said, 'Is he asleep?' He
heard you and last night, he did not sleep. This morning he does not
want to see anyone; he turns his head away; he is angry. You do not
know what these children want; one cannot judge them; one is not
sure of them. When he is sick, it is not the same as it is with the
other children. One does not care for him with medication. He is
very touchy; it is always necessary to please him, to talk to him."

Babacar (two and a half) is always in the arms of his mother, more
often seated on her knees. He is very thin with a wrinkled face; he
is profoundly sad. He pushes away all attempts to approach him; he
sighs or groans from time to time. His mother says, "He is annoyed
with us. I have carried him on my back very little since I became
pregnant. It is not good to carry the child when one is pregnant.
The one who is within is not pleased. He feels the warmth of the one
who is on my back; he thinks that he takes me completely away from
him. The one who is carried on my back is not content because he
senses the one within my belly. So, I do not carry him. . . ." The
child cries and she puts him on her back. I remark that "He is
pleased now. Perhaps he wants to depart because you do not put
him on your back often enough; he is alone, then he goes away. The
other one, within your belly, will not be jealous if he understands
that Babacar needs you." She smiles at my suggestions but in order
to please me, she will carry the child more often.

The Personal Problems of Fatou After she began to lose her children, she consulted the "pan" (mediums, healers) who can indicate from whence comes the evil, what sin has been committed, who in her blood line or within that of her husband ruined her fertility. "She is upset; this has done no good."

"Someone told her that she used to go out at night in order to throw out the garbage. This is forbidden to women. It is a very bad thing to do; to throw out the garbage at night is to create the "tji:d a paxer." one must not even sweep at night.

They also tell her that it is the same old man who does all of this. It is Pathé N'D · · ·, the father of her husband. He does it in order to punish her. He was not happy with his son, Gaït, the husband of Fatou. Gait did not respect him; she does not know why. She has been told a little about it, but if she has been hexed, she cannot tell. Pathé died before her marriage to Gaït. It was her father who asked for the marriage; but on her mother's side of the family, they did not agree. Her maternal uncle ("toker") was completely opposed; she does not know why, but after the marriage, he was in agreement."

Her husband is a poor peasant; he sweeps the mosque, and he kills the he-goats for the marriages. They gave him this work because he is very poor. He has three wives, but he has nothing. She is the first; the second had lost three children and she has two who are living. In her case, it is also the "tji:d a paxer." She would have liked to come to the hospital to speak of her situation. The third wife has not yet lost a child; she has only one, and she is pregnant. The three wives live on the same concession; each has her own hut and the husband has his. Beforehand, she lived with her husband at his brother's house but there was a dispute. There was a separation, and her husband himself built the huts. There is no good bed, no food, no clothing · · · there is no livestock.

"It is not good not to have children; one is not respected. If one speaks of children, she who has none cries. If they laugh at her, she cries; she thinks that if I have children, you will not do that to me. It is the same with her husband. He is not content and looks for other wives.

Bad things are happening to her. At night she dreams that she has sexual relations. If she is outside of the home, it is with her husband. If she is at home, she dreams of sleeping with her own father, with her maternal uncle, and sometimes with the men of the village. It happens frequently, but she cannot speak of it. Here at the hospital, the day before yesterday, it was with her brother; in the morning, she was ashamed, and she was ill. This has happened several times. All that, it is the child; both Moktar and Babacar are doing it; it is the same thing. The child transforms himself into her husband, her maternal uncle and, sometimes, other men who live in the village and whom the child knows. When she dreams of this, she is completely discouraged in the morning. It does not please her but she cannot refuse it. It does not enter her mind that she must refuse. The sexual act is completed; now it is happening every night. This upsets her greatly and worries her. It is the children who do this, and that is not good. They do it because they are going to depart; it is the time to die."

MEDICAL OBSERVATIONS

The two children are hospitalized with their mother. The elder, Moktar, has pyodermitis on both his legs which will be healed after several days of treatment.

The younger, Babacar, presents a state of severe malnutrition; he demonstrates the kwashiorkor syndrome. Treatment ameliorates this state fairly rapidly; his weight chart shows an upward climb the first week. Unfortunately, the child contracts the measles complicated by an ear infection. He quickly takes on again his former appearance, that of a little old man with a wrinkled face, annoyed, refusing all contact. His mother is not surprised. "It was meant to happen like this; it was the same for the one who preceded him. He was getting better and then he died." She makes these observations almost indifferent to the event.

One day she calls me. After greetings are exchanged, there is a long silence. Then she says, "Here at the hospital, you have done everything. You have given medicines, you have done everything, you have gone to too much trouble for my sake. Even if the child dies, I thank you." The interpreter explains: "She no longer trusts the child; she wants to give thanks before the child dies. She is now sure that he is going to die. That is why she thanks us. That is the custom among our people; one give thanks before the death."

Interpretation

The long story of Fatou, rich in anthropologic and cultural data, exempts us from a long commentary on it.

THE SOCIOCULTURAL FRAMEWORK

Expressed in this case history, which could have been that of numerous other African women, are several notions intertwined in a contradictory fashion that are too imprecise for our need for clarity and for our sense of logic.

Dialectic of Life and Death, Transcendence, Messages from the Spirit Beyond (the "numinose"). Life and death are poorly separated; the boundary line is imprecise. The dead continue to exist, and the living have, all during the course of their terrestrial existence, experiences of symbolic death [5]. There are cycles, more or less complex, that assure the passage of the living among the dead and of the dead among the living. The fate after death follows three fundamental models: a cyclic model with actual reincarnation; a linear model with nominal or formal reincarnation; and a mixed model which has elements taken from the two others.

The system of the Serers belongs to the first model. God, supreme force, generator of all life, has created for man two bodies: one for the world of the living and one for the world of the dead. The one that is in the world of the dead functions as the matrix. All of the stigmas that mark the body in the world of the living ("anda") also mark in the same way its double in the world of the dead ("alarira"). Children who depart quickly are marked in order to be recognized upon their return. A part of the ear or finger is cut, a cut is made on the cheek or chest or a thorn is planted in the child's foot. Although, for all, the body of the child will decay in the earth, the double within "alarira" will bear the same mutilations and the new body that it will engender will bear them also.

In regard to what interests us here, the passage from "alarira" (world of the dead) into "anda" (world of the living) begins well in advance of birth. The process begins with the state of "da:l" (which is that of the individual with his matrix and vital force being in the world of the dead); it is followed by the state of "pangol" (a word which also means serpent), a transitory state along the pathway of reincarnation. The passage to and the position of the state of "pangol" are linked to its functions: (1) it is the ancestor and hence the object of worship; it can reincarnate itself or remain "pangol"; (2) it is the companion of each individual, more or less a constituent of the visible person ("okin"); (3) it is the matrix of the person and therefore becomes the "tji:d," that is, a violent force, a whirlwind in search of a woman's belly. In order that a human being be born, three conditions are necessary: the "tji:d," the belly of a woman, and the sperm of a man. The "tji:d" also has a certain quality of the "pangol" that the child possesses at birth and which gradually becomes weaker. Before a name is given (on the eighth day), the child is not yet involved in being his own self; when he has been named, he will exist socially in so far as the reincarnation of an ancestor whose name he bears. Upon leaving, before acquiring language, the child had knowledge of the ancestors and the "pangol." As he becomes part of the social structure by means of the language, he loses the qualities of the ancestor and of the "pangol" and the knowledge assignable to them. It is only as he approaches the age of six that he becomes a person in his own right. But in some instances, this "becoming a person" cannot be produced, and the child will remain "tji:d" or "pangol" all the rest of his terrestrial life which can be a long time. Two movements are combined in this genesis: (1) the movement of the matrix in which one form engenders the other without, however, there being a brutal or definitive separation with the possibility of an arrest; and (2) a movement of fusion and separation which links two forms or several forms (ancestor, "pangol", child) or separates them; the "pangol," when the child grows older, becomes his invisible companion. Within this movement of double dimension, the situations are often ill defined; cessation, progression, or regression are set into motion by the will of transcendental forces which animate all things that live and by the varied experiences of individual existence.

By means of this ancestor-pangol which contains him in the double sense of the word, since it contains and finally becomes his companion, the individual is in constant relation with the spirit beyond (the "numinose"). He is obliged to observe the rules and the rituals in order to comply with the will of the ancestors. Voluntary, conscious transgression or unconscious and involuntary transgression calls for a penalty. When the penalty is manifested by the repeated deaths of children, the mother asks herself what the meaning of this message is. The meaning of the message will often be found with the aid of a medium (oracle) whose relations with the "numinose" are much closer.

The Child Who Returns The "tji:d", within the system of the Serers, is a moment of the "pangol," a moment which consecrates the fusion of the two elements by a third: the ancestor. The "tji:d" can depart during pregnancy, immediately after birth, very often at the time of weaning, especially if the mother is pregnant again, or later at the time of an important event in the existence of the person. He is called "tji:d a paxer," or evil spirit, because he takes away from the woman all possibility of assuming her social function of fertility.

The expression, in its meaning, is rather ambiguous. It is generally applied upon the return of the same one (the same "tji:d," the same child, the same ancestor, the same "pangol") until the moment when a conjuration, a sacrifice, or the identification of the one who is returning has put an end to this evil cycle.

The anthrologists have been able to compare the "tji:d a paxer" to the "nit-ku-bon" of the Wolofs,[3] that is, literally to the "evil person." In the case of the "nit-ku-bon" child [2, 9], there is no notion of the same one returning; but the psychopathologic picture is rather similar. The "nit-ku-bon" child is marked with the same ambiguity in regard to his situation in the world of the living. He can leave at any time. Who is he? Is he a person or an ancestral spirit, that is to say, already "nit" (a person) or refusing to become it and to engender the "nit"?

The interpretations of the child who returns vary somewhat according to the culture. In particular, the names that are given in order to keep the children and the messages addressed to the spirit beyond (the "numinose") in exchange for those it has sent vary greatly. These names make allusion to the phenomenon, indicate that the child is recognized, mark a disinterest, annihilate the human being or objectify it. The aim is always the same: to turn away the transcendental forces or to make an alliance with them.

THE PSYCHOPATHOLOGIC SYNDROME AND THE MOTHER-CHILD RELATIONSHIP

For the doctor, the case of Babacar is commonplace; it is an example of the kwashiorkor (KWK) syndrome of severe protein

[3]The Wolofs are the ethnic majority of Senegal.

deficiency due to dietary deficiency around the time of weaning. The KWK may receive other explanations. Recent studies have emphasized its psychologic and social dimensions [3,4, 7]. The KWK evokes, in effect, the well-known picture of children brutally separated from a mother with whom they had an exclusive, close, and difficult relationship.

The etymology refers to this interpretation. The word probably comes from the language of Ghana (ga) and probably has a psychological meaning: When a new child arrives, the one who has preceded him has the "kwasioko," that is to say, a state of jealousy with respect to a rival who wants to share his food, his mother, his parents. The word as a whole probably refers to the dynamics of the first child/second child. A passer-by says to a child who is crying, "Is your mother pregnant? Have you caught the *kwasioko*?" [1]

The studies made in the urban environment in Dakar confirm the psychosomatic meaning of the KWK that could then be interpreted as an expression of a more or less brutal modification of the mother-child relationship. In this perspective, the KWK might be a mental anorexia developed on a foundation of chronic malnutrition. As a matter of fact, it is observed especially in the second child of recently urbanized women for whom is posed the problem of adapting to a new relationship with the child. Under these conditions of urbanization, the woman, isolated from the collective family system that used to sustain her within her function of vector of the traditional cultural models, carries out with difficulty an essentially dual relationship. Her frustration, anguish, and aggressiveness are then borne by the child [7].

The same situation may be found in a rural environment in a state of familial impoverishment or severe economic restraints which dislocate the group. In the case of Fatou, the familial environment is very poor and the economic situation is very precarious.

A more personal psychological problem presents itself through the story and the dreams of Fatou. Dreams having a sexual content appear frequently in the country of the Serers (an ethnic group which is still matrilineal in spite of the influence of Islam). Her maternal uncle, father-substitute within the Oedipal triangle, is the chosen partner. What does this mean to Fatou—the upset blood line which merges in the same person the "tji:d-pangol" child, her husband and men of her maternal lineage (her father and her maternal uncle)? The guilt which is attached to this total form of incest is attenuated by the message which it contains. How does one describe the message of death and this sexual act with multiple partners supported by the same phallus which is also at the same time that of the child and that of the ancestors and . . . perhaps also that of Fatou?

FATOU AND THE DEATH OF THE CHILDREN.

The death of Babacar is expected; that of Moktar is also because they depart in two's. They leave, that is, they change status; they return from whence they came to go upon the earth; they become again the ancestors whom they had not stopped being.

The linear vision does not take into account an infinitely more complex representation in which the contrary aspects are not only in opposition to themselves but are also involved in the movements participating in both the dynamics of the matrix and of the fusion-separation dynamics. What relation is there between this representation and definitive annihilation, a common image of death among the western cultures; there was and there no longer is.

It is hardly possible for us to explore the experience of this mother who seems only wearied by what is happening to her, who is trying to understand the message that the ancestors are sending her through the death of the children. She has tried to decipher this message; she has not succeeded, nor have the mediums. She has resigned herself. If these two children die[4] and if with them, the third one who is within her belly dies—since it is a matter of the same one, she will be left with two children and some possibilities of fertility.

In the course of my investigation in the country of the Serers, the women always answered "yes" to the question: "Are you sad at not having had as many children as you would like?" This answer underlines the importance of the infant mortality rate and at the same time, expresses the function of the woman who wants to be fertile. The sadness and guilt are linked to fertility and to the social order more than to the problem of the individual facing death.

Bibliography

1. Autret, M., Reflections concerning the kwashiorkor syndrome, *L'enfant en Milieu Tropical*, 18 (1964), 3–13.

[4]She will leave the hospital with Moktar, Babacar, dietary advice and a little hope.

2. Collomb, H., Psychiatry and cultures (some general considerations), *Psychopathologie Africaine,* 2 (1966), 251–274.
3. Collomb, H., Valantin, S., Mattei, J. F., Dan, V., and Satge, P., Circumstances surrounding the appearance of the kwashiorkor syndrome in patients hospitalized in the pediatric service of the university hospital at Dakar *Bulletin de la Société Médicale d'Afrique Noire de Langue Française,* 14 (1969), 809–820.
4. Collomb, H., Diop, B., and Valantin, S., Protein deficiency in children, *Bulletins et mémoires de la Faculté Mixte de Médecine et de Pharmacie de Dakar,* 18 (1970), in press.
5. Collomb, H., Death in Africa, *Revue de Neuro-psychiatrie infantile,* 18 (1970), 827–836.
6. Houis, Maurice, *The Names of Individuals Among the Mossis,* Ifan, Dakar, 1963.
7. Mattei, J. P., Valantin, S., and Collomb, H., Familial environment of children attacked by the kwashiorkor syndrome, *Bulletins et Mémoires de la Faculté Mixte de Médecine et de Pharmacie de Dakar,* 18 (1970), in press.
8. Verger, P., The society "egbé orun des abiku": The children who are born to die many times, *Bulletin de l'Institut Fondamental d'Afrique Noire Dakar,* 30 (1968), 1448–1487.
9. Zempleni, A. and Rabain, J., The "nit ku bon child: A traditional psychopathological picture among the Wolofs and the Lebous of Senegal, *Psychopathologie Africaine,* 1 (1965), 329–441.

Discontinuity in the Female Role Within the Traditional Family in Modern Society: A Case of Infanticide

Phyllis Palgi, M.A. (Soc. Sc.) Doctorant (Israel)

Introduction

The richness of the cultural complexity of Israel's population, the dynamic growth and development of social institutions, the high commitment of most of the population to the declared ideals and ethos of the new State are features which both fascinate and puzzle people from many different parts of the world.

Professional persons visiting the country interested in the nature of stress accompanying human adaptation during periods of rapid change invariably pose two basic questions. Almost always one of the questions seeks an explanation for the strong feeling of solidarity in the country in spite of the diversity of family types and their obviously different modes of socialization. Usually the second question follows, namely, that in spite of the cohesive nature of Israeli society, surely, it is maintained, there must be some evidence of stress or cultural confusion which will find its expression in family pathology or conflictual behavior.

I shall first deal briefly with the social development leading to the cohesiveness of the country. The diversity and its concomitant

453

problems of acculturation will be illustrated later in this paper
through a case history of a seemingly well-integrated Yemenite family where all members were shocked back to traditionalism when
faced with their unmarried daughter's "immoral behavior" leading
to the stark act of infanticide.

The Phenomenon of Israelization

The basis for the solidarity of contemporary Israeli society was
laid down by the early pioneers in the 19th century who were motivated by a complex ideology tempered by much pragmatism. The
ideology grew out of a unique synthesism of revolt and preservation
of tradition. The revolt was at least twofold. It was against the acceptance by the Jews of the constant degradation imposed on them
as a religious minority group in Eastern Europe. The revolt was
equally against the life style in the ghetto built on religious orthodoxy
and a family structure which encouraged lasting dependencies of its
members each with their ascribed status and traditional role.

In the new country, the democratic family type became the
ideal. Innovations were not only a matter of principle but grew out
of the harsh conditions of frontier life. Children remained precious
as in the past but were encouraged to be physically tough and emotionally independent. In fact, the young people gained a new dimension of prestige for they were looked upon as the hope of the future,
a generation brought up in "normal" circumstances and with human
dignity. Thus developed the idea among the early pioneers that not
only must one meet life fearlessly but also die without fear. In
Eastern Europe death was surrounded by elaborate ritual and overt
public expressions of grief. The contrary became the ideal way of
behavior in Israel when a young person met his death in a way which
was regarded as "on behalf of the group," for example, if he died
from malaria while working in the infested fields or killed on guard
duty at some isolated settlement. The peer group was expected to
take the loss of one of their members in a stoic fashion, refrain from
expressing grief, and in particular disassociate the event from religious
or supernatural significance. As time passed and the state was established, parents were expected to behave in the same way when
following the hearse of their own son who fell in enemy action.

Religious ceremony and ritual in all spheres of life were deliberately thinned down by this group, but the power of the underlying mythos has remained till today as a driving and unifying force among all groups in the country. It is suggested here that this strange mixture of pragmatism and spiritual belief, the essential elements of the Israeli ethos, enabled the society to meet many of the diverse needs of the various groups constituting the population at different stages of its development. The veteran community continued to draw strength from this ethos and substantially sustained the high morale which diffused to all sections of the community who suffered alike from the loss of young lives due to three wars within two decades. In the same way, the holocaust survivors were given the strength and the belief in the future that it was worthwhile to rebuild their lives anew. Among other things, the middle-eastern immigrants learned that death and disease, particularly among children, can be fought and controlled.

These dynamic changes in the outer social system led to changes in the inner family relationships. Thus, in spite of the rich diversity in family structure and relationships, there is, in Israel today, an identifiable trend towards homogeneity, a convergence of the various family types starting at different points but moving centripetally towards a common type—the new Israeli family. This concept of the new Israeli family is more an ideal model than an actual one, but it is a conscious model in the minds of many, and in its incipient form may be described and analyzed. If to refer to its value system only, two main features are identifiable: one is the relative lack of bitterness between the generations, in other words, parents want for their children what the children want for themselves; second, both generations are strongly identified with the major components of the Israeli ethos.

This refers in general terms to the overall normative situation. However, while no acculturative process is free of social or psychological danger points during this process of change, some family forms are more vulnerable than others. Certain inherent features which are functional in the old culture may precisely be the ones which are a potential source of disturbance during the process of modernization, particularly for the traditional societies.

The Yemenite Community—A Traditional Culture

As a community, the Yemenites were culturally the furthest away from modern democratic society than any of the other immigrant groups. Before the establishment of the State there were about 50,000 Jews living scattered throughout 1000 villages in remote Yemen. Both Muslims and Jews, compared to other middle-eastern groups were fanatically orthodox in their religious beliefs. In both cases, religion sanctified the family structure based on a strict dichotomy between male and female roles. The sexual purity and modesty of the woman was a focal point of emotional involvement. Overtly the woman was in a subordinate position but, in fact, she was a source of dangerous power for she could pollute the entire family and even endanger the community if she violated any of the numerous taboos placed on her.

To sum up the situation, her correct sexual behavior was controlled through family structure, sanctified by the religious legal code, and reinforced by fear of supernatural powers, such as evil spirits, ghosts, and the evil eye. In Yemen, there was no difficulty in perpetuating this family structure and rigid relationships. While the Jews suffered serious disabilities as a minority group, in this area there was complete harmony between them and the ruling Muslim community.

With the establishment of the State, 45,000 Yemenites were brought on the famous "Magic Carpet" airlift to Israel. It was a severe shock for this traditional community when they arrived in the Holy Land and saw men with uncovered heads and girls dressed in shorts with exposed arms (a part of the body considered in the Middle East as especially erotic). It must have been much more incredible and startling to them than a performance like "Hair" or "Oh! Calcutta" is to anyone of the older generation now in the Western world. Like many immigrant communities in shock, the Yemenites developed their own techniques of coping with the threat to their very existence. They reacted by clinging together and so managed to preserve the traditional self-image that they were a very special people—"the people of the Book", as they were called in Yemen. At the beginning, their religious leaders protested against the Israeli laws which made polygamy and childbride marriages illegal. They also fought against compulsory education which was

introduced for girls as well as for boys. They claimed that only a
Yemenite could understand another and to this day they have the
highest rate of intra-ethnic marriages in Israel. They prefer to send
their children to religious schools and only a small proportion of
girls join the army obtaining exemption on religious grounds, low
educational level, or early marriage. Their emphasis on ethnicity is
very much against the social ideology of the country but, nevertheless, they were, by and large, rewarded by the general public with a
positive stereotype. Even those who termed them "primitive" felt
that they were a special and even a precious group.

The Attitude to Death in the Yemenite Culture

The ideal self-image of the Yemenite was that they were God-
fearing, living close to the way and spirit of the Biblical days with
their own unique cultural style. Thus, with regard to their attitude
to death, they not only accepted the religious precept that it is an
act of God but particularly emphasized the aspect of "judgment
upon sin." This was considered especially true of a death which
took place under distressing circumstances. Yemenites use an expression indicating that a home in which a recent death has taken
place is a home which has been temporarily denigrated by God.

In view of the reality that all men alike, "good" or "evil" are
immortal, the punishment concept is highly flexible in the way it is
interpreted. If a learned and just figure dies, then the community is
blamed. It will be pointed out at his funeral that the Lord took him
away because of the immorality within the group. In the ordinary
case when someone dies, it is understood that he sinned like all
mortals and would be judged accordingly in the next world. In all
cases, loud weeping and lamentations were and, to a large extent,
still are considered the appropriate behavior at funerals and for the
first three days following the burial. In Yemen there were special
women keeners for the occasion. The young generation in Israel is
already feeling uncomfortable with this behavior and often implore
their parents to restrain themselves. This was noted particularly
when a soldier son was killed.

In Yemen, the infant mortality rate was very high and culturally
constituted defense mechanisms were developed to cope with the
situation. The Jewish law that one must not mourn for a neonate

was taken very literally. In fact, according to the law, an infant which dies within 30 days after birth is placed in a special category called "Nefel." This concept implies that it is not a complete human being as it is not endowed with a soul. A great deal of folklore, as well as religious deliberations, developed around the concept of the soul and its significance in all Jewish communities. In Yemen, it was felt that a "Nefel" would not be among those qualifying for resurrection when the Messiah comes.

The passive manner in which Yemenite mothers, in the early days of mass immigration, accepted the death of an infant shocked the Western-trained medical personnel. It was not realized that a religious belief was applied in a highly adaptive manner so as to enable the family to face a harsh reality without too much damaging anxiety or guilt.

Acculturation and Its Pressures

During the last 22 years, in spite of their clannishness, many features of Israelization were absorbed, some through choice, some of necessity, and others by law. As a result we see more and more families slowly freeing or helping to free their children to participate fully in the wider society. This applies particularly to those who succeed in the academic sphere. But what is happening to those young people who are caught in a state of partial adjustment? I am referring, in particular, to the young teen-age girls who daily go out to work who are part and parcel of the modern industrial system, yet are tied and controlled by the traditional home.

I am suggesting here that there is a strain on these young people, who are caught in a state of conflict, not because of the authoritarianism of the home, per se, but because of the disharmony between the different roles which they are fulfilling, simultaneously, in their day to day life. The severity of the conflict will thus depend on the degree of incompatibility of behavior associated with the different roles and the degree of dissatisfaction which they derive from them respectively. The case which shall be presented today shows how an adolescent teenager, maneuvered into extremely incompatible roles, was brought to get rid of her newborn illegitimate baby by killing it with the help and collusion of her family. When faced with the devastating situation of a premarital pregnancy in the family, every adult member reverted to the traditional way of handling this stressful situation, namely, first denial and then infanticide.

The Case of Sara—Stress and Cultural Confusion

When I met, in the jail, this fragile, delicate looking 17-year-old girl with large stricken eyes, it was hard to associate her with the report which I had read of the brutal details of how the baby had been killed.[1]

Up to this event, this young girl, Sara, was regarded as a member of a very well-established Yemenite family. Her parents had arrived as penniless immigrants in 1948. In 1970 we see the father, the head of the household, in a well-paid skilled occupation; the mother running an efficient household; the son in the army and this daughter, Sara, in regular employment; the smaller children were attending school. A flash back enables us to trace the family development leading up to this tragic event. I shall start with the mother who was arrested together with her daughter.

The mother told how in Yemen she was married at the age of 13½ to a man who severely mistreated her. Through her unusual strength and determination, she managed to persuade her parents to obtain a divorce for her and later she became the second wife to an older, quieter man. She told how on the first night of her wedding, she unexpectedly began menstruating. She was so afraid that her husband, in his stimulated state, might touch her when she was ritually impure that she urged him to go upstairs to his first wife and spend the night there. She added that, by this move, she earned the respect both of the husband and her co-wife.

With regard to the father, he proudly explained how in Israel he was mastering his two main roles in life. At work, he had an image of himself as a successful foreman in a large modern factory while at home he was the undisputed patriarchal head. Further investigation, however, revealed that if he had any trouble at work, his anxiety became so great that once, by the time he got home, he passed out in a faint. He also suffered from repeated asthma attacks. It was he who described his wife as "primitive" and said she "knew nothing of life outside the home." But his description of her did

---

[1] The regional psychiatrist, Dr. Z. Yermelowitz, considered anthropological consultation essential in this case.

not fit at all with the strong-willed woman described above. In fact, it was she who was capable of explaining this apparent contradiction. Being in jail for some time, awaiting trial and, as she said, having to eat at the same table with prostitutes, the mother dropped her facade and for the first time exposed the cultural myth that the father was the strong patriarchal figure at home. In fact, she explained that she was the real power but behind the scene. All working members of the family handed their entire salary to her, and she thus had power over them all. She even managed to have the first wife eased out of the house and placed in a room in another neighborhood.

Let us now turn to the tragic figure of the daughter, Sara. She completed eight years at an ultraorthodox school for girls. Her school report stated that she is quiet, highly disciplined, sociable, but totally apathetic about studying. At the age of 16, her father found work for her in the same factory where he worked. She could thus be chaperoned by day as well as by night. However, she managed to joke with the male workers during coffee break, cautiously looking over her shoulder to make sure that her father could not see. She even dressed, from time to time, in slacks—behavior which was forbidden according to what she had learned at school. She was fully informed as to her rights, such as overtime pay, severance pay, etc. In other words, every day as she got on or off the bus, to and from work, she changed her role, as if she had an automatic switch, from an independent, worldly, industrial worker to an obedient, submissive daughter. Immediately on returning home, she helped her mother clean and cook and particularly served her older brother. At nights she sat with the elders of the extended family when they told legends and quoted from the Holy Books. Once, when her learned maternal uncle, the real authority figure in the family, told a story of how sinful people go to hell, Sara went into a faint. She would wake up at night terrified because of her bad dreams and then she would bribe her small brother with money to accompany her to the outside toilet. But what made Sara so anxious and apprehensive? On the surface it seems as if she suffered the same type of strain as her father. But, in fact, her situation was much more complicated. Her father felt the strain at work because he was a weak man and feared his boss who was a natural part of the modern world. When he came home, however, he could be himself for his wife played her role in such a way that he at least appeared as if he were the distant authority figure, an image which was pleasing and culturally prescribed for him. With regard to Sara, the actual work itself was no problem, she had low aspirations; but the atmosphere was fraught with danger because of the tempting nature of the free and easy relationship. She could not respond for her father was watching. At home there was little reward for her docile acceptance of the traditional role prepared for her. On the contrary, it was deeply threatening. Behind that subdued front was a highly stimulated guilt-ridden adolescent. But she played her role so well that even her astute mother thought she was so "innocent" that she allowed her to sleep in the same bed with her elder brother till the age of 13. In accordance with the cultural pattern, all sex instruction was forbidden except that she was told in no uncertain terms that a girl must be a virgin at the time of marriage. When her elder step-sister married, the principle was demonstrated by showing to Sara the blood stains on the sheets. Because of her inner turmoil she did everything to avoid gaining the slightest knowledge of biological development through the informal system. She even turned away when her girl friends gossiped about such things.

This was the emotional and social climate of Sara's life on the night when, for the first time, through chance events, she went alone to a friend's wedding, presumably chaperoned by the neighbors. A series of forbidden deeds followed. First, she disloyally responded to the approaches of a young man who was known to belong to a family with which her family was engaged in a long-standing bitter feud. Second, she left the wedding alone with him. From this point on, her story is confused. At the time of the trial she claimed this man threatened to kill her if she did not submit to his sexual advances. However, that night when she came home she was aware of one fact only—that she had lost her virginity. The stain on her underclothes was the damning evidence for her. To what extent it was seduction or not was irrelevant. She could not tell anyone about this incident. It was impossible to speak about it. There was little doubt in her mind that her father would kill the boy or perhaps her as well. She utilized to the fullest the traditional technique of denial at this moment, the moment of distress. She wiped out the event as if it had never happened and carried on with her daily routine. One Friday afternoon, nine months later, just before the Sabbath was ushered in, Sara became terribly ill with an acute stomach ache. To the total disbelief of Sara and her mother the doctor who was called in diagnosed labor pains and gave a note for admittance to the hospital.

Realizing the implications of the situation, he left saying that he would alert the social worker to arrange for adoption. But neither the mother nor the daughter was able to accept the situation and act appropriately. They played for time, apparently hoping for some magic solution to save them. In the meantime, the mother kept the father occupied in the main room assisting him with the usual Friday night prayers. Sara gave birth alone in the room under the bed so that her cries would not be heard. The mother returned, saw the child, and in a fury placed a knife in the daughter's hand, saying: "You brought this on us, you will get rid of it," and left the room because she could not bear to see more. Sara was as if paralyzed until the baby sneezed and then she killed it. When the brother came home that night, he was given a wrapped up bundle and together with his uncle told to bury it and ask no questions. In their confusion they were not very efficient; the next day it was discovered and mother and daughter were arrested.

The father first threatened to kill himself and the daughter and then he fell ill. Later he said he could not understand what had happened; perhaps something supernatural caused the pregnancy. If not, it was rape by design—this other feuding family of the boy wished to have revenge on him. Furthermore, he stated categorically that a child produced from rape is dirt, a sinful object, and must be destroyed. In Yemen the authorities would have no problem in understanding this, he claimed. The mother remained bitter and angry although she agreed that it would have been impossible for her daughter to tell what had happened that night. She felt cheated that she had always managed her family, and life in general, so successfully and now events had been stronger than her. It appears as if the family held council and it was decided that the mother would change her evidence. It was not her idea to kill the baby, she now maintained; the daughter was solely responsible. The daughter apparently obligingly changed her evidence accordingly. The rationale was simple: The mother was needed at home to look after her husband and small children. And in any case it was only Sara who really felt guilty. She told how she had sat opposite the baby, not seeing it until it sneezed. Suddenly she was confronted with the concrete evidence of her sin which she had denied for nine months and so blindly plunged with the knife to destroy it and, perhaps, all her bad thoughts as well. In other words, her real guilt was associated with her sex life and not with the killing of the baby.

Both parents maintained that nobody in the family should be punished by the Court of Law. They did what had to be done in the circumstances! As a rule in Yemen, the Jewish community was not actively punitive towards those who acted in a deviant fashion. Delinquent behavior was usually considered as a violation of religious laws. Thus one's own shame at being discovered was usually considered sufficient punishment on this earth for the wrongdoer. If necessary, he would receive his punishment in the next world. Only Sara who had studied in an orthodox Israeli school said she knew that there was no place for her in the hereafter.

Conclusion

This is an extreme case highlighting the rigid aspects of the Yemenite culture which was manifested during the process of acculturation. In Western society, cases of infanticide are usually associated with actual mental illness of the mother. In this instance, a number of members of the family were involved, directly or indirectly, in the killing which took place in the throes of a cultural crisis. This particular family, seemingly so well integrated, managed to maintain its homeostasis as a unit in Israel as long as each member rigidly conformed to his or her roles as prescribed. The rigor, with which each role was defined, allowed for no resilience so when faced with a new situation which violated a key value of theirs, they reverted to traditional behavior in its extreme form.

The case of Sara demanded a multidisciplinary approach. She had her own intrapsychic problems, the particular family dynamics needed to be interpreted but, above all, it was essential to know and understand the cultural values and functioning of the society in which she grew up.

Dying and Death: Some Hindu Cultural Rules and Paradigms

R. S. Khare, Ph.D. (U.S.A.)

The Quality of Death: A Cultural Theme

The biological death is a natural and necessary consequence (and a complementary opposite) of life. However, while the specific conception of this inevitable event may vary between cultures, there must be an internal logical correspondence between what a group of people believe about death and what they actually do about it. This structural consistency among ideas, actions, objects, and relationships is central to our discussion, for our aim here is not only to point out a set of appropriate Hindu cultural features but also to show their internal paradigmatic arrangements (between ideas and actions) that help cope with the crisis produced by death.

Generally, the attention accorded to the problem of death logically corresponds with dominant themes and purposes of life. An illustration of this point is provided by the Hindus (a cultural system that concerns us here) because it variously weaves the concept of death around life, and of life around death.[1]

The Hindu culture offers us a system that "feeds" on a complex and pervasive preoccupation with the thought and event of death, because one of the basic systemic principles is: what one receives in this life flows from one's previous lives (i.e., separated by one or more events of death), and what one gives (or does) in this life returns to those in the future (again the separation by death being inevitable). Thus, whatever be the particular philosophical system of Hinduism (or Bhuddhism or Jainism), a heavy preoccupation should be evident with either "conquering" or disregarding or transcending the barriers of death (for some comparative remarks, see Jung [12], for another anthropological study from South India, see Gough [8]). Under the (historically) later devotional emphasis, one's death became one's moment of truth. For to be able to die with "God's name on one's lips" (for example, Mahatma Gandhi died this way) means a release from the Hindu cycle of birth and death and is accordingly called "a perfect death." The belief in, and the emphasis on, "perfect death" is a major cultural theme for the contemporary Hindu. But since this death is not easily attainable by the commoner (or so the popular conception goes), a common death is more normally conceived of as a "gate way" to rebirth to continue on the cycle of transmigration.

Worldly Attachment and Death

These two conceptions of death emerge from a more basic cultural theme which lays down that death, whether of a sinner or a holy man, is always an opportunity for bettering one's next birth [12]. A death for a Hindu therefore becomes the means to a more enduring

---

[1]It is necessary that the reader be made aware of certain empirical limitations of this inquiry. Although most of the remarks remain general enough to hold for northern India, we do allude to some case specific data to illustrate the higher-caste cultural rules. These data are primarily drawn from my field researches (since 1958) in northern India in a village (Gopalpur) and among such caste groups as the Kanya-Kubja Brahmans, the Thakurs, and Kayasthas. Additionally, being an Indian and a Hindu, my cultural background should also play a role in my mode of exposition. The account is particularly incomplete with regard to lower-caste variations since we seriously lack information in this area (for the Camārs of northern India, see Cohn [2], who alludes to the presence of certain important distinctions in the lower-caste conception of afterlife). Statements in quotes, not specified otherwise, are taken from my field notes.

spiritual goal—the welfare of one's soul in the succeeding life. This interpretation of death in terms of future lives explains the Hindu's emphasis on death itself.

But the exact meaning of any particular case of death can always remain uncertain because if some of the most impure persons (sinners) have been known to die a perfect death (at least mythologically), the holiest of holy men have accidentally missed it. This enormous element of chance may be culturally "minimized" (but never eliminated). One specialized way is to attempt a symbolic "prediction" of death either of one's own or of somebody else's (see Khare [13]). But the normative procedure requires that one should be increasingly more religious, detached, pious, and devout as one advances in age so that when one's death arrives, one should feel fulfilled and should "cast off his old body like a tattered clothing" in favor of the new one, without fear or regret.

Thus the five cardinal principles that variously interrelate to govern the conception and domain of death for the contemporary Hindu are the principle of "action" (*karma*), the principle of absolute moral order (*dharma*), the principle of renunciation (*sannyāsa*), the principle of the God's grace (*kripā*), and the principle of spiritual liberation (*moksha* or *mukti*). Ideally, an increased pursuit of the first four principles results in spiritual liberation (i.e., freedom from death); but this result is avowedly difficult to obtain in practice. Only a few among thousands are supposed to achieve "good" death—like good life.[1] Out of these principles emerges a paradigm that is widely followed among the Hindus: the quality of one's death is directly related to, and is in a large measure determined by, one's emotional involvement (*samsarga*) in worldly affairs.[2] Let us follow it up.

---

[1]The preceding is an extremely simplified indication of the point that the Hindus, over the centuries, have evolved several competing and even contradictory systems of thought that conceptualize the place of death in life, whether in this world or in the realms beyond. The reader should note that the observations made so far refer towards the ideal scheme of the Hindus.

[2]It is a very comprehensive category under the Hindu thought, including all mundane aspects of life and life processes.

Death for the Householder and the Monk

Death does not mean the same thing to different members of the same society. Unlike the biological reality, the cultural conception of death becomes loaded with different values and social relationships. Feifel [5] conveyed this point by quoting " 'Death is terrible to Cicero, desirable to Cato, and indifferent to Socrates.' "

The Hindu system also postulates a "typology" of death based essentially on the distinctions of age, sex, kinship, caste, and "involvement" with worldly affairs. First, a distinction appears along the differences between the householder and the monk. The first lives a normal worldly life while the second renounces it; one leads a group life while the other wanders solitary. Accordingly, the death of a householder causes ritual pollution and mourning. Actually, a monk does not "die" but he just passes on, ideally, once and for all beyond the cycle of rebirth. The terms "dying" and "death" do not apply to him which is only logical under the conceptual scheme. If the monk symbolizes the freedom from worldly attachments, the householder symbolizes the opposite. However, it is the householder who represents the social majority and we need to consider him further.

Child's Death

But, whether a monk or a householder, everyone first passes through childhood and we must, therefore, begin our consideration with two questions that concern children and death. First, how is a child's death rated under the Hindu system? Second, what does the death mean to children? These questions should be answered in the background of the social and cultural place that the children are awarded under the Hindu culture. Against the basic Hindu rule on worldly involvement, children are found to stand only "on the fringe." A child's dependence on its parents for physical, social, and emotional security does *not* count as worldly involvement because these characteristics are regarded as part of the child's instinct [a product of ignorance, the absence of "true knowledge" (*jnana*), under the Hindu system], rather than a part of volitional behavior. Children's actions remain the responsibility of their parents. If a child is seriously ill or dies, it is predominantly because of the previous bad deeds of the parents. A child is not held morally, ritually, or socially responsible for what it does until it has grown into adolescence. But among the children, the sexual difference is not uniformly significant under various contexts, except the fact that the male children are generally prized over females.

It should be clear in terms of the worldly involvement why the Hindu regards a child's death to be not as ritually polluting as that of an adult. A child's death produces insignificant mourning when compared with the normal ten-day period for the adult. However, the mourning period increases with a child's transition into adolescence which is marked by a series of rites that successively announce his increased worldly involvement. Orenstein [17] recently noted this feature in textual (*shāstric*) studies as well. (However, it should be pointed out that my emphasis remains on empirical findings rather than on textual propositions, particularly since the two versions may sometimes contradict each other.)

The death of a child is not ritually differentiated along the lines of sex although the loss of a son is *felt* more in a society which assigns numerous important roles to a male person. This lack of recognition of sexual dichotomy for the child's death relates with other cultural features. For example, a dead child is not cremated in northern India, it is either buried in a safe place or (depending on the "cause" of death) it is consigned to a river. (A dead monk's body, let us note, also does not get cremated.) A child's body does not have to be treated with those numerous mortuary rites that appear at the death of an adult, and normally the path that a child's soul takes is not clearly specified. The heaven, the specified worlds of ancestors and manes and the domains of "tortured spirits" (*bhūta, prêta,* and *jinn*) are not clearly mentioned in the context of a child's death. No obsequies are therefore required for the child that help lodge the spirit of an adult person in the "world of ancestors."

The above characteristics require that we answer two questions: What happens to a child's soul under Hindu system? Why is the child's soul treated so differently from that of an adult? In answer to the first question, since the principle of transmigration must go on, the child's soul, I am told by my informants, returns to that cycle. It automatically happens with the child because it does not become entangled in the worldly affairs. It is because of the latter,

I was told, that a child's soul does not have to go either "up" (i.e., in heaven) or "down" (i.e., in the domain of tortured spirits), but it must simply be reborn.

The second question is also answered in the same terms but with a further elaboration of the fundamental principle. A child, unlike an adult, not only remains free from the worldly attachments but is also free from the emotional attachment (*moha*) to its own body. It is either unaware or only partially aware of its physical existence. This difference between the child and the adult is held responsible for the different modes of body disposal. An adult's soul hovers over his dead body for some time and the cremation is regarded necessary to destroy this bondage. A child's soul, on the other hand, being free of this attachment does not require that its erstwhile "abode" (body) be destroyed through fire.

Although the indigenous scheme consistently explains the above characteristics of a child's death in terms of the "principle of attachment," we may also allude to some underlying logical relationships that relate with wider data. First, we note that a child is conceived of as standing only on the "fringes" of both life and death (although one must first be aware of life to be aware of death) providing support to the observation that one's awareness about life and death proceeds hand in hand and that death receives increasing conscious attention as one (which is at least true in the case of a Hindu) gets older. The duration and complexity of rites are accordingly minimal (or absent) with stillborn children and miscarriages. This feature is also noted by Hertz [11], and Diskin and Guggenheim [3] for other societies. However, there seems to be very little attention given to studying a child's death and we need more systematic information from other societies before we can rigorously compare it with the Hindu scheme. For example, a limited contrast between the Hindu and the American societies is suggested when we are told that a loss of a child is found to be greater by the Americans because a high value is placed by them on having a full life, according to Glaser and Strauss [7].[1]

---

[1] Although more work is required, one might conjecture that a low ritual concern expressed by the Hindus on a child's death may be, at least in part, related to the demographic fact of high infant mortality coupled with a higher fertility rate. Losing a child becomes a necessary fact of married life although it is true at the same time that a great ritual concern is shown to keep a child alive. But once dead, the simplified procedures for physical and spiritual disposal apply to a child producing a logical congruence with the larger scheme of handling death.

The Child's Conception of Death

When we come to study the child's discovery and conception of death, we are disadvantaged in another way. The Hindu culture does not provide any widely shared detailed or systematic explanation to account for this aspect. A child is considered to be surrounded by "unawareness" and ignorance (*ajñāna*). Before a child's role is directly linked with mortuary rites [which is only after the initiation (for the boys) or the marriage (for the girls) for the twice-born caste groups], little information is provided on how a child's images and conceptions about death grow. If some such information exists, empirical research is needed to bring it out. In contrast, a great deal of attention is being given to this topic in the west, a point that becomes evident after reading Nagy [15, 16], Grollman [10], Anthony [1], Feifel [4], Gorer [9], Gartley and Bernasconi [6], and Vernon [18]. These studies suggest that the child in western cultures gradually starts to formulate and consolidate his conception of death (of others and of his own), working around a set of appropriate cultural symbols (e.g., sleep, lying, breathing, closed eyes, immobility, coffin, journey, mass, graveyard, purgatory, mourning procession, etc.), first in a matter-of-fact manner and later on with explicit emotions.

It is not hard to guess that there must exist a comparable scheme marking the emergence and growth of the Hindu child's conception of death. Since there is no specified and overt mode of learning and socializing about the death among the children (as they are normatively kept "away" from the dying, the dead, and the death-related ceremonies, until they are sufficiently grown-up), it should be useful to find out how the idea of death takes shape among the higher caste as against the lower-caste children. Some very tentative observations that emerge from my field work in a north Indian village (Gopalpur) indicate that lower-caste children are found to use more freely the words related to "death" and dying while speaking to their playmates. It may be partly because these children "receive" such verbal expressions from their elders when being scolded or punished. This linguistic behavior could be symptomatic of other substantive cultural experiences that a lower-caste child comes face to face with during and after each death, especially since a lower-caste child is not as strictly excluded from the dead and his mourning as is the one of higher caste. A very common analogy that is employed to "explain" to children (both of high and low caste) the disappearance of a dead person consists in saying that so-and-so has "journeyed to heaven." If the children ask more, they are either dismissed or are provided with a distraction. A discussion of death (like sex) is considered both inappropriate and unnecessary in front of children. Thus, we may note that the "ignorance" (as defined by the culture) of a child is employed to "explain" both the cultural significance of a child's death and the psychological attitude toward a child's awareness about death.

Adaptive Mechanisms for Coping with Dying

We will here consider the questions: How does a Hindu prepare himself to face death? How does he attempt to improve the quality of his (or one of his kith or kin's) death? However, before we consider some specific adaptive mechanisms, we must note that cultural adaptation normally corresponds with cultural "causation" of death. Normal deaths call for normal modes of adaptation whereas abnormal causes of death call for specialized adaptations. Very briefly, therefore, we must further recognize different "types" of deaths among the Hindus.

There is a basic distinction recognized between the "timely" (*kāla*) and "untimely" (*akāla*) deaths of adults. However, one's chronological age is not the sole determinant for such a concept of "timely" death. For example, the death of a woman (however young in chronological age) while her husband is alive is always a timely death; actually, it is a moment of rejoicing (as the funeral procession indicates) because it averts for her the possibility of becoming a widow (a status full of hardships). On the other hand, when a man dies at a ripe old age, his death is considered timely.

Untimely deaths are produced when a person dies through what the Hindus call "unnatural" means which include all violent deaths (either self-inflicted or those inflicted by others), accidental deaths, and deaths of such indirect means as poisoning. A great deal of attention is paid under the Hindu ideological system to discourage such deaths for they are supposed to bring about spiritual degradation. But the practice, as always, differs from the ideal.

Unless the death is sudden, preparing a dying person to accept death in a ritually appropriate condition is as important under the Hindu system as it is to offer mortuary rites afterwards. Adaptive mechanisms may be primarily classified for our purposes in terms of two interrelated aspects—social and religious and ritual. For the lack of space we will summarize them under the following points:

(A) SOCIAL ASPECT

As soon as a person is determined to be irreversibly sick, telegrams and "express-delivery" letters go out to most important kin (usually to brothers, sisters, sons, and daughters) to hurry home to be at the bedside of the dying relative. (Such letters may be sent out after one of their four corners is torn or cut—a symbolic means of announcing the death.)[1] In more symbolic language, the kinship network tightens itself at the apprehension of losing a "link." It also is evidently a psychological preparation for the individual (whether he is the one dying or he is the one who is surrounding the dying). It is the time when appreciation of the dying person's social performance begins to be glorified "within his earshot," with all his lapses of the past being overlooked (the similar point is expressed in Latin for the western culture: *dē mort'uis nil nisibon'um.*   Despite the religious emphasis on detachment, the dying person appreciates being surrounded by his relatives, and the coming together of relatives and sharing the grief of death for ten days constitute the major mechanism for social adaptation. New social roles are carved out; property inheritance questions are decided; and appropriate emotional adjustments are made.

B. RELIGIOUS AND RITUAL ASPECT

1. Sacred Surroundings The immediate physical surroundings of the dying person are purified. He is "brought down" from the bed (a symbol of "returning the dying to the earth") and is placed on the ground plastered with cow-dung paste (a purifying substance under the Hindu system) and sprinkled with water from the Ganges. The enclosure where the dying is placed is emptied of other material goods. The entire house is also adapted to the imminent death: the cooking and eating is brought to a complete halt, the fire of the

[1] Such customs are regional and group-specific, and I am reporting it for the Kayasthas of Uttar Pradesh. The custom may actually be wider in distribution in northern India. In order to study the Hindu death it should be useful to know such comparative modes of communication (with symbolisms involved in them) under birth, marriage and death.

hearth (a symbol of normal life) is put out, and the family deities
are sent to a temple (for the house will get polluted as soon as the
death has occurred). All sacred, auspicious, and normal activities
are instantaneously stopped. Now clothes are not to be washed nor
are the clean or new ones to be worn for the specified mourning
period. Finally, the children are hustled and sent to a neighboring
family (except of course the infants who must remain with their
mothers) for the reasons already provided; and all the adults, men
and women, come to surround the dying person (or they remain
nearby) with a division on the basis of sex, all men and all women
form two exclusive groups almost imperceptibly (see also Khare [14].

2.   *Sacred Gifting* The dying person, whether conscious or unconscious, may be also called upon to give several gifts (*dān*) in
quick succession to a Brahman priest who recites the appropriate
sacred verses. These pious acts (see the *karma* notion presented
earlier) are supposed to help accrue some further religious merit for
the dying person, "for such acts are one's only true companion in
the other world." The gifts given away on such occasions clearly
fall under symbolic and substantive categories. The gifting of a cow
and of gold, silver, and money are considered especially efficacious.
But since the poor cannot afford these costly items, they may give
only symbolic or token gifts.

3.   *Purifying the Dying* The religious and ritual preparations
around, and in relation to, the dying person start simultaneously.
The sacred scriptures (particularly the Gītā and the Rāmāyana) are
brought out and loudly recited until moments before the death.
(Once the death has occurred, these sacred objects cannot be touched
because of the ritual pollution brought about by the death). It is
done in the hope that the sacred words will enter the dying person's
"ears" (consciousness) and will help him attain a "quality" death.
A priest or a relative performs this religious act. If the family belongs to Vaishnavism (a religious sect), the use of such symbols of
purity as water of the river Ganges and *tulsi* (Oscimum sanctum) leaf
is made. Both of these items are dropped in the dying person's mouth
since the mere contact of these objects is supposed to help the dying
person's body and soul. Briefly, therefore, an attempt is made to
create a highly religious environment so that all the major senses of
a dying person may become simultaneously engaged in the religious

domain and help him in his spiritual welfare.

Adaptive Mechanisms after Death

As the above preparations proceed, anxiety gives way to grief and grief to loud weeping and crying as soon as the death has occurred. Symbolically, then, in a sense, "the normal time passage stops," at least until the corpse is taken out to the cremation ground, and even the immediate neighborhood may drop cooking and eating for that period. When considering symbolisms that either directly represent or become associated with death, the Hindu culture draws upon physical, biological, social, and astrological dimensions to produce a consistent system of symbolic communication. If death is something not to be discussed openly, it can always safely remain imminent through this "code" language. Thus the symbols may be taken from colors (black), geographic directions (south), natural events (storms and lightning), edibles ("bitter rice," whole *Urd* lentils), astrological signs (falling stars; inability to see the north star), social acts and events (breaking of a mirror or a utensil; journey, and demolition of a house); signs of senescence (gray hair, weak limbs, failing senses), and certain birds and animals (crow, vulture, jackal, etc.).

Regaining social and ritual normalcy, however, begins almost at the same time the death occurs. The main stages of recovery are taking out of the dead body to the cremation ground, the cremation, the bath on return by the cremators, the vigil by the chief mourner, and most importantly, the ten-day *reconstruction* of the dead's "essential body" (*sukshma déha*) in the other world by offering him rice balls through the priest-presided ancestral rites (*srāddha*).[6] However, the passage of each day is a milestone in the recovery for both the dead and the alive. After ten days, the dead passes from the most insecure stage of wandering spirits (*prêta*) into that of an ancestor (*pitra*), and the kin of the dead after performing the ten days

---

[6] The following sequence is recognized for the "reconstruction" of the dead's body: the rice balls offered on the first day are supposed to form the dead person's head; second day, neck and shoulders; third day, chest and heart; fourth day, back; fifth day, navel area; sixth day, waist, hips, and sexual organs; seventh and eighth days, thighs and legs; and ninth and tenth days, hunger and thirst. Let us here note that the normal eating pattern returns to the kin of the dead as soon as the latter is able to "eat" in the other world. For these ten days, the mourners subsist, usually eating only once in 24 hours.

of mortuary rites regain their normal cooking and eating (and some other normal social) activities. Some restrictions may, however, persist for one full year.

Implication

Being as complex as the Hindu death rites are, the above is barely an indication of the kinds of rules and paradigms that explicitly or implicitly exist to help accept the fact of death. Much more systematic work, however, remains to be done to fully understand the significance and limitations of the indigenous scheme in terms of the findings of modern psychology and psychiatry. Little is known about those aspects of the Hindu death that the culture does not formalize but only keeps entailed or implicit. Such features may exist at both the conscious and unconscious levels and collective and individual levels, and we need to study the problem at all of these levels before we can hope to discover a more complete system of thought and action that surrounds the event of death among the Hindus.

Bibliography

1. Anthony, Sylvia, *The Child's Discovery of Death*, Harcourt, New York, 1940.
2. Cohn, Bernard, Changing Traditions of a Low Caste, in *Traditional India: Structure and Change*, Milton Singer, Ed., American Folklore Society, Philadelphia, 1959.
3. Diskin, Martin and Guggenheim, Hans, The Child and Death as Seen in Different Cultures, in *Explaining Death to Children*, Earl A. Grollman, Ed., Beacon Press, Boston, 1967.
4. *The Meaning of Death*, Herman Feifel, Ed., McGraw-Hill, New York, 1959.
5. Feifel, Herman, Death, in *The Encyclopedia of Mental Health*, Vol. II., Albert Deutsch and Helen Fishman, Eds., Franklin Watts, New York, 1963.
6. Gartley, Wayne and Bernasconi, Marion, The concept of death in children, *J. Genet. Psychol.*, CX (1967), 71–85.
7. Glaser, Barney and Strauss, Anselm, The social loss of dying patients, *Am. J. Nurs.*, LXIII (1964), 119–121.
8. Gorer, Geoffrey, *Death, Grief and Mourning*, Doubleday, New York, 1965.
9. Gough, Kathleen, Cults of the Dead Among the Nāyars, in *Traditional India: Structure and Change*, Milton Singer, Ed., American Folklore Society, Philadelphia, 1959.
10. Grollman, Earl A., The Ritualistic and Theological Approach of the Jew,

in *Explaining Death to Children*, Earl A. Grollman, Ed., Beacon Press, Boston, 1967.

11. Hertz, Robert, *Death and the Right Hand*, Cohen and West, Aberdeen, England, 1960.

12. Jung, Carl G., *Psychology and Religion: West and East*, translated by R. F. C. Hull, Pantheon Books, New York, 1958.

13. Khare, R. S., Prediction of death among the Kanya-Kubja Brahmans: a study of predictive narrative, *Contributions to Indian Sociology, New Series*, (1967), 1–25.

14. Khare, R. S., The Perennial Food: Symbolic and Substantive Structures of the Hindu Culinary System, unpublished manuscript, 1972.

15. Nagy, Maria, *The Child and Death*, Brenz, Budapest, 1936.

16. Nagy, Maria, The child's theories concerning death, *J. Genet. Psychol.*, LXXIII (1948), 3–27.

17. Orenstein, Henry, Death and kinship in Hinduism: structural and functional interpretations, *American Anthropologist*, 72 (1970), 1357–1377.

18. Vernon, Glenn M., *Sociology of Death: An Analysis of Death-Related Behavior*, Ronald Press, New York, 1970.

The Reaction of Peruvian Families
to the Disablement of the Father[1]

Renato Castro de la Mata, M.D. (Peru),
Maria A. Silva de Castro, M.D. (Peru),
Alegria Majluf, M.S. (Peru), and Luis Estrada, Ph.D. (Peru)

This chapter is based on a study of family functioning carried out between 1959 and 1962 on Peruvian families [1, 2, 3, 4]. It was thought that a situation that placed a family under heavy stress would offer good opportunities for examining role function and family homeostasis. From previous research experience with Canadian families a sudden and severe disablement of the father was selected as the stressful situation likely to yield the most information.

Selection of Families

The families were selected on the basis of the following criteria: intact families containing at least one child; the absence of overt psychiatric symptoms in any of the members; the presence of a sudden and severe physical disablement of the father with a less than 75% recovery of his previous capacity. Disablement in this series included hemiplegias quadriplegias, double detachment of the retina, and traumatic amputation of limbs. The families came from three socioeconomic classes: Indians (the lowest group), Obreros

[1] This study was made possible by a Grant from the Foundation's Fund for Research in Psychiatry.

(the next lowest), and Empleados (the middle class).[2] The term "Obreros" is roughly equivalent to "blue-collar worker" and "Empleados" to "white-collar worker." A total of 21 families, comprising 135 individuals, were studied, made up of six Indian, eight Obreros, and seven Empleados families.

Methodology

I. THE CLINICAL STUDY

A.   Personal interviews with each family member carried out whenever possible at home and aimed at eliciting as complete biographical data as possible.

B.   Visits to the home in order to observe the family in interaction.

Conducting the inquiry within the home helped to diminish the formal aspects of the doctor-patient relationship. The total number of hours spent with the family varied greatly, but no less than 50 hours were given to direct study of the family and the individual family members.

II. THE PSYCHOLOGICAL STUDY

A.   Adults were tested by the TAT, the Michigan Picture Test (MPT), the SACKS (a specially designed questionnaire), and a Sentence Completion Test. (With the Indians, the Rorschach was used in place of the MPT.)

B.   Children were tested by the Draw-a-Family, the Draw-a-Person, the MPT, and structured doll play (SPD). (With Indian children, the CAT and story telling were substituted for the MPT and the SPD.)

The reason for not using certain tests with Indians related to the test material being incompatible with Indian culture and therefore conducive of cultural artifacts.

---

[2]It is not possible to speak of "Indian" from a racial point of view. Intermixing between Indian and Spaniard took place from the time of the conquest and continued for a long time. Today, the term "Indian" refers to a "mestizo" of white and Indian blood and is used to denote someone originating in a rural area, possessing physical features that are predominantly Indian, speaking only the Indian language, or, if bilingual, speaking this at home, manifesting certain psychological characteristics generally associated with this particular group, dressing in a distinctive fashion different from the urban style, habitually chewing coca leaves, and residing in small rural communities.

Findings

This study of Peruvian families has made it abundantly clear that when dealing with family dynamics in a large geographical area, one has to think in terms not of one but of several cultures, each with their own ethnic, social, and economic characteristics.

I. TYPES OF FAMILY FUNCTIONING

The investigation has disclosed three main types of functioning in the Peruvian family labeled according to the paternal attitude: the despotic family, the patriarchal family, the companionate family.

A. *The Despotic Family.* In the despotic family, the father provides, makes decisions, sets the discipline for the family, and demands absolute submission from it. The mother dispenses love and physical attention to the family. The children are objects on whom the father exerts authority and to whom the mother dispenses love and are potential helpers. At the unconscious level, the father demands unilateral and unconditional love and admiration without any inclination to give anything in return. The mother demands security and an opportunity to give and the children expect love and security. At the conscious level there is good complementarity of roles. Fathers are submitted to, mothers dispense love, and children submit to the father and receive love from the mother. The roles are clear-cut, well recognized and accepted. It would seem that on an individual basis, the deeper wishes of the members are at least partially met: fathers get cared for, mothers obtain some measure of security and an opportunity to give, while children find love in the mother. However, in the functioning of the family *as a whole* and in the interaction of roles, there are profound sources of dissatisfaction. The father's punishing and threatening behavior pushes the family away from him; he expects love but provokes fear. The mother does not give freely but is forced to do so, and she cannot defend the children against the father. The children are loved by the mother but threatened by the father and since the mother submits to him and cannot defend them they are left basically frustrated. As a result, there is internal strife within the family and strong undercurrents of hate and divisiveness with the father on one side and the mother and children aligned against him on the other, the total picture being one of general insecurity.

B. The Patriarchal Family. In the patriarchal family, the father provides, makes decisions, and sets the discipline. The mother dispenses love and physical attention to the family. The children submit to the father and are loved by the mother; they are also regarded as objects of self-realization and potential help by both parents. Unconsciously, the fathers demand love and admiration but with a certain readiness to give; the mothers demand security and an opportunity to give; and the children expect love and security. At the conscious level there is good complementarity and roles are clear-cut, well recognized, and accepted. At the unconscious level, there is also a relatively large measure of good complementarity; fathers are cared for, mothers have a measure of security and an opportunity to give, and children find love in the mother and a certain amount of love in the father. In the functioning of the family *as a whole,* there are fewer sources of dissatisfaction than with the despotic family. The father's behavior, tinged with some readiness to give, gets him, if not love, at least respect. The mothers can give more freely and can defend the children, and the children can feel more secure. The family begins to become a goal in itself, and there is greater readiness among the members to feel part of the group with a history and tradition behind them and a purposeful future in front of them. Members are not fragmented by individual reactions, satisfying and frustrating each other, but interact more widely to the satisfaction of the group as a whole. In this sense, they are better off than the despotic family. Hate is better managed and less in evidence and so there is less strife, insecurity, and splitting up.

C. The Companionate Family. In the companionate family, the father provides, but decisions and discipline are the result of the father-mother team. The mother dispenses love and attention and the children are objects of family realization. Unconsciously, the father demands love but is ready to give as much in return; mother asks for security and opportunities to give; and children expect love and security. Consciously and unconsciously there is a good complementarity of roles and role interactions are satisfying to the members. Father and mother both give love and obtain love and children feel secure. The family is a goal in itself and its members feel part of a solid group without splitting. There is little strife and a large measure of security.

II. OUTSIDE AFFILIATIONS IN RELATION TO FAMILY TYPE

The behavior of nuclear family groups toward agencies external to them reflects the behavior of members within the family.

A. The Despotic Family and Outside Affiliations. Despotic families are singularly isolated; the family as a group does not relate to outside agencies while individual members do. Friends are friends of the father or of the mother but not of the family as a group. Religious worship is a matter for the individual or for the preservation of a family front; membership in a community organization is also related to individual incentive rather than to family action. The fathers often use outside agencies to escape from closer contact with the family. The status of the group is very much centered around the figure of the father in terms of his accomplishments and his financial position. The weakness in external solidarity as manifested in affiliations within the extended family and in respect for ancestors reflects itself in the weakness of internal ties so that children at adolescence tend to break away from the family and to sever relationships with each other and with the parents. Often, the only contact that remains is with the mother who serves as a cohesive factor, and when she has gone, the family splits itself up into its constituent members.

B. The Patriarchal Family and Outside Affiliations. Patriarchal families are also isolated from outside agencies. The same relationship described above for the despotic family is equally true for this type of structure. However, the home is more of a point of reference for family members than in the other case and there is more group consciousness. The father is still psychologically distant and the family still revolves around the father's interests as if it were his possession. He tends to be rather proud of it and to show it off for which the family is grateful to him. Status is achieved not only by what father can do himself but also by what father can do through the family. The relationship towards ancestral and contemporary families is also better, and stronger ties are maintained than in the previous group. The mother is, again, the cohesive factor but the family does not split wide open in her absence.

C. The Companionate Family and Outside Affiliations. Companionate families relate well to outside agencies. Friendships, religious worship, community groups, and outings are family affairs and not those of individual members. The home is the point of reference for family members. The family is not a possession of the father but shared among the members. Status is a cooperative characteristic and one and each member contributes to it. The relationship to ancestral and contemporary families is close and both parents add to the cohesiveness of the group.

III. FAMILY OUTLOOK AND FAMILY TYPE

Outlook on life, Weltanschauung, and time orientation also reflect intrafamily relationships.

The world of despotic families is a dreadful one in which life is hard, progress constantly hampered by evil forces, and the future is ominous. The world of patriarchal families is less terrible because although life is hard, it is worth fighting for and the future depends on one's efforts. The world of companionate families is a pleasant one since life can be conquered and the future is very promising. Distrust pervades the relationships of despotic families, misgivings those of patriarchal ones, and optimism those of companionate families. Despotic families are present oriented whereas patriarchal and companionate families are future oriented.

In summary, one could say that the father in the despotic family does not appear to care for his family; that the father in the patriarchal family seems to own his family; and that in the companionate type, the family is not a possession of the father but a corporation of members.

IV. SOCIOECONOMIC CLASS AND FAMILY TYPE

The Peruvian families that we have studied roughly range themselves along this dynamic spectrum extending from the unintegrated despotic type to the highly integrated companionate type, with the patriarchal variety at some point between them on this scale of interaction. The despotic type was the only one found among Indians, the patriarchal one was prevalent among Obreros families, and the companionate type was observed only among Empleado families. Elements of the patriarchal attitude in the father were beginning to appear in two Indian families, the only ones in the upper economic bracket of their class.

The relationship between types of family dynamics and socioeconomic class is summed up in Table 1.

Table 1 Relation between Family Dynamics and Socioeconomic Class

	Indian N = 6		Obrero N = 8		Empleado N = 7	
	Rich	Poor	Rich	Poor	Rich	Poor
Despotic	0	4	3	3	0	2
Patriarchal	2	0	2	0	1	1
Companionate	0	0	0	0	2	1

This indicates that a better integrated type of family tends to occur in the higher socioeconomic class but that poorly integrated families may be found in all socioeconomic groups.

There is a highly significant feature with regard to acceptance of these patterns of family dynamics. The despotic type is accepted by the subcultural Indian, reluctantly so by the subcultural Obrero, and frowned upon by the subcultural Empleado, not only in terms of the members of the subculture but also by the members of the family. The Indian family expects the father to behave that way, the Obrero family complains about the father's behavior, and the Empleado family condemns the father when in all three cases the father shows a despotic disposition. Indian families, for instance, do not consider that playing with children is appropriate behavior for the father. Furthermore, only fathers of Empleado families ever acknowledge the fact that they behave badly towards their family.

How can one explain the role played by socioeconomic factors in the emergence of subcultural types of family functioning? The answer may lie in the fact that attitudes are learned in childhood, mainly through interaction with the parents, and are thus perpetuated from generation to generation. A man who has learned his role of father from a despot and who, at the same time, yearns to be loved, will try to obtain love through force. A woman who has learned her role from a submissive mother and who yearns to feel love and security, will submit in order to obtain both. The result could be that in each case there is a frustration of the basic wishes; care is obtained but not love and this would inevitably lead to resentment and family strife.

If the woman had an opportunity to demand love and security because she is free to choose the man who can best give them to her, this might well force the man to modify his attitude, lessen his demands, and give more. This would be more likely to gratify both their basic wishes; the man would obtain love and care and the woman love and security on a more genuine basis and with less resentment and family strife.

Large urban centers give the woman better opportunities to prepare herself for her life struggle, a clearer awareness of her status, and a chance to challenge the man to give more and ask for less. This soon develops into a self-perpetuating mechanism that becomes the approved pattern of family functioning for a given subculture and this, in turn, gives children an opportunity to test parental behavior against the cultural background. A dissatisfying parental role will tend to provoke negative identification and when the cultural checks are added, the self-perpetuating mechanism gains momentum.

This last fact may explain the companionate behavior of the two fathers who descended from despotic families and whose wives were "hard to get." On the other hand, the two despotic fathers from the Empleado group were married to women who were not prepared for the life struggle and were essentially passive.

V. THE DISABLED FATHER IN RELATION TO FAMILY TYPE

The response of the family to a disabled father varied in the different types of families.

A.   The Disabled Despotic Father. Despotic fathers identify themselves and are identified by the family solely as providers. They themselves stress this particular aspect, paying little attention to the role of dispensing of love, counsel, and support. Hence, when they become disabled and lose the capacity to provide, they are unable to identify themselves within the family nor can they be identified by the other members within the family. They are gradually pushed out of the family with the members explicitly stating their wish to get rid of them. Those who are compelled to assume the father's lost role do so under protest since they inherit the feeling of being used and abused.

There is another point worth mentioning. Despotic fathers who after disablement change their previous attitude and begin to approach the family in a more positive way are accepted, and family functioning may improve to a level better than before disablement. But, in general, a despot who does not provide is not tolerated by the family.

B.   The Disabled Patriarchal Father. Patriarchal fathers who, in addition to providing, are ready to give some measure of counsel and

support are likely to be better accepted when they become disabled. Since providing is not the only aspect of his role, the father can re-identify himself within the family and be better identified by its members. Nevertheless, members of the family who are forced to assume the role of providers tend to do so with resentment.

C.   *The Disabled Companionate Father.* Companionate fathers have no difficulty in identifying themselves within the family after disablement nor does the family experience any difficulty in accepting them. Since no special emphasis has been placed on the partial role of provider, when this is lost the other partial aspects of the paternal role allow the family to accept him as a functioning member. Members of the family who have to take on the task of providing do so without difficulty. The family may express this in words to the effect that "you did your share and now it is our turn."

The study also brought out the relationship between self-esteem and role function. In the last analysis, the father's basic role is to provide and when this is lost, he may become depressed. This is of importance for rehabilitation programs since the family's attitude may lessen or increase the father's feelings of inadequacy and depression and, in the long run, may determine the success or failure of rehabilitation. Fathers who solely identify themselves and are identified by the family with providing are much less able to tolerate any diminution in their capacity to earn and, hence, they adopt an "all or nothing" attitude towards rehabilitation as does the rest of the family. This may lead to a refusal to accept rehabilitation and therefore to a reduced work capacity.

Bibliography

1. Castro de la Mata, R., Impact of a sudden severe disablement of the father upon the family, *The Canadian Medical Assoc. J.*, 82 (1960).
2. Castro de la Mata, R., *Dynamics of the Peruvian Family*, Proceedings, III World Congress of Psychiatry, 1961.
3. Castro de la Mata, R., Aspectos psiquiatricos de la rehabilitacion, *Revista del Cuerpo Medico*, Hospital, Obrero, 1962.
4. Castro de la Mata, R., Dinamica de la familia peruana, *Revista de Ciencias Psicologicas y Neurologicas, Facultad de Medicina*, U. N. M. S. M., Lima, (1964).

Symposium: The Dying Child in an African Hospital

Death of a Child in Nigeria

T. Asuni, M.D. (Nigeria)

Clinical Case Presentation

A ten year old boy, S. F., sustained a 40% burn accidentally and was rushed to the Aro Hospital in Abeokuta in Nigeria. He appeared to be responding to treatment but then took a sudden turn for the worse after several months in hospital and died 5½ months after the injury in July, 1971.

S. F. was the third of six children in his family, the ages ranging from two to 16 years. The two older ones, both girls, were away at boarding school so S. F. was the oldest child living at home. There had been one previous death in the family of a second-born son at the age of eight months. The father, age 43, was a clerical worker whose job necessitated him working in a different town over a 100 miles away. Mother, age 40, lived alone with the four remaining children and engaged in small trading. The relationship between the parents was reported to be good even though they lived apart. S. F. was apparently an average Nigerian boy who was said to get on well with his peers.

The accident took place on the thirteenth of January. The mother said that she had intended to stay at home on this particular day for some inner reason that she could not disclose. A naming ceremony for a newborn baby of another tenant in the house was scheduled for this day, but this was not her reason for staying at home from work. One of her neighbors, Mrs. X, had twice asked her why she had not gone to work, and she felt vaguely uneasy about this question. A ram was being barbecued when S. F. inadvertently was sprinkled with kerosene and was set on fire. Only his mother was around to help him, but later Mrs. X helped to rush him to hospital. The mother reported that her co-tenants seemed hardly affected at all by the incident and later only a few of them visited S. F. in hospital.

During the terminal period in hospital, S. F. had several nightmares, possibly part of a delirium, during which he called out Mrs. X's name imploring her to release him. With the sudden change in his condition for the worse the hospital stopped mother from visiting for a while. She was declaring that S. F. had been bewitched.

This belief was derived from a male relative on the father's side, a 42-year-old man, also a clerical worker, who said that the witchcraft affecting S. F. had been revealed to him in a dream. He sought permission from the hospital to take S. F. home for traditional treatment by healers who would be able to counteract the witchcraft. He believed that as long as this was working, the medical treatment in hospital would be ineffectual.

After S. F.'s death, mother consulted a herbalist who confirmed that death had taken place through witchcraft. There seemed to be no other reason for the fatal change in the boy's condition. Mother then recalled that Mrs. X had seemed jealous over S. F.'s progress in school where he was doing much better than her own child whom she frequently punished for his poor academic performance. S. F.'s mother was disturbed by this invidious comparison and the relation between the two women became strained although they continued to be superficially pleasant to each other until the accident occurred. After S. F.'s death, Mrs. X, a small trader and wife of a teacher, moved out of the house and this was regarded by S. F.'s mother as an indication of guilt. Both she and her husband had become increasingly anxious and concerned about the safety of their other children and had also been considering a move to some other area.

The staff nurse in charge of the ward confirmed that S. F. had been responding to treatment initially but had then started to refuse his food especially when his mother was left alone to feed him.

The nurse felt that because of mother's anxiety and nervousness, S. F. played up with her. Her visits generally managed to disturb her son who seemed an intelligent child, and he would become "hysterical" when she was around him. The nurse supposed that S. F. must have been told tales about Mrs. X. before the fire accident and that this carried over to his delirium. During his conscious periods he would talk of Mrs. X's envy and the nurse thought that his preoccupation with this must have been derived directly from his mother.

The autopsy disclosed cortical necrosis of the liver and bronchopneumonia.

Comment

There is no doubt that he had been receiving the best treatment possible in this teaching hospital and was responding in a satisfactory manner until the sudden change in his condition took place. Presumably, the medical staff must have had an adequate explanation for the sudden deterioration, but to the relatives it must have been mystifying. To what extent the doctors or nurses were able to clarify this unexpected situation for the relatives in understandable medical terms is uncertain but whatever was said, it was obviously not enough to satisfy them so that they had recourse to their own magical interpretations.

Culturally determined paranoia of this kind is quite common in this country where accidents, mishaps, illnesses, and death are frequently ascribed to malevolent forces stimulated by human envy, jealousy, avarice, etc. As in the case of a paranoid patient, a pseudo-community of suspected people is rapidly built up and anecdotes are recalled to substantiate the suspicion. S. F.'s mother, for example, interpreted Mrs. X's question about her staying at home on the day of the accident in a paranoid manner but only *after* the accident; and similarly, the resentment she felt about Mrs. X's carping comparisons between the school performance of S. F. and her son became subsequently invested with paranoid feeling. Because of this and because it rankled in the mother's mind, Mrs. X became an obvious suspect in the case. If Mr. X had been polygamous, one of his other wives might well have been accused of witchcraft.

The traditional healers fully exploit this cultural tendency to paranoid interpretation. And it was, therefore, not at all surprising that the herbalist immediately confirmed what his client was suspecting. It would have been anticultural for him to have concluded that the inexplicable change in S. F.'s condition was due to natural causes.

The uncle's dream together with S. F.'s delirious ravings lent further support to the supernatural intervention. As the oldest male child, S. F.'s success in school could have been a source of great pride to his parents as well as anxiety since it would stimulate an overconcern for his welfare. His preciousness would sensitize them to his possible loss. Mrs. X's envy would certainly have activated this source of anxiety and made her anxious and nervous in her dealings with S. F. He, in turn, would assimilate this anxiety and come to regard Mrs. X as a threatening agent. Under conditions of delirium this nuclear preoccupation on the part of mother and son could well be released.

The departure of Mrs. X and her children from the house was interpreted in typical fashion by the mother as a reflection of guilt, but it is more than likely that the atmosphere of accusation and insinuation gave Mrs. X no alternative but to move away from the unpleasantness. The reason for S. F.'s family deciding to move could be related to the cultural belief that a curse settles not only on the individual but also on the house and that further calamity can only be prevented by leaving the premises. On the other hand, it cannot be altogether ruled out that the family felt unconsciously guilty at accusing an innocent person and generating much ill feeling. The parents might also have felt guilty about taking insufficient care to prevent such an accident to one of their children. Last, the family might have thought it best to move to assuage the anxious apprehension of the remaining children who, under the circumstances, could easily have gained the impression that they too could become victims of witchcraft. Frequently, rituals can be performed to counteract the curse on the family of the house or to prevent the dead child from attracting others to the world of the dead.

Discussion

L. A. Hersov, M. D. (England)

The account of this unfortunate child's accident, illness, and death and his family's response raises several issues for discussion among which sociocultural factors are especially important. The family was very probably members of the Yoruba people, possibly of the Egba subtribe, living either in a village or in the city of Abeokuta in the Western region of Nigeria. These people are hardworking and diligent and the particular circumstance of a father separately engaged in clerical work away from his family while the mother worked as a petty trader at home is very common. The emphasis on education for the children leading to better jobs is very typical shown by the fact that the other children were at boarding school. Among the Yoruba, children are much valued and it is very likely that S. F. occupied a particular place in the family as the only surviving son and the eldest at home. With the death of another son in infancy, S. F. may have been the focus of anxiety and protection until his survival was assured so that his accident and unexpectedly sudden death must have been especially difficult for his mother to bear as her traditional task was to protect him from harm.

The account describes in some detail the family's attempt to cope with events by recourse to explanations bringing in unseen forces, malignant supernatural influences, and misfortune, illness, and death caused by magical means, especially witchcraft. There is mention that S. F.'s success at school had aroused envy in Mrs. X. This sentiment is considered potentially dangerous by the Yoruba because those more fortunate are then susceptible to misfortune and to harm from others through magical means. We are told that S. F. had nightmares when he talked of Mrs. X's envy. He was possibly influenced by his mother's beliefs, yet he also refused food offered by her as if she might also be potentially dangerous to him. "Bad dreams" are one of the many symptoms thought to be due to witchcraft so the setting in which the deterioration in S. F.'s condition occurred was ripe for the projection of blame and paranoid interpretation of events which is so often emphasized in descriptions of psychological mechanisms among the Yoruba.

S. F.'s mother also remarked how her co-tenants seemed little affected by the accident and that only few of them visited him later in the hospital. This could be taken as further evidence of paranoid feelings, but an alternative explanation might be that her comment reflected her feeling of lack of support from her social group, support which is very important in a world where there is always potential danger from one's fellows who may have been antagonized or made envious. Mother seems to have been much influenced by the male relative of her husband whose dream of witchcraft appears to have set in train the search for a magical explanation by malevolent forces. In the absence of her husband the opinion of this member of the extended family would naturally have carried great weight with her.

A further issue is the apparent absence of any grief reaction or evidence of depression in the mother which might have been expected from a Western mother in similar circumstances. Many authorities have observed that the depressive syndrome occurs less frequently among the Yoruba; indeed there is some difficulty in finding a word in the Yoruba language to describe depression. There is typically the absence of guilt and self reproach even when depressive phenomena occur which is usually among the more highly westernized Yoruba. The account we are given only describes the immediate response of the family so that we do not know whether later observation would have shown evidence of depression and mourning. The whole account does appear to show that the behavior of the mother was culturally typical for the circumstances of the child's death and not a deviant response.

Anna Pipineli-Potamianou, Ph. D. (Greece)[1]

Dr. Asuni's observation certainly opens up some very interesting perspectives on the interrelationships between physiological, psychological, and sociocultural factors in the study of a case. A physical injury as significant as the one sustained by this particular child is only too likely to provoke a wide variety of connected responses in the psychosomatic and social spheres. It is, therefore, regrettable that the author opted for a presentation in which the total emphasis is placed on a single aspect of the case, namely, the information derived from the interprojections of the people involved.

[1] Translated by E. James Anthony, M. D.

Dr. Asuni is, without doubt, better qualified than us to decide whether the occurrence of a serious accident in a child can activate the emergence of mechanisms habitually used in a Nigerian environment to understand and master reality although even with regard to this, the simple equation between magical thinking and paranoid projection, of which we see less in our own culture, might have provided matter for discussion.

It is fairly easy to see why the way in which the family, and particularly the mother, approached the situation should have stimulated the appearance of very primitive fears in the boy responding as he was to the unconscious communications emitted by the mother. There is also no problem in understanding how the implicit and even explicit tensions aroused by the accident could trigger off a sequence of reactions that might then bring about affective changes in the relationships of the household and its neighborhood.

On the other hand, what seems less clear is the position taken up by the author with regard to his exposition of the case.

Does he find the information he has presented to us sufficient for the evaluation of the factors concerned? He tells us, for example, that the patient received the best possible treatment for the kind of hospital in which he was; consequently, the worsening of his condition to the point of death becomes difficult to explain, especially since he had initially given a positive response to the therapy. But this, obviously, by no means excludes the possibility of the medical procedures, the blood transfusions (if they were given), or even a subsequent infection being the cause of the diffuse hepatic lesions, a lowered resistance of the organism providing the necessary precondition following the severe traumatic shock; this would also explain the impact on the bronchopulmonary system.

Furthermore, no mention is made of any explanations to the family to account for the deterioration of the boy's condition, and one could suppose an unconscious complicity of beliefs linking, on a deep level, the hospital personnel to the indigenous cultural group causing them to resent the situation as much, to be as mystified, and to have the same difficulty with regard to clarification.

Finally, in the case in question, the mother is reported as being "devoted" to her children. This brings up the question: On what kinds of observations was this conclusion based? Because, as we well

know, devotion thrives on the registration and reception of many
different but profound attitudes.

One is struck by the fact that the mother remained at home on
the day of the accident prompted by an impulse that seems to have
provoked in her some feeling of guilt, and we do not know how it
happened that the boy was splashed with kerosene. His reaction to
Mrs. X, if we see her in the light of a displacement, makes it doubtful whether such a displacement could have operated unless the previous mother-son relationship had not in some way facilitated the
mechanism. The behavior of the child, when alone with his mother,
would seem to indicate that the displacement was operating when he
asked Mrs. X to "leave him alone." Indeed, it is when his mother is
present that he becomes disturbed and it is with her that he refuses
to eat which could be either because he is afraid of taking in her
"badness" or because he is reacting to hospitalization and separation
from her.

It is understandably very difficult to assemble all aspects of a
case in a short report of this type or even to convey some awareness
of its complexity. This is why we should be grateful to Dr. Asuni
for disclosing at least some part of the picture.

Jean Pouillon (France)[1]

Beneath its apparent neutrality, this observation discloses a total
inability on the part of physicians who are European, or European
in orientation, to understand the way in which disease is conceptu-
alized in numerous African societies including, it would seem,[2] the
one to which S. F. belongs. Let me say at once that in my opinion
the African conception is less dogmatic and less exclusive than the
"modern" counterpart subscribed to by the doctors of the Aro
hospital.

Under the direction of the latter, one notes that the illness took
a fatal turn when the boy, influenced by his mother, believed himself to be bewitched suggesting that this subjective credence rendered
(or helped to render) the objective medical treatment ineffectual.

[1] Translated by E. James Anthony, M. D.

[2] In the absence of ethnographic information, I cannot be more definite.

One goes further and interprets the uncle's demand for traditional intervention as a pure and simple repudiation of modern medicine tacitly assuming that the veto was warranted and in fact justified by the findings at autopsy. One, therefore, implicitly concludes that the traditional conception must be rejected as incompatible with the scientific practice of medicine.

In reality, neither the boy nor his family were guilty of refusing the treatment offered but, undoubtedly, they regarded the illness as doubly determined and hence calling for double treatment, both medical and ritualistic. In fact, every kind of disease results from physical causes while, at the same time, reflects a particular social situation (witchcraft is not only a matter of faith, but also a particular configuration of interpersonal relationships), and so one must take both into account. The traditional approach operates on two levels: On one level, it is based on proper medical care and the use of drugs; and on the other, according to practices varying from one society to the next, on a "neutralization" of the sorcerer and the restoration of the social order. Put differently, the sickness is conceived both as an evil and brought about by an evil spell and, therefore, if the treatments which counteract the evil are without effective action against the spell, one is forced to believe that the latter will nullify the former. The two aspects are inextricably linked but yet distinct; this is why an African patient can admit the superiority of modern techniques over the traditional pharmacopoeia without giving up the use of countersorcery.

The mistake of the Aro hospital physicians lies, then, in a unilateral conception both of traditional as well as scientific medicine that they practice (and which also involves a certain amount of ritual). They believed that the family of S. F. rejected the physical treatment (or doubted its validity) and they failed to understand that they were the ones who rejected the sociological treatment.

This observation also shows, without intending to, the need for a sociosomatic medicine.

Reimer Jensen, Cand. Psych. (Denmark)

Only the mother was around to help the boy when he was sprinkled with kerosene and was set on fire. Was she actually responsible for the accident by doing something which she could neither

understand herself nor explain to others? Did she afterwards struggle with the feeling that she had caused the accident by not preventing it? If so, her own irrational aggressive impulses towards the boy
might have been unbearable for her and therefore projected onto
Mrs. X to whom she then ascribed the capacity to influence and
even kill by witchcraft.

Why did the first boy in this family die at the age of eight months?
Are the boys of this mother in danger simply by the fact that they
are boys? What kind of inner reasons might she have had for not
going to work on the day of the accident that she was unable to disclose? Could she have been struggling with some internal fantasies
and/or delusions about danger, killing, witchcraft, and so on? We
cannot tell from the information given in the presentation, but the
mother herself might have been able to reveal some of the unknown
and hidden factors that inaugurated the tragic developments beginning on January thirteenth. Or was this development only taken
into its fatal phase on that day? Are there any other boys in the
remaining group of three children in the family and is the next one
in danger after the death of S. F.?

These are some of the questions stimulated in me by the case.
Unfortunately, the question marks have to remain as we do not
know enough of the mother's possible psychopathology to answer
the questions.

Epilogue

We have surveyed the universal experience of disease, disability, dying, and death as they affect the child in his family in different countries across the world. Although on the manifest level the individual and cultural differences appear to be large, below the surface there is a surprising similarity.

We have also seen that the mechanisms of adaptation to catastrophic experiences vary from individual to individual, from family to family, and from culture to culture but, once again, the transcultural differences begin to dissipate when the situations are explored in depth. We have looked at the primary notions of disease and death through the eyes of observers from different countries who have come up with developmental trends and dynamic epistemologies that would suggest that certain core experiences remain basic for all people irrespective of differing cultural institutions. All roads lead to death and along this path we are all fellow travelers imbued with the same existential anxieties.

Tolstoy, in one of his profoundest stories, made the point that the style of dying depends very much upon the style of living and that, therefore, our mode of dying may be diagnostic of the way that we have lived. He goes even further with the notion that dying can in some respects become therapeutic for a disturbed life. When Ivan Ilyitch lies dying after an empty, futile life, surrounded by empty, futile people, he suddenly becomes aware that his real illness is not physical but psychological. He ceases pretending and begins a "primal scream" that lasted for three days during which he learned to care for others and, for the first time, to love, and at that point, death loses its terror. It is not surprising that the story was a central inspiration for Heidegger. In many of the cases recorded in these pages, the young patients seem all of a sudden to surrender their illusions and to stop pretending and from then onward, death is no longer an accident but a necessity.

Piaget has described two moralities of childhood. One morality, for the younger child below the age of seven, is authoritarian and outer directed governed by absolute, inflexible laws, and crime is punished unmercifully according to the lex talonis. The second morality is autonomous, inner directed and practiced democratically. Laws are made by and for the people and punishment is considered only in the context of mitigating circumstances. There are also two moralities of death. In the earlier morality, death is not due to natural causes but is a punishment for disobedience or a retaliation for aggressive or sexual wishes. The child believes, consequently, that the bad must die before the good and that the good return to life but that the bad remain dead. Fundamentalist religious beliefs may reinforce this first morality of death so that death anxiety grows with age. The older and more benign morality of death views it in natural, nonpunitive terms and as part of a biological cycle. Psychological life is deemed to end with death and romantic concepts of afterlife are eschewed. Rochlin has made the interesting suggestion that the first morality, that also functions as a psychological defense against the reality of death, persists as a hard core of beliefs deep in the emotional life of the individual and apparently not altering to any extent throughout life. As Rochlin [7] puts it: "The concept of death fused with its amalgam of defenses is established as a core around which a knowledge of the facts of life is wrapped. The knowledge will vary considerably in people and in different societies and cultures, but neither the core nor the defenses differ in any appreciable way. The core seems to be irreducible and unaltered." He points out that in times of life-threatening crises, intellectual concepts are swept away and the elemental core concepts of the first morality are brought into play. This is one reason why children and adults, as illustrated in these pages, seem to function so much alike in the dying situation.

Although the majority of mankind is comparatively thanatophobic, there are cultures and there are individuals including children who seem preoccupied with death. For instance, death is celebrated in feasts in Mexico and during the festivities, death heads are eaten as confectionery, houses decorated with skulls, loaves of bread are shaped like bones, and firework displays illuminate skeletons. In some parts of Brazil, the death of a child is greeted with joy in marked

contrast to the sadness attending an adult funeral. The child is regarded not as a sinner but as an angel that God is calling back to
him.[1]

An adult's preoccupation with death is generally a product of
hypersensitivity and chronic illness. A good example would be the
author Marcel Proust [6] who was an ailing child with asthma and
a highly sensitive and imaginative mind. Toward the end of his great
work, *Remembrance of Things Past,* he wrote: "The idea of death
took up its permanent abode within me as does love for a woman.
Not that I loved death, I detested it. But, doubtless because I had
pondered over it from time to time as over a woman one does not
yet love, now the thought of it adhered to the deepest stratum of
my brain so completely that I could not turn my attention to anything without first relating it to the idea of death and even if I was
not occupied with anything but was in a state of complete repose,
the idea of death was with me as continuously as the idea of myself."

The thanatophobic child may play, almost compulsively, the game
of death. The games extend across cultures and are stimulated often
by personal experiences. Reverting again to Brazil, Montoya related
a typical story of a little boy's response to the extreme idealization
of the dead child. The boy was taken to view the funeral of one of
his playmates whose body was covered with a wonderful display of
flowers. After the funeral, the boy constantly begged his father to
let him die and spent many hours in a death game in which he was
the corpse. In desperation the father said to him: "My son, if God
wants you to die, then His will will be done." In hearing this, the
child said: "Very well, Father, I am going to die now," and he took
to his bed and died. This strange type of death has also been recorded among primitive people such as Australian aborigines. After the
Aberfan disaster in which a large number of children were buried
under a landslide, some of the survivors began playing "being buried
alive" games. Mitchell [4] described a four-year-old boy who had
watched the death of Winston Churchill on television and had then
played "being dead like Sir Winston," lying in a box quite still with
his eyes tightly shut. He refused to come alive even for cocoa time
at the nursery and was carried in "still dead." In a case seen by the
present commentator, a four-year-old boy entered a room where he

---

[1] Cultural details furnished by Dr. Serge Lebovici.

found his mother giving mouth-to-mouth artificial respiration to her father who had just dropped dead from a heart attack. The mother was lying on top of the grandfather and there was no doubt that the boy utterly misconceived the scene. For months after, he compulsively repeated the same situation, lying on his back, clutching a pillow and breathing deeply in and out all the time. He had been told that his grandfather had died. Another child, also aged four, had been troubled by death and began to play a counterphobic game as reported by her mother (Belsley [1]). She would lie down on the kitchen floor and tell her mother that she was dead. She remained quite still. Her mother, in trying to make it playful, would say: "Oh, Karen's dead! What an awful thing that she doesn't move." and would pretend to grieve over her. The little girl would then get up and announce that she was not really dead but was only fooling. However, she apparently enjoyed playing the game. Bierman [2] reported a case of a 13-year-old Negro boy who had been present when his 26-year-old sister died from stomach cancer. She had been very much a mother figure for him and he had cried almost continually for two weeks. Subsequently, anything that reminded him of his sister would start him crying. He developed insomnia, sleep walking, nail biting, headaches, and refused to attend school. He threatened to jump off the roof when his brother told him to pick up some papers he had thrown on the floor. Following his visit to the funeral home, he became intensely interested in the undertaker business. He started to visit other funeral parlors and would place long distance calls asking undertakers how their business was doing. He wrote to mortuary colleges for catalogs. At home he typed letterheads marked "John S's Funeral Home," complete with mock service charges. He read the obituary column daily and attended all the funerals he possibly could. At home he talked only about undertakers, embalming techniques, funerals, and costs of caskets. There was no doubt that his activity went beyond what could accurately be called play since he had lost his ability to stop voluntarily and had become fixated to one phase of play in a phobic defense. It seemed that his sister's illness and death were traumata that he could not assimilate. In the "undertaker" game he was an active controlling agent. Apart from playing with death and playing at death, small children will sometimes experiment with death, and the Scupins's [8] reported this sort of experimentation in their son Ernie at the age of five. One day he crushed a fly at the window and was greatly amused over it until his mother told him that the poor mother fly would come and find her child dead and would cry about it. Ernie became very distressed and said that if another fly child came along he would not kill it. Later he felt a pain in his finger and believed that the mother fly had hurt him when she found her child dead. Sometime after, he saw a dead fly on the window ledge and this appeared to incite him to catch another fly and to squeeze it with his fingers until it lay just as still as the other. Following this, he looked very embarrassed and guilty at what he had done. When another fly hovered near, he wondered whether this was the baby fly and asked if it were crying because it thought that its mother was dead.

The vulnerability of the children to the death experience varies with age but in any group of small children, one or two seem to stand out as particularly sensitive. Mitchell [4] has a small vignette that illustrates this very well. A mixed group of children around about seven years of age watched a small bird fly into the room through an open window and dash itself on the glass. The children decided to look after it and arranged a sickbed. All of a sudden a boy shouted "Oh look!" and the bird's head had dropped. For a moment there was silence and then the same boy said "He's dead" and wandered off. The rest insisted on a funeral and collected flowers. A question arose as to whether there should be a lid to the coffin and one of the girls insisted that there had to be one and that it must be nailed down. One of the girls said: "It's awful for it to have a lid. It's awful to be shut up." A boy answered her: "Don't be silly. It's dead, isn't it?" and the girl who had insisted on a lid added: "How would you like to be buried in a coffin without a lid with all that soil over your face?" A little later a rather quiet little boy aged seven came in and asked what had happened about the bird (he had taken no part in the burial rituals and had been the only one who had verbalized his sorrow at the death of the bird). Rather curiously, he asked: "Who is that bird?" and the teacher asked him in turn: "Who are you?" After a moments hesitation, he answered: "I am my name." Then he went on: "I wonder if there is a part of the bird that comes out invisible and flies away" and still later he said: "If I came back and heard that bird chirping again, I'd jump for joy all over the field!"

"I'd jump for joy all over the field!" How beautifully he expresses the relief from his death tensions. Here we have developing
in a vulnerable child the beginnings of the death ideations that haunt
certain individuals over the life cycle creating existential crises during
certain phases of change. It appears to be based on an exquisite sensitivity to all the nuances of life against death, to all the pains of
loss and anticipated loss of self or of loved objects, to numerous
identifications with the helpless, passive and finally immobilized
creature, and to all the vivid internal representations of the death
concept in terms of wishes and fears. In such children, to use
Proust's [6] language, the idea of death takes up its permanent abode;
and from such vulnerable children one can learn in depth about the
impact of the death and dying processes on the human personality.

E. James Anthony

Bibliography

1. Belsey, J., personal communication.
2. Bierman, J. S., Necrophilia in a thirteen-year-old boy, *Psychoanal. Q.*, 31 (1962), 329–340.
3. Freese, G., *Maitres Esclaves*, Gallimard, Paris, 1955.
4. Mitchell, M. E., *The Child's Attitude to Death*, Schocken Books, New York, 1967.
5. Paz, O., Labyrinthe de la solitude, *Esprit*, July, 1953.
6. Proust, M., *The Past Recaptured*, translated by F. A. Blossom, Modern Library, New York, 1932.
7. Rochlin, G., How Younger Children View Death and Themselves, in *Explaining Death to Children*, E. Grollman, Ed., Beacon Press, Boston, 1967.
8. Scupin, E. and Scupin, G., *Bubi From the Fourth to the Sixth Year*, Basel: Grabel, 1910.

Index

Aberfan disaster, 355–356
"Accidental crisis" (Erikson), 129
Accidents in childhood, 24
Acknowledgment in anticipatroy mourning, 130–131
Adaptive mechanisms for coping with death, 472–476
Adolescents who kill, 334–336
  potential for homicide in, 320
  predisposing factors in, 336
  triggering factors in, 336
Affective deficiency syndrome, 390
Affirmation of life in mastery operations, 13
Analysis of a survivor's child, 363–364
Anticipatroy mourning, 130–131
  acknowledgment in, 130–131
  detachment in, 131
  grieving in, 131
  memorialization in, 131
  reconciliation in, 131

Bereavement, 393–438
  in Britain, 423–438
  despair and, 435
  grief and, 435
  process of, 402–403
  refusal to mourn in, 435
Body concept, 88–90
  genesis of, 88–90
  and hypochondriasis, 90
Brain damage in children, 34

Catathymic crisis, 337
Children's capacity for mourning, 225–231
Children's conception, of death, 471–472
  of physical illness, 90–93
Children's reaction to doctor and hospitals, 33

Congenital heart disease, 75–83
  emotional effects in, 77–79
  mother-child relationship in, 79–80
  parental attitudes in, 81–82
  psychometric data in, 76–77
Criminal children, 316–317
Cystic fibrosis, 34, 37–47, 49–57
  appearance in, 39
  child's view of himself in, 40
  defensive and coping styles in, 41, 55–56
  demographic data in, 38–39
  emotional health of children in, 43
  intellectual functioning in, 39
  psychological study of patients in, 49–57

Death, 11, 12–16, 26, 191–264, 423–476
  adaptive mechanisms after, 475–476
  attitude in Yemenite culture to, 457–458
  in Britain, 423–438
  child's conception of, 12–16, 471–472
  existential crisis in relation to, 11
  family's reaction to, 25–27
  grandparent's response to, 26
  in India, 465–477
  quality of, 465–466
  in Senegal, 439–452
  sibling's reaction to, 26, 195–209
  wishes and fears in relation to, 26
  worldly attachment and, 466–464
"Death man," 10
Death on an adolescent pediatric ward, 211–218
  dreams associated with, 212–218
  mourning associated with, 191–264
  nursing staff and, 211–218
Developmental models in hypochondriasis, 87–88
Developmental-transactional model in family studies, 4–5, 8–9

Diabetes in children and adolescents, 59–
64
personal-social adjustment in, 60–64
psychosomatic factors in, 59–60
somatopsychic factors in, 60
Disability of fathers affecting families, 479–
487
congenital heart disease and, 32, 75–83
convalescent syndrome and, 17
cystic fibrosis, 34, 37–47
diabetes and, 16, 32, 59–64
epilepsy and, 35
family's reaction to, 21–24
hemophilia and, 16, 32
magic-phenomenistic theories connected
with, 32
muscular dystrophy and, 34
nephropathy, 32, 65–74
polio and, 34
pulmonary tuberculosis and, 17
rheumatic heart disease and, 16, 32
Dying children, 99–188, 244–250, 472–
476
adaptive mechanisms for coping with,
472–476
anticipatory mourning of parents of,
130–131
clinicians and, 124–125, 145–157, 162–
164
communicating with, 105–119
crisis and adaptation in families of, 127–
144
cultural differences in dealing with, 159–
161
fear of death in, 121–124
"life space" interviews with, 107
management of terminal phase of, 164–
168
mastery operations of, 132–136
medical attitudes to, 162–164
needs of, 250–251
parents and professionals with regard to
parent's participation in care, 248–
250
patient-staff communications with
respect to, 110–113
process of adaptation in, 129
reactions, to death of, 117–118
to over-concern and indulgence of,
116–117

secrecy in relation to, 153–155, 244–248
self-diagnosis of, 113–116
treatment reactions in, 109–110

Epilepsy in childhood, 35
"External" family, 8

Family process, 3–9, 25–26
cognitive levels and, 7
communicative aspects of, 7
"external" aspects of, 8
homeostatic mechanisms in, 9
identity and likeness in, 6
"internal" aspects of, 8
psychopathological aspects of, 6
psychosexual aspects of, 7
Psychosocial aspects of, 7
Family's response, to death, 25–27
anticipatory mourning in, 25
denial as, 25
depression as, 26
divorce as outcome of, 26
guilt and mourning as, 25
from leukemia, 25
pregnancy as outcome of, 27
religious aspects of, 25
resignation as, 25
to disease, inadequate coping in, 22
by theorizing, 23

Grandparent's reaction to death in the
family, 26

Hiroshima disaster and children, 353–355
Homicide in adolescence, *see* Adolescents
who kill
Hypochondriasis in childhood, 85–95
body concept in, 88–90
developmental models pertaining to, 87–
88
neurophysiological model for, 86
psychodynamic model for, 87
sociodynamic model, 87

Infanticide, 453–463
"Israelization" and, 454–455
Yemenite community and, 456–458

Kwashiorkor (K.W.K.) in children, 449–450

Leukemia children, 24, 105–119, 127–144, 145–168, 195–209
communications with, 105–119
doctor and, 145–157, 162–164
families of, 127–144
in hospital, 159–168
impact on siblings of, 195–209

Matricide, 320–333
incidence of, 323–325
maternal deprivation and, 331
mythology of, 320
psychiatric literature on, 321–323
sado-masochistic mother-child relations and, 333
Models, 4–5, 8–9, 86–87
in family studies, 4–5, 8–9
in hypochondriasis, 86–87
Mourning, 130–132, 191–264, 435
anticipatory in parents of dying children, 130–132
child's capacity for, 225–231
need for, 129–224
pathological, 233–243
psychic loss and, 255–264
refusal to undergo, 435
who undertakes it when a child dies, 245–254
Mythology and parricide, 320

Nephropathy in childhood, 65–74
child's reaction to, 66–68
chronic hemodialysis in, 72
communication problems in, 72
doctor-patient relationships in, 70–72
parental reactions to, 68–70
stresses involved in, 65
Parricide, by children and adolescents, 270–272, 320–338
involving fathers, 333–338
involving mothers, 320–333
Patricide, *see* Parricide
Primal crime, *see* Parricide
Psychotic illness in parents, 255–264
effects on children of, 255–263
mourning with, 255–264
psychic loss through, 259–263
Psychic loss through mental illness in parents, 255–264
"Psy function," 146–149

Renal disease in children, *see* Nephropathy

Role theory in family studies, 7

Sadism in children, 272–273, 308–313
genesis of, 310–313
torturing in relation to, 308–310
Schizophrenic crime, 330
Sibling death, 26, 195–209
death fears and wishes in relation to, 26
effect on siblings of, 195–209
Suicide, 267–297, 299–306
childhood parent loss and, 275–297
ideation and behavior as antecedents in, 275–297
impact on child of father's, 299–306
psychoanalytic studies in, 278
retrospective studies in, 276–278
Survivors, 363–415
Aberfan disaster and, 355–356
affective deficiency syndrome and, 390
analysis of child of, 363–367
children of, 375–377
concentration camps and, 379–384
family systems of, 405–407
Hiroshima disaster and, 353–355
hypothesis and methodology in studies of, 411–415
parental attitudes in, 390–391
parental disequilibrium in, 388–389
as parents, 375, 403–405
Symposium, 171–188, 491–500
dying child, in an American hospital, 171–188
in an Nigerian hospital, 491–500

Thanctophobia in children, 503
Transcultural experiences of disability, dying and death, 25, 299–306, 419–487
Africa (Senegal) and, 439–452
Britain and, 423–438
France and, 25
India and, 465–477
Israel and, 299–306, 453–463
South America (Peru) and Yemenite community and, 479–487

Undertaker games, 503–504

Vulnerable child syndrome, 16

Yemenite community reactions to infanticide, 453–463